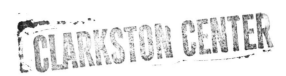

Principles & Practice of Public Health Surveillance

Principles & Practice of Public Health Surveillance

Third Edition

Lisa M. Lee, PhD
Steven M. Teutsch, MD, MPH
Stephen B. Thacker, MD, MSc
Michael E. St. Louis, MD

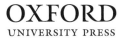

OXFORD
UNIVERSITY PRESS

2010

OXFORD
UNIVERSITY PRESS

Oxford University Press, Inc., publishes works that further
Oxford University's objective of excellence
in research, scholarship, and education.

Oxford   New York
Auckland   Cape Town   Dar es Salaam   Hong Kong   Karachi
Kuala Lumpur   Madrid   Melbourne   Mexico City   Nairobi
New Delhi   Shanghai   Taipei   Toronto

With offices in
Argentina   Austria   Brazil   Chile   Czech Republic   France   Greece
Guatemala   Hungary   Italy   Japan   Poland   Portugal   Singapore   South
Korea   Switzerland   Thailand   Turkey   Ukraine   Vietnam

Published by Oxford University Press, Inc.
198 Madison Avenue, New York, New York 10016
www.oup.com

Library of Congress Cataloging-in-Publication Data

Principles and practice of public health surveillance. — 3rd ed. / [edited by]
Lisa M. Lee ... [et al.].
p. ; cm.
Rev. ed. of: Principles and practice of public health surveillance / edited by Steven M. Teutsch,
R. Elliott Churchill. 2nd ed. 2000.
Includes bibliographical references and index.
ISBN 978–0–19–537292–2   1. Public health surveillance. I. Lee, Lisa M.
[DNLM: 1.   Population Surveillance—methods—United States.   2.   Data Interpretation, Statistical—United
States.   3.   Disease Outbreaks—prevention & control—United States.
4.   Models, Statistical—United States.
WA 950 P9565 2010]
RA652.2.P82P75 2010
614.4—dc22
2009049403

9 8 7 6 5 4 3 2 1
Printed in the United States of America
on acid-free paper

Foreword

The first edition of this book traced the history of surveillance back to the origins of human history through the critical contributions of Alexander Langmuir at the Communicable Disease Center. The second edition was expanded to explore five other aspects of surveillance—the basic role of surveillance in public health practice, risk factor surveillance, the public health approach of observing all of life to separate out the patterns that lead to pathology and those that lead to wholeness, the then emerging digital revolution, and the trends of globalization provide compelling reasons for developing useful and workable surveillance networks.

This edition examines further the developments in public health surveillance following the bombing of the World Trade Center in New York City, enhanced surveillance for disease determinants, and environmental tracking. Public health preparedness has both challenged and strengthened public health surveillance; new chapters in this edition outline the important relationship between these two public health priorities. In addition, expansion of the tools of informatics and access to data from sources outside of public health have both increased dramatically the potential for better surveillance and forced us to look at the changing role of public health surveillance in the context of the demand for situation awareness in close to real-time.

Throughout this edition, the editors collect strong evidence that in the midst of many changes and opportunities, public health surveillance has maintained its foundational disciplinary integrity, while adapting to the needs of an increasingly complex field of public health. This third edition provides an excellent framework for all of us to strengthen public health by collectively improving the surveillance foundation. Our thanks to the editors for that effort.

William H. Foege, MD, MPH
David Sencer, MD, MPH

Preface

When the first and second editions of *Principles and Practice of Public Health Surveillance* were published in 1994 and 2000, there existed few fundamental resources on public health surveillance. Since then, a handful of graduate schools of public health have developed courses on surveillance methods, primarily driven by faculty interest in the topic. A number of textbooks have been published about specific topic areas in public health surveillance. Still, in 2010, there remains only one comprehensive text on the science of public health surveillance, and here we offer the third edition of that text.

In the decade since the second edition, many developments have transformed the landscape of public health surveillance. There have been increasing demands on surveillance data, resulting in rapid growth of the field. These developments include the addition of preparedness- and response-related surveillance; enhanced surveillance for disease determinants, including social, behavioral, risk factor surveillance; and environmental tracking. In addition, surveillance methods have been used in a variety of non-public health settings, such as health-care practices to provide a way of ranking or grading services, blurring the lines between methods and practice. The broader use of surveillance methods has brought us back to the table to consider the definition of public health surveillance—to remind ourselves of first principles of routine collection, analysis, and communication of data *for public health action*.

Surveillance information has played an increasingly important role in decision making—from funding appropriation and allocation to program development and evaluation. Exacerbated by the events of September 11, 2001, there has been increased demand for "health situation awareness" that requires public health officials to possess broad knowledge of health status indicators across the health horizon, keeping a keen eye for emerging threats, natural or otherwise. These events changed the context in which public health surveillance is practiced. They have required public health departments at all levels to consider properly locating and understanding the contributions of public health surveillance amidst emergency management organizations. Additionally, the monumental advances in information technology and the emerging field of informatics have the potential to reshape the way health data are collected, collated, managed, analyzed, distributed, and communicated. Leveraging efficiencies in this arena will be critical for limited public health surveillance budgets.

Even with an agile response to the numerous changes listed above, challenges for public health surveillance remain. How does public health surveillance as a discipline fit under the most broadly conceived umbrella of comprehensive "health awareness?" How is public health surveillance different from the unstructured scanning and data-mining of electronic databases, or is it? Are all health data collections "surveillance?" If not, what is the common vocabulary or taxonomy for characterizing public health data collections? How is surveillance different from research? What protections should be afforded data collected by public health surveillance systems? Answers to these questions are incomplete, but the chapters in this text provide a thoughtful start to the field's movement forward.

What has remained constant is the foundational science of public health surveillance. These principles can be described in five overarching domains of public health surveillance methods: *(1)* system development and data collection; *(2)* data management and information integration; *(3)* data analysis and interpretation; *(4)* communication of findings for public health action; and *(5)* evaluation of the surveillance system itself. Each of these domains makes use of a variety of scientific disciplines from traditional fields like epidemiology and laboratory sciences to more recent additions to the public health repertoire like economics and informatics.

This edition touches on each of these important factors—the history, principles, practice, and future challenges of public health surveillance. The sections of the text are arranged around these ideas, providing updated chapters on ethics and evaluation, a new chapter outlining the economic and policy justification for public health surveillance, and a new section on the practice of public health surveillance, which includes chapters that demonstrate the principles in action. We conclude the text by outlining some of the remaining challenges.

We express our deepest appreciation to the authors and editors of the first and second editions of the text who laid the foundation for this updated and expanded edition. We are eternally grateful to the contributors and authors to this edition, without whose time and expertise this project would not have been possible. We thank the Centers for Disease Control and Prevention's (CDC) Chief Science Officer, Dr. Tanja Popovic, for her support of this project. We recognize numerous colleagues at the Los Angeles County Department of Public Health and throughout CDC who served as our "laboratories" for many of the ideas contained in the book; in particular, we thank members of CDC's surveillance and situation awareness work group—Henry Falk, Rita Helfand, Rima Khabbaz, Denise Koo, Steve Solomon, Daniel Sosin, and Kathleen Toomey. Finally, we extend our appreciation to public health surveillance colleagues in state and local health departments and ministries of health across the globe who carry out this critical and challenging work.

Lisa M. Lee, PhD	*Atlanta, Georgia, USA*
Steven M. Teutsch, MD, MPH	*Los Angeles, California, USA*
Stephen B. Thacker, MD, MSc	*Atlanta, Georgia, USA*
Michael E. St. Louis, MD	*Atlanta, Georgia, USA*

March, 2010

Contents

Contributors

At the U.S. Centers for Disease Control and Prevention, Atlanta, GA

Joseph L. Annest, PhD, MS
Director, Office of Statistics and
    Programming
National Center for Injury Prevention
    and Control

Lorraine C. Backer, PhD, MPH
Team Leader
National Center For Environmental
    Health

Scott F. Dowell, MD, MPH
Director, Division of Global Disease
    Detection and Emergency Response
Center for Global Health

Robert R. German, DrPH, MPH
Lead Epidemiologist, Cancer
    Surveillance Branch
Division of Cancer Prevention and
    Control
National Center for Chronic Disease
    Prevention and Health Promotion

Richard A. Goodman, MD, JD, MPH
Co-Chief, Public Health Law Branch
Office for State, Tribal, Local, and
    Territorial Support

M. Kathleen Glynn, DVM, MPVM
Veterinary Epidemiologist
National Center for Emerging and
    Zoonotic Infectious Diseases

Samuel L. Groseclose, DVM, MPH
Chief, Statistics and Data Management
    Branch

Division of STD Prevention
National Center for HIV/AIDS, Viral
    Hepatitis, STD, and TB Prevention

Charles M. Heilig, PhD
Lead Methodologist
Division of TB Elimination
National Center for HIV/AIDS, Viral
    Hepatitis, STD, and TB Prevention
and
Senior Advisor for Human Research
    Ethics
Office of the Associate Director for
    Science

Robin M. Ikeda, MD, MPH
Deputy Director, Noncommunicable
    Diseases, Injury and Environmental
    Health
Office of the Director

Denise Koo, MD, MPH
Acting Director
Scientific Education and Professional
    Development Program Office
Office of Surveillance, Epidemiology,
    and Laboratory Services

**Ramesh S. Krishnamurthy,
PhD, MPH**
Senior Informatics Advisor
Global AIDS Program
National Center for HIV/AIDS, Viral
    Hepatitis, STD, and TB Prevention

Lisa M. Lee, PhD
Chief Science Officer
Office of Surveillance, Epidemiology,
    and Laboratory Services

Cara T. Mai, MPH
Public Health Analyst
National Center on Birth Defects and
    Developmental Disabilities

Matthew T. McKenna, MD, MPH
Chief Medical Officer
National Center for Chronic Disease
    Prevention and Health Promotion

Verla S. Neslund, JD
Vice President for Programs
CDC Foundation

Peter Nsubuga, MD, MPH
Chief, Capacity
    Development Branch
Division of Global Public Health
    Capacity Development
Center for Global Health

Helen Perry, PhD
Public Health Educator
Division of Emerging Infections and
    Surveillance Services
National Center for Preparedness,
    Detection, and Control of Infectious
    Diseases

Chesley Richards, MD, MPH
Acting Director, Office of Prevention
    through Healthcare
Office of the Director

Daniel M. Sosin, MD, MPH, FACP
Acting Director
Office of Public Health Preparedness
    and Response

Michael E. St. Louis, MD
Associate Director for Science
Center for Global Health

Patricia Sweeney, MPH
Epidemiologist
Division of HIV/AIDS Prevention
National Center for HIV/AIDS, Viral
    Hepatitis, STD, and TB Prevention

Stephen B. Thacker, MD, MSc
Deputy Director for Surveillance,
    Epidemiology, and Laboratory
    Services
Office of the Director

Herman D. Tolentino, MD
Director, Public Health Informatics
    Fellowship Program
Scientific Education and Professional
    Development Program Office
Office of Surveillance, Epidemiology,
    and Laboratory Services

Chris A. Van Beneden, MD, MPH
Medical Epidemiologist
Respiratory Diseases Branch
Division of Bacterial Diseases
National Center for Immunization and
    Respiratory Diseases

Henry T. Walke, Jr., MD, MPH
Chief, Program Development Branch
Division of Global Public Health
    Capacity Development
Center for Global Health

Mark E. White, MD, FACPM
Medical Officer
Center for Global Health

G. David Williamson, PhD
Director, Division of Health Studies
Agency for Toxic Substances and
    Disease Registry

At Other Organizations

Janet B. Arrowsmith, MD
Consultant
Arrowsmith Consulting, LLC
Ruidoso, NM

Guthrie S. Birkhead, MD, MPH
Deputy Commissioner, Office of
   Public Health
New York State Department of Public
   Health
New York, NY
and
Professor, Department of
   Epidemiology and Biostatistics
School of Public Health, University at
   Albany
Albany, NY

M. Miles Braun, MD, MPH
Global Head of Epidemiology and
   Associate Vice President
sanofi pasteur
Lyon, France

Thomas P. Gross, MD, MPH
Office of Surveillance and Biometrics
Center for Devices and Radiological
   Health
Food and Drug Administration
Silver Spring, MD

James G. Hodge, Jr., JD, LLM
Lincoln Professor of Health Law and
   Ethics
Sandra Day O'Connor College of Law
Arizona State University
Tempe, AZ

Richard S. Hopkins, MD, MSPH
Acting State Epidemiologist
Bureau of Epidemiology
Florida Department of Health
Tallahassee, FL

Ruth Lynfield, MD
State Epidemiologist
Minnesota Department of Health
St. Paul, MN

**Sharon M. McDonnell, BSN, MD,
MPH**
Associate Professor
Department of Community and
   Family Medicine

Dartmouth Medical School & The
   Dartmouth Institute for Health
   Policy and Clinical Practice
Hanover, NH

Christopher M. Maylahn, MPH
Program Research Specialist
Office of Public Health Practice
New York State Department of Health
Albany, NY

John P. Middaugh, MD
Director, Division of Community
   Health
Southern Nevada Health District
Las Vegas, NV

Ali H. Mokdad, PhD
Professor, Global Health
Institute for Health Metrics and
   Evaluation
University of Washington
Seattle, WA

James F. Murray, PhD
Senior Director, Global Health
   Outcomes
Center for Epidemiology and Health
   Services Research
Global Health Outcomes, Eli Lilly and
   Company
Indianapolis, IN

David E. Nelson, MD, MPH
Director
Cancer Prevention Fellowship Program
National Cancer Institute, National
   Institutes of Health
Bethesda, MD

Roy Gibson Parrish, II, MD
Peacham, VT

David B. Rein, PhD
Economist, Public Health Economics
   Program
RTI International
Atlanta, GA

Patrick L. Remington, MD, MPH
Professor and Associate Dean for
    Public Health
Department of Population Health
    Sciences
University of Wisconsin, School of
    Medicine and Public Health
Madison, WI

Paul J. Seligman, MD, MPH
Director
Latin America Office, Office of
    International Programs
Food and Drug Administration
San Jose, Costa Rica

Patrick S. Sullivan, DVM, PhD
Associate Professor, Department of
    Epidemiology
Rollins School of Public Health
Emory University
Atlanta, GA

Steven M. Teutsch, MD, MPH
Chief Science Officer
Los Angeles County Department of
    Public Health
Los Angeles, CA

Lance A. Waller, PhD
Rollins Professor and Chair
Department of Biostatistics and
    Bioinformatics, Rollins School of
    Public Health
Emory University
Atlanta, GA

Principles & Practice of Public Health Surveillance

1

Historical Development

STEPHEN B. THACKER

You can observe a lot just by looking.

—Yogi Berra

The definition for public health surveillance most often used by the Centers for Disease Control and Prevention (CDC) is "the ongoing systematic collection, analysis, and interpretation of health-related data essential to the planning, implementation, and evaluation of public health practice, closely integrated with the timely dissemination of these data to those who need to know. The final link in the surveillance chain is the application of these data to prevention and control" (*1*). A surveillance system includes the functional capacity for data collection, analysis, and timely dissemination of information derived from these data to persons in public health programs who can undertake effective prevention and control activities. Although the core of any surveillance system includes the collection, analysis, and dissemination of data, the process can be understood only in the context of specific health events (e.g., hazards, exposures, risk factors, and outcomes).

BACKGROUND

The idea of observing, recording, and collecting facts; analyzing them; and considering reasonable courses of action stems from Hippocrates (*2*). However, the first real public health action that can be related to surveillance probably occurred during the period of bubonic plague (early 1300s), when public health authorities boarded ships in the port near the Republic of Venice to prevent persons ill with plague-like illness from disembarking (*3*). Before a large-scale organized system of surveillance could be developed, however, certain prerequisites needed to be fulfilled. First, a semblance of an organized health-care system in a stable government had to exist; in the Western world, this was not achieved until the time of the Roman Empire. Second, a classification system for disease and illness had to be established and accepted; such a system only began to be functional in the 17th

The findings and conclusions in this report are those of the author(s) and do not necessarily represent the views of the Centers for Disease Control and Prevention.

century with the work of Thomas Sydenham. Finally, no adequate measurement methods were developed until that time.

Modern concepts of public health surveillance have evolved from public health activities developed to control and prevent disease in the community. In the late Middle Ages, governments in Western Europe assumed responsibility for both health protection and health care of the population of their towns and cities (4). A rudimentary system of monitoring illness led to regulations against polluting streets and public water, construction for burial and food handling, and the provision of certain types of care (5). In 1766, Johann Peter Frank advocated a more comprehensive form of public health surveillance with the system of police medicine in Germany. It covered school health, injury prevention, maternal and child health, and public water and sewage (4). In addition, Frank delineated governmental measures to protect the public's health.

The roots of analysis of surveillance data can also be traced to the 17th century. In the 1680s, Gottfried Wilhelm von Leibniz called for establishment of a health council and the application of numeric analysis in mortality statistics to health planning (2). At approximately the same time in London, John Graunt published a book, *Natural and Political Observations Made Upon the Bills of Mortality*, in which he attempted to define the basic laws of natality and mortality. In his work, Graunt developed certain fundamental principles of public health surveillance, including disease-specific death counts, death rates, and the concept of disease patterns. In the next century, Achenwall introduced the term *statistics*, and during the next decades vital statistics became more widespread in Europe. A century later, in 1845, Thurnam published the first extensive report of mental health statistics in London.

Lemuel Shattuck and William Farr are two prominent names in the development of the concepts of public health surveillance activities. Shattuck's 1850 report of the Massachusetts Sanitary Commission was a landmark publication that related death, infant and maternal mortality, and communicable diseases to living conditions. Shattuck recommended a decennial census, standardization of nomenclature of causes of disease and death, and a collection of health data by age, sex, occupation, socioeconomic level, and locality. He applied these concepts to program activities in the areas of immunization, school health, smoking, and alcohol abuse and introduced related concepts into the teaching of preventive medicine.

William Farr (1807–1883) is recognized as one of the founders of modern concepts of surveillance (6). As superintendent of the statistical department of the Registrar General's office of England and Wales during 1839 through 1879, Farr concentrated his efforts on collecting vital statistics, on assembling and evaluating those data, and on reporting both to responsible health authorities and the general public.

In the United States, public health surveillance has focused historically on infectious diseases. Basic elements of surveillance were evident in Rhode Island in 1741, when the colony passed an act requiring tavern keepers to report contagious diseases among their patrons. Two years later, the colony passed a broader law requiring the reporting of smallpox, yellow fever, and cholera (7).

Activities associated with disease reporting at the national level did not begin in the United States until 1850, when mortality statistics based on death registration and the decennial census were first published by the federal government for the entire country (8). Systematic reporting of disease in the United States began in 1874, when the Massachusetts State Board of Health instituted a voluntary plan for physicians to provide weekly reports on prevalent diseases, using a standard postcard-reporting format (9,10). In 1878, Congress authorized the forerunner of the Public Health Service (PHS) to collect morbidity data for use in quarantine measures against such pestilential diseases as cholera, smallpox, plague, and yellow fever (11).

In Europe, compulsory reporting of infectious diseases began in Italy in 1881; in Great Britain, it began in 1890. In 1893, Michigan became the first U.S. jurisdiction to require reporting of specific infectious diseases (9). Also in 1893, a law was enacted that provided for collection of information each week from state and municipal authorities throughout the United States (12). By 1901, all state and municipal laws required notification (i.e., reporting) to local authorities of selected communicable diseases, including smallpox, tuberculosis, and cholera. In 1914, PHS personnel were appointed as collaborating epidemiologists to serve in state health departments and to telegraph weekly disease reports to PHS.

In the United States, however, all states did not begin participating in national morbidity reporting until 1925, after markedly increased reporting occurred associated with the severe poliomyelitis epidemic in 1916 and the 1918 through 1919 influenza pandemic (13). A national health survey of U.S. citizens was first conducted in 1935. After a 1948 PHS study led to revision of morbidity reporting procedures, the National Office of Vital Statistics assumed the responsibility for reporting morbidity. In 1949, weekly statistics that had appeared for years in *Public Health Reports* began being published by the National Office of Vital Statistics. In 1952, mortality data were added to the publication that was the forerunner of the *Morbidity and Mortality Weekly Report* (*MMWR*). As of 1961, responsibility for this publication and its content was transferred to the Communicable Disease Center (now the Centers for Disease Control and Prevention).

In the United States, the authority to require notification of cases of disease resides with state legislatures. In certain states, authority is enumerated in statutory provisions; in others, authority to require reporting has been assigned to state boards of health; still other states require reports both under statutes and health department regulations. Conditions and diseases to be reported vary from state to state, as do time-frames for reporting, agencies to receive reports, persons required to report, and conditions under which reports are required (14).

The Conference (now Council) of State and Territorial Epidemiologists (CSTE) was authorized in 1951 by its parent body, the Association of State and Territorial Health Officials (ASTHO), to determine what diseases should be reported by states to PHS and to develop reporting procedures (15). Officially incorporated in 1955, CSTE meets annually and, in collaboration with CDC, recommends to its constituent members appropriate changes in morbidity reporting and surveillance, including what diseases should be reported to CDC and published in the *MMWR*.

DEVELOPMENT OF THE CONCEPT OF SURVEILLANCE

Until 1950, the term *surveillance* was restricted in public health practice to monitoring contacts of persons with serious communicable diseases (e.g., smallpox) to detect early symptoms so that prompt isolation could be instituted (*16*). The critical demonstration in the United States of the importance of a broader, population-based view of surveillance was made after the Francis Field Trial of poliomyelitis vaccine in 1955 (*17,18*). Within 2 weeks of the announcement of the results of the field trial and initiation of a nationwide vaccination program, six cases of paralytic poliomyelitis were reported through the notifiable-disease reporting system to state and local health departments; this surveillance led to an epidemiologic investigation, which revealed that these children had received vaccine produced by a single manufacturer. Intensive surveillance and appropriate epidemiologic investigations by federal, state, and local health departments identified 141 vaccine-associated cases of paralytic disease, 80 of which represented family contacts of vaccinees. Daily surveillance reports were distributed by CDC to all persons involved in these investigations. This national common-source epidemic was ultimately related to a particular lot of vaccine that had been contaminated with live poliovirus. The Surgeon General requested that the manufacturer recall all outstanding lots of vaccine and directed that a national poliomyelitis program be established at CDC. Had the surveillance program not been in existence, many, and perhaps all, vaccine manufacturers would have ceased production for vaccines against polio.

In 1963, Alexander Langmuir advocated limiting the use of the term *surveillance* to the collection, analysis, and dissemination of data (*19*). Langmuir, the chief epidemiologist at CDC for more than 20 years, made pivotal contributions to public health surveillance that ultimately defined modern practice throughout the world (*20*). This construct did not encompass direct responsibility for control activities. In 1965, the Director General of the World Health Organization (WHO) established the epidemiologic surveillance unit in the Division of Communicable Diseases of WHO (*21*). The Division Director, Karel Raska, defined surveillance much more broadly than Langmuir, including "the epidemiological study of disease as a dynamic process." In the case of malaria, he saw epidemiologic surveillance as encompassing control and prevention activities. Indeed, the WHO definition of malaria surveillance included not only case detection but also the obtaining of blood films, drug treatment, epidemiologic investigation, and follow-up (*22*), akin to what is defined currently as *biosurveillance* (described in Chapter 14).

In 1968, the 21st World Health Assembly focused on national and global surveillance of communicable diseases, applying the term to the diseases themselves rather than to the monitoring of persons with communicable disease (*23*). After an invitation from the Director General of WHO and with consultation from Raska, Langmuir developed a working paper, and in the year before the 1968 Assembly, he obtained comments from throughout the world on the concepts and practices advocated in the paper. At the Assembly, with delegates from approximately 100 countries, the working paper was endorsed, and discussions on the national and global surveillance of communicable disease identified three main features of surveillance that Langmuir had described in 1963: *(a)* the systematic collection of pertinent data, *(b)* the orderly consolidation and evaluation of these data, and *(c)* the prompt dissemination of results to those who need to know—particularly those in position to take action.

The 1968 World Health Assembly discussions reflected the broadened concepts of epidemiologic surveillance and addressed the application of the concept to public health problems other than communicable disease *(22)*. In addition, epidemiologic surveillance was said to imply ". . .the responsibility of following up to see that effective action has been taken."

Since that time, multiple health events (e.g., lead poisoning among children, leukemia, congenital malformations, abortions, injuries, adverse reactions to vaccines, and behavioral risk factors) have been placed under surveillance. In 1976, recognition of the breadth of surveillance activities throughout the world was made evident by the publication of a special issue of the *International Journal of Epidemiology* devoted to surveillance *(24)*.

SURVEILLANCE IN PUBLIC HEALTH PRACTICE

The primary function of the application of the term *epidemiologic* to surveillance, which first appeared in the 1960s in association with the newly created WHO unit of that name, was to distinguish this activity from other forms of surveillance (e.g., military intelligence) and to reflect its broader applications. Use of the term *epidemiologic*, however, engenders both confusion and controversy. In 1971, Langmuir noted that certain epidemiologists tended to equate surveillance with epidemiology in its broadest sense, including epidemiologic investigations and research *(16)*. He found this "both epidemiologically and administratively unwise," favoring a description of surveillance as "epidemiological intelligence."

What are the boundaries of surveillance practice? Is *epidemiologic* an appropriate modifier of surveillance in the context of public health practice? To address these questions, we must first examine the structure of public health practice. One can divide public health practice broadly into surveillance; epidemiologic, behavioral, and laboratory research; service delivery (including program evaluation); and training. Surveillance information should be used to identify research and service needs, which, in turn, help to define training needs. Unless this information is provided to those who set policy and implement programs, its use is limited to archives and academic pursuits, and the material is therefore appropriately considered to be health information rather than surveillance information. However, surveillance does not encompass epidemiologic research or service, which are related but independent public health activities that might not be based on surveillance. Thus, the boundary of surveillance practice excludes actual research and implementation of delivery programs.

Because of this separation, we do not use *epidemiologic* to modify surveillance *(25)*; rather, the term *public health surveillance* describes the scope (surveillance) and indicates the context in which it occurs (public health). It also obviates the need to accompany any use of the term *epidemiologic surveillance* with a list of all the examples this term does not cover. Surveillance is correctly—and necessarily—a component of public health practice and should continue to be recognized as such.

PURPOSES AND USES OF PUBLIC HEALTH SURVEILLANCE DATA

Purposes

Public health surveillance information is used to assess public health status, track conditions of public health importance, define public health priorities, evaluate programs, and develop public health research. Surveillance information aids the health officer in identifying where the problems are, whom they affect, and where programmatic and prevention activities should be directed. Such information can also be used to help define public health priorities in a quantitative manner and also in evaluations of the effectiveness of programmatic activities. Analysis of public health surveillance data also enables researchers to generate hypotheses to identify areas for further investigation (26).

The basic analysis of surveillance data is, in principle, simple. Data are examined by measures of time, place, and person. The routine collection of data about reported cases of congenital syphilis in the United States, for example, reflects not only numbers of cases (Fig. 1–1), geographic distribution, and populations affected but also reflects the steady decline of congenital syphilis since the early 1990s, with a less consistent pattern in primary and secondary syphilis in those years, partly because of a resurgence in the disease in men who have sex with men. Examination of routinely collected data reveals rates of salmonellosis by county in New Hampshire and in three contiguous states. Mapping these data illustrates the pattern of the occurrence of disease across state boundaries (Fig. 1–2). Examination of homicide-related death certificates identifies groups at high risk and demonstrates that the problem has reached epidemic proportions among young adult men (Fig. 1–3).

Uses

The uses of surveillance are illustrated in Table 1–1. Portrayal of the natural history of disease can be illustrated by the surveillance of malaria rates in the United States since 1930 (Fig. 1–4). In the 1940s, malaria was still an endemic health problem in the southeastern United States to the degree that persons with febrile illness were often treated for malaria until further tests were available. After the Malaria Control in the War Areas Program led to the virtual elimination of endemic malaria from the United States, rates of malaria decreased until the early 1950s, when military personnel involved in the conflict in Korea returned to the United States with malaria. The general downward trend in reported cases of malaria continued into the 1960s until, once again, numbers of cases of malaria increased, this time among veterans returning from the war in Vietnam. Since that

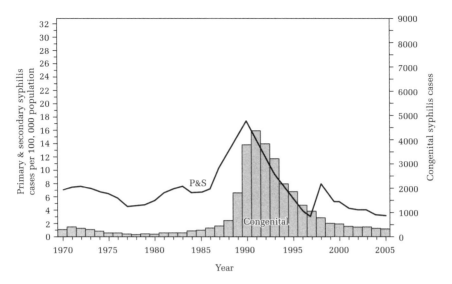

Figure 1–1 Reported cases of congenital syphilis among infants aged 1 year and rates of primary and secondary (P&S) syphilis among women—United States, 1970–2005. Note: the surveillance case definition for congenital syphilis changed in 1989.

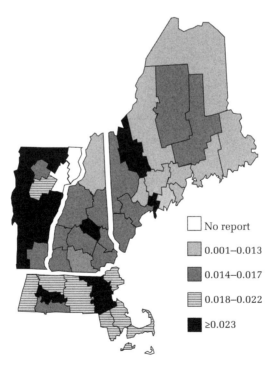

Figure 1–2 Rates of *Salmonella* infection in New Hampshire and contiguous states, by county. Cases per 100,000 population.

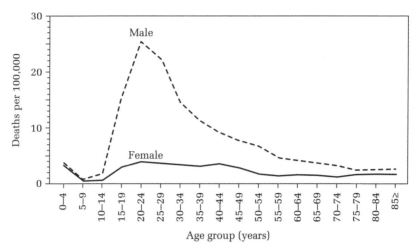

Figure 1–3 Homicide rate, by age and sex of victim—United States, 2004. Cases per 100,000 population.

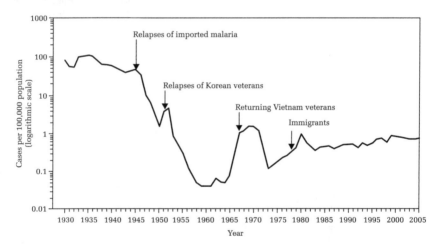

Figure 1–4 Malaria rates, by year—United States, 1930–2005. Cases per 100,000 population.

time, we have continued to see increases in numbers of reported cases of malaria involving immigrant populations as well as U.S. citizens who travel abroad.

Surveillance information also can be used to detect epidemics. For example, during the swine influenza immunization program in 1976, a surveillance system was established to detect adverse sequelae related to the program (*27*). Working with state and local health departments, CDC was able to detect an epidemic of Guillain–Barré syndrome, which led rapidly to termination of a program in which 40 million U.S. citizens had been vaccinated. In fact, the majority of epidemics have not been detected by such analysis of routinely collected data but are identified through the astuteness and alertness of clinicians and community public

Table 1–1 Uses of Surveillance

- Quantitative estimates of the magnitude of a health problem
- Portrayal of the natural history of disease
- Detection of epidemics
- Documentation of the distribution and spread of a health event
- Facilitation of epidemiologic and laboratory research
- Generation and testing of hypotheses
- Evaluation of control and prevention measures
- Monitoring of changes in infectious agents
- Monitoring of isolation activities
- Detection of changes in health practice
- Planning of public health actions and use of resources
- Appropriation and allocation of prevention and care resources

health officials. From a pragmatic viewpoint, the key idea is that when someone notes an unusual occurrence in the health status of a community, the existence of organized surveillance efforts in the health department provides the infrastructure for conveying information to facilitate a timely and appropriate response. Laboratory data provide critical information about specfic pathogen and toxin characteristics (*28*); PULSENET, a national electronic laboratory reporting system for specific bacterial pathogens, has led to early detection of point-source outbreaks caused by *Escherichia coli* 0157:H7, salomonella, and shigella (*29*).

Distribution and spread of disease can be documented from surveillance data, as observed in the county-specific data regarding salmonellosis (Fig. 1–2). Cancer mortality statistics in the United States have also been mapped at the county level to identify selected geographic patterns that indicate hypotheses on etiology and risk (*30*). Recognition of such patterns can lead to further epidemiologic or laboratory research, sometimes using persons identified in surveillance as subjects in epidemiologic studies. The association between the periconceptual use of multivitamins by women and the development of neural tube defects by their children was documented by using children identified through a surveillance system for congenital malformations (*31*).

Surveillance information can also be used to develop and test hypotheses. For example, in 1978, PHS announced a measles elimination program that included an active effort to vaccinate school-age children. Because of this program and the state laws that excluded school students who had not been vaccinated, CDC anticipated a change in the age pattern of persons reported to have measles. Before the initiation of the program, the highest reported rates of measles were for children aged 10 through 14 years. As predicted, almost immediately after the school exclusion policy was implemented, not only did an overall decrease in the number of cases occur, but a shift in peak occurrence occurred from school-age to preschool-age children (Fig. 1–5). By 1979, the measles incidence was even lower, and age-specific patterns had been altered.

Surveillance information can be used in evaluating control and prevention measures. With information derived from routinely collected data, one can examine—without special studies—the effect of a health policy. For example, the

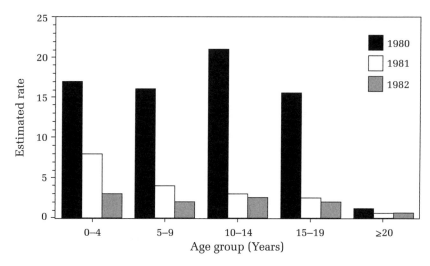

Figure 1–5 Reported cases of measles by age group—United States, 1980–1982. Reported cases per 100,000 population. Note: rates were estimated by extrapolating age from the records of patients with known age.

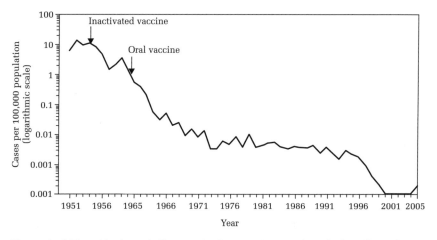

Figure 1–6 Logarithmic-scale line graph of reported cases of paralytic poliomyelitis— United States, 1951–2005. Reported cases per 100,000 population.

introduction of inactivated poliovirus vaccine in the United States in the 1950s was followed by a decrease in the number of reported cases of paralytic poliomyelitis, and the subsequent introduction in the 1960s of oral poliovirus vaccine was followed by an even greater decline (Fig. 1–6).

Efforts to monitor changes in infectious agents have been facilitated by using surveillance data. In the late 1970s, antibiotic-resistant gonorrhea was introduced into the United States from Asia. Laboratory and clinical practice-based surveillance for cases of gonorrhea enabled public health officials to monitor the rapid diffusion of multiple strains of this bacterium nationally, and surveillance

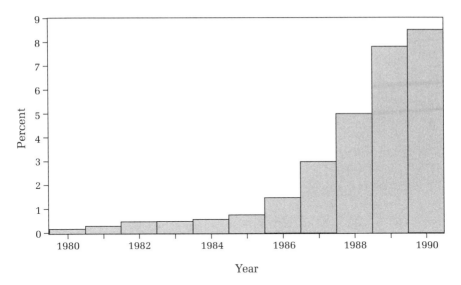

Figure 1–7 Percentage of reported cases of gonorrhea caused by antibiotic resistant strains—United States, 1980–1990.

facilitated prevention activities, including notifying clinicians of correct treatment procedures (Fig. 1–7). Similarly, the National Nosocomial Infections Surveillance System, a voluntary, hospital-based surveillance system for hospital-acquired infections, has been used to monitor changes in antibiotic-resistance patterns of infectious agents associated with hospitalized patients and is now integrated into The National HealthCare Safety Network (see Chapter 15).

As noted earlier, the first use of surveillance was for monitoring persons with a view of imposing isolation and quarantine as necessary. Although this use of surveillance is now rare in the United States, in 1975—with the introduction of a suspected case of Lassa fever—approximately 500 potential contacts of the patient were monitored daily for 2 weeks to ensure that secondary spread of this serious infection did not occur (*32*).

Surveillance information can also be used to good effect for detecting changes in health practice. The increasing use of technologies in health care has become a growing concern during the past decade; surveillance information can be useful in this area (*33*). For example, since 1965, the rate of cesarean delivery in the United States has increased from less than 5% to approximately 30% of all deliveries (Fig. 1–8). This kind of information is useful both in planning research to learn the causes of these changes and in monitoring the impact of such changes in practice and procedure on outcomes and costs associated with health care.

Surveillance information is useful for population health planning. With knowledge about changes in the population structure or in the nature of conditions that might affect a population, officials can, with more confidence, plan for optimizing available resources. For example, information about refugees who entered

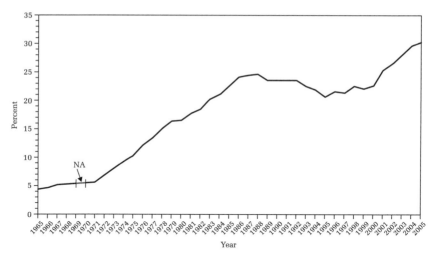

Figure 1-8 Cesarean deliveries as a percentage of all deliveries in the U.S. hospitals—1970–2005.

the United States from Southeast Asia in the early 1980s was broadly applicable; it told where people settled, described the ages and sexes of the population, and identified health problems that might be expected among that population. With this information, health officials were able to plan more effectively the appropriate health services and preventive activities for this new population.

Finally, data from surveillance systems are used for appropriation and allocation of billions of U.S. dollars each year for care, treatment, and prevention of a variety of conditions. HIV surveillance data in the United States is used by the U.S. Congress annually to allocate billions of dollars in care and treatment for persons living with HIV/AIDS through the Ryan White Care Act to state and local organizations that provide need-based care to millions of persons in all states in the county (*34*).

CURRENT ISSUES IN PUBLIC HEALTH SURVEILLANCE

During the 21st century, certain activities continue to contribute to the evolution of public health surveillance. First, use of the computer continues to revolutionize the practice of public health surveillance. In the United States, by the early 1990s, the National Electronic Telecommunications System for Surveillance (NETSS) had linked all state health departments by computer for the routine collection, analysis, and dissemination of information on notifiable health conditions (*35*). The Minitel system used in France has also demonstrated the essential utility of office-based surveillance for multiple conditions of public health importance (*36*). The transition to integrated electronic disease surveillance systems has continued to accelerate; by 2007, a total of 38 states and the District of Columbia were using secure, Internet-based systems for entry of notifiable disease reports that include an integrated data repository, electronic laboratory result reporting, and an Internet-based browser (personal communication, Scott Danos, MPH, CDC, 2008). Forty-one states and the District of Columbia receive laboratory test results through an automated electronic laboratory results system. The Internet-based system enables immediate data access by state and local health departments, as well as CDC; certain state systems automatically send e-mail and telephone messages to public health offices in the event of an urgent laboratory report (*37*).

A principle goal of both the National Electronic Disease Surveillance System (NEDSS) and the Public Health Information Network (PHIN) is the use of standard systems to exchange information between the clinical and public health practice sectors. Use of secure, Internet-based systems enables public health response 24 hours a day, 7 days a week. This improves state and local capacity to manage workloads and increases capacity during disasters and epidemics. Public health informatics is an emerging discipline that promotes sharing and use of health data through the rapidly evolving fields of information science, engineering, and technology (*38*) (*see* Chapter 5). Informatics contributions to public health surveillance include data standards, a communications infrastructure, and policy-level agreements on data access, sharing, and burden reduction (*39*). Along with epidemiology and statistics, informatics has become a critical science in the practice of surveillance, and the contributions of this emerging science are anticipated to be of increasing importance.

A distributed system of coordinated, timely, and useful multisource public health surveillance and health information can be readily developed. Integration of independently developed, disease-specific, or source-specific surveillance systems is a critical element in implementing such a system. Similar systems are used today in finance, travel, and retail marketing, but no such system is used routinely in public health practice in the United States. The technology and the majority of the necessary data are available; however, to make these data useful, our society must have sufficient commitment to develop and maintain such a distributed system for public health. This commitment must be underscored by the recognition and acceptance of the needs for both community health and individual privacy and confidentiality (*40*) (*see* Chapter 9).

The second area of renewed activity associated with surveillance is that of epidemiologic and statistical analysis. A byproduct of using computers is the ability to make more effective use of sophisticated tools to detect changes in patterns of occurrence of health problems. In the 1980s, applications and methods of time-series analysis and other techniques have enabled us to provide more meaningful interpretation of data collected during surveillance efforts (*41*). More sophisticated techniques such as geographical/spatial methods and space–time monitoring will no doubt continue to be applied in the area of public health as they are developed (*see* Chapter 6).

Until recently, surveillance information was disseminated as written documents published periodically by government agencies. Although paper reports will continue to be produced and the use of print media will continue to be refined, public health officials also use such electronic media as the *MMWR* for disseminating surveillance information (*42*). More effective use of electronic media and all the other tools of communication should facilitate use of surveillance information for public health practice. Meanwhile, ready access to detailed information related to individual persons will continue to provide ethical and legal concerns that might constrain access to data of potential public health importance (43).

The 1990s saw surveillance concepts applied to such new areas of public health practice as chronic disease (44), environmental (45) and occupational health (46), emerging infectious diseases (47), injury control (48), and risk behaviors (49). In 1998, recognition of the importance of surveillance in preventing intentional injuries was underscored by the publication of a special issue of the *American Journal of Preventive Medicine* devoted to firearm-related injury surveillance (50). Evolution and development of methods for these programmatic areas will continue to be a major challenge for public health practice. In addition, changes in the organization of medical practice (e.g., emergence of managed care in the United States) will affect the way data are collected and used in public health practice (51). A more fundamental principle that will underlie the ongoing development of surveillance is the increasing ability of people to view public health surveillance as a scientific endeavor (52). A growing appreciation of the need for high standards in the practice of surveillance will improve the quality of surveillance programs and will therefore facilitate the analysis and use of surveillance information. An important result of this more vigorous approach to surveillance practice will be the increased frequency and quality of the evaluation of the practice of surveillance (53).

Finally, and possibly most important, surveillance should be used more consistently and thoughtfully by policymakers. Epidemiologists not only need to improve the quality of their analysis, interpretation, and display information for public health use, they also need to listen to persons who are empowered to set policy to understand what stimulates the policymakers' interests and actions. In turn, policymakers as well as public health officials and researchers should describe their needs for surveillance information. This allows surveillance information to be crafted so that it is presented in its most useful form to the appropriate audience and in the necessary time-frame (*see* Chapter 7). As we maximize the utility of the concept of "data for decision making" and better understand what is essential to that process, we will raise the practice of public health surveillance to a new and higher level of importance.

Public health surveillance is a cornerstone of public health practice, providing accurate and timely data that are essential to informed decision making and action. Surveillance is the foundation of all public health practice, and we must continue to develop methodologically sound systems that yield high-quality, useful data that inform policy and practice. New technology, innovations in surveillance methods, informatics, renewed interest in redesign of the health system in the United States, and the focus on emergency response challenge us to be creative and thoughtful as we move surveillance science forward. In this effort, we must have rigorous evaluation of public health surveillance systems. To do this completely, one must understand fully the principles of surveillance and its role in guiding epidemiologic research and influencing other aspects of the overall mission of public health. Epidemiologic, statistical, and informatics methods must continue to evolve for application to public health surveillance practice; the most appropriate computer technology for efficient data collection, analysis, and graphic display must be applied; ethical, policy, and legal concerns must be addressed effectively; the use of surveillance systems must be evaluated routinely; and surveillance principles must be applied to emerging areas of public health practice.

REFERENCES

1. Centers for Disease Control. *Comprehensive Plan for Epidemiologic Surveillance.* Atlanta: US Department of Health and Human Services, Public Health Service; 1986.
2. Eylenbosch WJ, Noah ND. Historical aspects. In: Eylenbosch WJ, Noah ND, eds. *Surveillance in Health and Disease.* Oxford: Oxford University Press; 1988:3–8.
3 Moro ML, McCormick A. Surveillance for communicable disease. In: Eylenbosch WJ, Noah ND, eds. Surveillance in Health and Disease. Oxford: Oxford University Press; 1988:166–182.
4. Hartgerink MJ. Health surveillance and planning for health care in the Netherlands. *Int J Epidemiol* 1976;5:87–91.
5. Surveillance [Editorial]. *Int J Epidemiol* 1976;5:4–6.
6. Langmuir AD. William Farr: founder of modern concepts of surveillance. *Int J Epidemiol* 1976;5:13–18.
7. Hinman AR. Surveillance of communicable diseases. Presented at the *100th Annual Meeting of the American Public Health Association*, Atlantic City, New Jersey, November 15, 1972.
8. *Vital Statistics of the United States, 1958.* Washington, DC: National Office of Vital Statistics; 1959.
9. Trask JW. Vital statistics: a discussion of what they are and their uses in public health administration. *Public Health Rep* 1915;Suppl 12:30–34.
10. Bowditch HI, Webster DL, Hoadley JC, *et al.* Letter from the Massachusetts State Board of Health to physicians. *Public Health Rep* 1915;12(Suppl):31.
11. Centers for Disease Control. *Manual of Procedures for National Morbidity Reporting and Public Health Surveillance Activities.* Atlanta: US Department of Health and Human Services, Public Health Service; 1985.
12. Chapin CV. State health organization. *JAMA* 1916;66:699–703.
13. National Office of Vital Statistics. Reported incidence of selected notifiable disease: United States, each division and state, 1920–50. *Vital Stat Spec Rep (National Summaries)* 1953;37:1180–1181.
14. Chorba TL, Berkelman RL, Safford SK, Gibbs NP, Hull HF. The reportable diseases. I. Mandatory reporting of infectious diseases by clinicians. *JAMA* 1989;262:3018–3026.
15. Koo D, Wetterhall SF. History and current status of the National Notifiable Diseases Surveillance System. *J Public Health Manag Pract* 1996;2:4–10.
16. Langmuir AD. Evolution of the concept of surveillance in the United States. *Proc R Soc Med* 1971;64:681–684.
17. Langmuir AD, Nathanson N, Hall WJ. Surveillance of poliomyelitis in the United States in 1955. *Am J Public Health Nations Health* 1956;46:75–88.
18. Nathanson N, Langmuir AD. The Cutter incident: poliomyelitis following formaldehyde–inactivated poliovirus vaccination in the United States during the spring of 1955. *Am J Hyg* 1963;78:16–81.

19. Langmuir AD. The surveillance of communicable diseases of national importance. *N Engl J Med* 1963;268:182–192.
20. Thacker SB, Gregg MB. Implementing the concepts of William Farr: the contributions of Alexander D. Langmuir to public health surveillance and communications. *Am J Epidemiol* 1996;144:523–528.
21. Raska K. National and international surveillance of communicable diseases. *WHO Chron* 1966;20:315–321.
22. Terminology of malaria and of malaria eradication. Report for drafting committee. Geneva: World Health Organization, 1963.
23. National and global surveillance of communicable disease. Report of the technical discussions at the Twenty-First World Health Assembly. A21/Technical Discussions/5. Geneva: World Health Organization, May 1968.
24. *Int J Epidemiol* 1976;5:3–91.
25. Thacker SB, Berkelman RL. Public health surveillance in the United States. *Epidemiol Rev* 1988;10:164–190.
26 Thacker SB. Les principes et la practique de la surveillance en santé publique: l'utilisation des données en santé publique. *Santé Publique* 1992;4:43–49.
27. Retailliau HF, Curtis AC, Starr G, Caesar G, Eddins DL, Hattwick MA. Illness after influenza vaccination reported through a nationwide surveillance system, 1976–1977. *Am J Epidemiol* 1980;111:270–278.
28. Bean NH, Martin SM, Bradford H Jr. PHLIS: an electronic system for reporting public health data from remote sites. *Am J Public Health* 1992;82:1273–1276.
29. Swaminathan B, Barrett TJ, Hunter SB, Tauxe RV, CDC PulseNet Task Force. PulseNet: the molecular subtyping network for foodborne bacterial dissease surveillance, United States. *Emerg Infect Dis* 2001;7:382–389.
30. Pickle LW, Mungiole M, Jones GK, White AA. *An Atlas of United States Mortality.* Hyattsville, MD: US Department of Health and Human Services, National Center for Health Statistics; 1996.
31. Mulinare J, Cordero JF, Erickson D, Berry RJ. Periconceptional use of multivitamins and the occurrence of neural tube defects. *JAMA* 1988;260:3141–3145.
32. Zweighaft RM, Fraser DW, Hattwick MAW, *et al.* Lassa fever: response to an imported case. *N Engl J Med* 1977;297:803–807.
33. Thacker SB, Berkelman RL. Surveillance of medical technologies. *J Public Health Policy* 1986;7:363–377.
34. Ryan White Comprehensive AIDS Resources Emergency (CARE) Act Ryan White Care Act, Ryan White, Pub.L. 101-381, 104 Stat. 576, enacted August 18, 1990.
35. Centers for Disease Control. Current trends: National Electronic Telecommunications Systems for Surveillance—United States, 1990–1991. *MMWR Morb Mortal Wkly Rep* 1991;40:502–503.
36. Valleron AJ, Bouvet E, Garnerin P, *et al.* A computer network for the surveillance of communicable diseases: the French experiment. *Am J Public Health* 1986;76:1289–1292.
37. Centers for Disease Control and Prevention (CDC). National Electronic Disease Surveillance System. Atlanta, GA: US Department of Health and Human Services, CDC. http://www.cdc.gov/nedss. Accessed January 10, 2008.
38. Broome CV, Loonsk JW. A standards-based approach to integrated information systems for bioterrorism preparedness and response. U.S. Department of Health and Human Services Data Council Meeting, February 13, 2003. Atlanta, GA: CDC, 2003.

39. Morris G, Snider D, Katz M. Integrating public health informatics and surveillance systems. *J Public Health Manag Pract* 1996;2:24–27.
40. Thacker SB, Stroup DF. Future directions for comprehensive public health surveillance and health information systems in the United States. *Am J Epidemiol* 1994;140:383–397.
41. Stroup DF, Wharton M, Kafadar K, Dean AG. Evaluation of a method for detecting aberrations in public health surveillance data. *Am J Epidemiol* 1993;137:373–380.
42. Centers for Disease Control and Prevention. Notice to readers update: availability of electronic *MMWR* on Internet. *Morb Mortal Wkly Rep* 1995;44:757–759.
43. Fairchild AL, Bayer R, Colgrove J. *Searching Eyes: Privacy, the State, and Disease Surveillance in America*. Berkeley, CA: University of California Press; 2007.
44. Thacker SB, Stroup DF, Rothenberg RB, Brownson RC. Public health surveillance for chronic conditions: a scientific basis for decisions. *Stat Med* 1995;14:629–641.
45. Thacker SB, Stroup DF, Parrish RG, Anderson HA. Surveillance in environmental public health. *Am J Public Health* 1996;86:633–638.
46. Baker EL, Melius JM, Millar JD. Surveillance of occupational illness and injury in the United States: current perspectives and future directions. *J Public Health Policy* 1988;9:198–221.
47. Centers for Disease Control and Prevention. Preventing emerging infectious diseases: a strategy for the 21st century; overview of the updated CDC plan. *Morb Mortal Wkly Rep* 1998;47(No. RR-15):1–14.
48. Graitcer PL. The development of state and local injury surveillance systems. *J Safety Res* 1987;18:191–198.
49. Centers for Disease Control and Prevention. Behavioral Risk Factor Surveillance System operational and user's guide, Version 3.0. Atlanta, GA: US Department of Health and Human Services, CDC; 2004.
50. Rosenberg ML, Hammond WR. Surveillance the key to firearm prevention. *Am J Prev Med* 1998;15(Suppl 1):1.
51. Rutherford GW. Public health, communicable diseases, and managed care: will managed care improve or weaken communicable disease control? *Am J Prev Med* 1998;14(3 Suppl):53–59.
52. Thacker SB, Berkelman RL, Stroup DF. The science of public health surveillance. *J Public Health Policy* 1989;10:187–203.
53. Centers for Disease Control. Guidelines for evaluating surveillance systems. *Morb Mortal Wkly Rep* 1988;37(Suppl No. S-5):1–20.

2

Considerations in Planning a Surveillance System

STEVEN M. TEUTSCH

While few people plan to fail, many fail to plan. The outcome is the same.
                                                                —Anonymous

Surveillance systems evolve in response to ever-changing needs of society in general and of the public health community in particular. To understand and meet those needs, an organized approach to planning, developing, implementing, and maintaining surveillance systems is imperative. The sections below discuss approaches to the planning and evaluation processes that are presented in more detail elsewhere in this book. Appendix 2A provides a description of a single surveillance system. Table 2–1 demonstrates the steps in planning a system.

OBJECTIVES OF A SURVEILLANCE SYSTEM

Planning a surveillance system begins with a clear understanding of the purpose of surveillance—that is, the answer to the question, "What do you want to know?" In the context of public health, surveillance might be established to meet a variety of objectives, including assessment of public health status of a health condition, establishment of public health priorities, evaluation of programs, and allocation of resources. Surveillance data can be used in all of the following ways (*see* Chapter 1):

- to estimate the magnitude of a health problem in the population at risk
- to understand the natural history of a disease or injury
- to detect outbreaks or epidemics
- to document the distribution and spread of a health event
- to generate hypotheses about etiology
- to evaluate control strategies
- to monitor changes in infectious agents
- to monitor isolation activities

Table 2–1 Steps in Planning a Surveillance System

1. Establish objectives.
2. Develop case definitions.
3. Determine data source or data collection mechanism (type of system).
4. Develop data collection instruments.
5. Field-test methods.
6. Develop and test analytic approach.
7. Develop dissemination mechanism.
8. Ensure use of analysis and interpretation.

- to detect changes in health practice
- to assess the quality of health care
- to assess the safety of drugs, devices, diagnostics, or procedures
- to identify research needs and to facilitate epidemiologic and laboratory research
- to facilitate planning

Surveillance is inherently outcome-oriented and focused on various outcomes associated with health-related events or their immediate antecedents. These include the frequency of an illness or injury, usually measured in terms of numbers of cases, incidence, or prevalence; the severity of the condition, measured as a case fatality ratio, hospitalization rate, mortality rate, or disability rate; and the impact of the condition, measured in terms of cost or surrogate measures. Where risk factors or specific procedures are incontrovertibly linked to health outcomes, it is often useful to measure them because they are often more frequent (and hence more precisely ascertainable) than the health outcomes and can be linked to public health interventions. For example, mammography with suitable follow-up is the major prevention strategy for reducing mortality associated with breast cancer. The level of use of mammography by women can be regularly monitored and should be a more timely indicator of the impact of public health prevention programs than measurement of mortality from breast cancer. Surveillance data should also provide basic information on the use of mammography services by age and race/ethnicity of recipient, allowing better targeting of prevention efforts on the population sectors with the lowest use. In addition, over-use by some parts of the population (e.g., women under age 40 years, who do not have other risk factors) might stimulate efforts to reduce unnecessary procedures.

High-priority health events clearly should be under surveillance. However, determining which events should be considered high-priority events can be a daunting task. Both quantitative and qualitative approaches can be used in a selection process. Some quantitative factors are shown in Table 2–2. In addition, criteria based on a consensus process to identify high-priority problems might identify emerging issues or problems that otherwise might not be considered. The consensus process leading to the Year 2010 and anticipated for the Year 2020 Health Promotion and Disease Prevention Objectives in the United States is an example of a mechanism for identifying high-priority conditions, types of behavior, and interventions that require ongoing monitoring (*1*).

Table 2–2 Criteria for Identifying High-Priority Health Events for Surveillance

---

- Frequency
  - incidence
  - prevalence
  - mortality

- Severity
  - case-fatality ratio
  - hospitalization rate
  - disability rate
  - years of potential life lost
  - quality-adjusted life years lost

- Cost
  - direct and indirect costs

- Preventability
- Communicability
- Public interest

Public health surveillance is also used to drive action in urgent health situations where timely information is required for effective intervention. The global SARS outbreak in 2002 to 2003 (2), numerous disease surveillance activities during Hurricane Katrina (3), and novel H1N1 influenza in 2009 (4) are examples of agile public health surveillance addressing new or unusual circumstances, driving public health interventions to identify pathogens, contain transmission, and manage population health.

Because public health surveillance in the United States is driven by the public health need to be cognizant of diseases and injuries in the community and to respond appropriately, surveillance is inherently an applied science. Therefore, as surveillance has evolved, it is generally undertaken only when there is reasonable expectation that appropriate control measures will be taken. For many conditions, the link between surveillance and action is obvious (e.g., meningococcal meningitis prophylaxis for contacts of patients diagnosed as having meningitis). For emerging conditions, such as eosinophilia-myalgia syndrome or West Nile Virus, there is a compelling public health need to identify cases (delineate the magnitude of the problem), identify the mode of spread, and take appropriate action. For indicators of health-care quality, surveillance can be used to identify services that need improvement and also to guide the purchase of health care and prevention services.

Surveillance data are often augmented by additional studies to determine more precisely the causes, natural history, predisposing factors, and modes of transmission associated with the health problem. Yet undertaking surveillance exclusively for research purposes is less often warranted. Research needs are often better served by other, more precise (and often more costly) methods that facilitate more detailed data collection and tracking of cases. For example, longitudinal follow-up of type I diabetes cases might have value for surveillance but are justified primarily because they fill research or quality-of-care needs. The ongoing public health application of these data is more limited. Scarce public health resources and the efforts of health-care providers to report cases need to be focused on problems for which the public health importance and the need for public health action can be readily recognized.

A primary role of surveillance is the assessment of the overall health status of a community. One approach to this issue is the development and identification of a set of indicators that measure major components of health status. Such a set has been developed in the United States to be used at national, state, and local levels (5, 6). Another approach is to examine the most frequent, severe, costly, and preventable conditions in the community by examining the most frequent causes of death, hospitalization, injury, disability, infection, worksite-associated illness and injury, and major risk factors for all the preceding items. This information can be obtained in most communities in terms of age, race/ethnicity, gender, and temporal trends. Regular assessments of the information can form the basis for educating the community about its major health problems and for identifying specific conditions that merit more intensive surveillance and intervention.

METHODS

Once the purpose of and need for a surveillance system have been identified, methods for obtaining, analyzing, disseminating, and using the information should be determined and implemented (*see also* Chapters 4, 6, and 7).

Because surveillance systems are ongoing and require the cooperation of many individuals, careful consideration must be given to issues of evaluation discussed in Chapter 8. The system adopted must be feasible and acceptable to those who will contribute to its success; it must be sensitive enough to provide the information required to do the job at hand, while having high positive predictive value to minimize the expenditure of resources on following up false-positive cases. A surveillance system should be flexible enough to meet the continually evolving needs of the community and to accommodate changes in patterns of disease and injury. It must provide information that is timely enough to be acted on. All of these considerations must be carefully balanced to design a system that can successfully meet identified needs without becoming excessively costly or burdensome.

System Development, Data Collection, and Management

Case Definitions

Public health surveillance is heavily dependent on clear case definitions that include criteria for person, place, and time and that are potentially categorized by the degree of certainty regarding diagnosis as "suspected" or "confirmed" cases (7). These have been documented for notifiable diseases (8). Clear "case definitions" are important for risk behaviors and environmental exposures as well.

Although high sensitivity and specificity are both desirable, generally one comes at the expense of the other. A balance must be struck between the desire for high sensitivity and the level of effort required to follow-up false-positive cases where necessary. In addition, case definitions evolve over time. During periods of outbreaks, cases epidemiologically linked to the outbreak cases may be accepted as cases, whereas in non-epidemic periods, serologic or other more specific information may be required. Similarly, when active surveillance is used, such as in measles control programs, the number of cases identified tend to rise.

As our understanding of a disease and its associated laboratory testing improves, alterations in case definitions often lead to changes in sensitivity and specificity. As new systems complement old ones (e.g., as a morbidity system supplements a mortality system for injury surveillance), the reported frequency and patterns of conditions change. These changes must be taken into account in analysis and interpretation of secular trends in the frequency of reporting. It is all too easy to define cases of various conditions with such different criteria that it is difficult to compare the essential descriptors of person, place, or time. For example, in surveillance of diabetes, one could determine the prevalence of diabetes from surveys (self-reported), from surveys using glucose determination (laboratory-confirmed), or from reviews of ambulatory or hospital records (physician-diagnosed). Each method provides a different perspective on the problem. Self-reports are subject to vagaries of recall and variation in interpretation (patient may be under treatment, may have "a touch of diabetes"—or impaired glucose tolerance—or may have a history of gestational diabetes). Determinations of glucose levels allow detection of previously undiagnosed diabetes. Medical records identify only patients who are currently receiving medical care.

Case definitions should include criteria for person, place, time, clinical or laboratory diagnosis, and epidemiologic features.

Active and Passive Systems

Primary surveillance systems have traditionally been classified as passive or active. For example, most routine notifiable-disease surveillance relies on passive reporting. On the basis of a published list of conditions, health-care providers report notifiable diseases to the local health department on a case-by-case basis. This passive system has the advantage of being simple and not burdensome to the health department, but it is limited by variability and incompleteness in reporting. Although the completeness of reporting can be augmented by efforts to publicize the importance of reporting and by continued feedback to communications media representatives, passive reporting systems might not be representative and might fail to identify outbreaks. To obviate these problems, more active systems are often used for conditions of particular importance. These systems involve regular outreach to potential reporters to stimulate the reporting of specific diseases or injuries. Active systems can validate the representativeness of passive reports, assure more complete reporting of conditions (9), or be used in conjunction with specific epidemiologic investigations. Because resources are often limited, active systems are often used for brief periods for discrete purposes such as the measles elimination efforts.

Limited Surveillance Systems

Some surveillance efforts may not require long-term solutions. Surveillance to deal with specific problems might be needed to address problems for which all cases must be identified to assess the level of risk. Such programs can be conducted to resolve specific problems and then be terminated (*10*). Similarly, for logistic and economic reasons, it may not be feasible to mount a surveillance system across large geographic areas, and representative populations may need to be selected. Sentinel providers can also provide information on common conditions or conditions of particular interest to them.

Data Security and Confidentiality

Data security and confidentiality are of critical concern in a public health surveillance system. In most circumstances in the United States, data are being collected under the authority of state or local laws and do not require consent or notification (*see* Chapters 10 and 18). Often data are personal and private in nature; often they are associated with identifiers, or persons can be indirectly identified by their demographic characteristics. Public health data are protected by state law, but these protections lack standardization and vary substantially by state (*11*). Each system must carefully consider policies and protections for identifiable personal data. Model public health laws, which include strong privacy safeguards, were developed in the 1990s (*12*), but adoption across states has been difficult. Still, the model legislation provides specific actions a program can take to ensure security and confidentiality of public health data (*see* Chapter 10).

Field Testing

The careful development and field testing of surveillance systems and procedures is important to facilitate the implementation of feasible systems and to minimize making changes as systems are implemented on a broad scale. The frustration engendered by a new and poorly executed system may undermine efforts to improve or use existing systems for the same or other conditions. As new surveillance systems or new instruments and procedures are developed, field tests of their feasibility and acceptability are recommended. These field-test projects can demonstrate how readily the information can be obtained and can detect difficulties in data-collection procedures or in the content of specific questions. Analyses of this test information may also identify problems with the information collected. Model surveillance systems may facilitate the examination and comparison of a variety of approaches that would not be feasible on too large a scale and might identify methods suitable for other conditions or other settings.

The data to be collected by a surveillance system, the data sources and collection methods, and the procedures for handling the information should be developed and tested.

Data Collection

Information on diseases, injuries, and risk factors can be obtained in many ways. Each mechanism has characteristics that must be balanced against the purpose of the system (*see* Chapter 4). Time is of the essence for frequently fatal acute conditions such as plague, rabies, or meningococcal meningitis. Rapid provider-based disease-reporting systems are most appropriate for such potentially catastrophic conditions with high and urgent preventability requirements. Conversely, detailed information on influenza strains or Salmonella serotypes must come from laboratory-based systems. Long-term mortality patterns are available through vital records systems.

Often, existing data sets can provide surveillance data. Such sets include vital records, administrative systems, and risk factor or health interview surveys. Some examples of administrative systems that can provide needed data are hospital discharge data, medical management information and billing systems, electronic health records, police records for violence, and school records for disabilities or injuries among children. In addition, with some modification, an existing system might provide necessary data more economically or efficiently than a newly initiated system. Although existing data sets can be used for surveillance, they are not surveillance systems in and of themselves. Surveillance is a larger process that requires analysis, interpretation, and use of the data. These steps are not components of most data systems.

Existing registries or surveys might collect information on defined populations. To the extent that the condition of interest is uniformly distributed, the population under study is reasonably representative, and the information collected is available on a timely basis, such systems can be valuable data sources. Although many registries are established for research or quality-improvement purposes, they often provide valuable data for surveillance purposes. In particular, cancer registries have been widely used (*13*).

Sentinel providers can also constitute a network for collecting data on common conditions, such as seasonal influenza; more specialized providers can provide data on less common conditions (e.g., ophthalmologists who provide information on treatment of patients for diabetic retinopathy).

Standardization

Data-collection instruments should use generally recognized and, where suitable, computerized formats for each data element to facilitate analysis and comparison with data collected in other systems (e.g., census and other surveillance data). Careful consideration should be given to collection of personal identifiers, minimizing the private identifiable information held by a system (*14*) (*see* Chapters 4 and 9). Although additional assurances of confidentiality and privacy considerations will be required, the ability to link data to other systems, such as through the National Death Index, may enhance the value of the system, arguing for striking a balance on this issue.

Analyzing and Interpreting Data

Data Analysis

A determination of the appropriate analytic approach to data should be an integral part of the planning of any surveillance system. The data needed to address the salient questions must be assessed to assure that the data source or collection process is adequate. Analyses might prove to be as simple as an ongoing review of all cases of rare but potentially devastating illnesses, such as plague. For most conditions, however, an assessment of the crude number of cases and rates is followed by a description of the population in which the condition occurs (person), where the condition occurs (place), and the period over which the condition occurs (time). These basic analyses require decisions as to the information that needs to be collected. The level of detail required varies substantially from condition to condition. For example, one might need more detailed information regarding the population that is not receiving prenatal care than on the one that is exposed to meningococcal disease, because the nature of the intervention for the former is likely to be more complex and to require an understanding of socioeconomic factors. Similarly, how one will collect data on geographic areas will depend on whether the data will be examined at the county, state, or census tract level.

Most contemporary surveillance systems are maintained electronically (see Chapter 5). Highly integrated computer systems and networks are widely available. Surveillance systems can be operated on personal computers and over the Internet. Software is now widely available to meet most basic analytic needs for surveillance, including statistical analyses, mapping, and graphing. The analytic approach often suggests a basic set of analyses that are performed on a regular basis. These analyses can be designed early in the development of the system and incorporated into an automated system, which can then be run by support personnel. The availability of easy-to-use computerized statistical software has increased the complexity and usefulness of analyses that can be performed on surveillance data, yielding more sophisticated uses of data in recent years (see Chapter 6).

The adequacy of the data collection system and the processing mechanisms should be assured.

Dissemination and Communication of Data

Information resulting from analyses of public health surveillance data must be presented in a compelling manner so that decision makers at all levels can readily see and understand its implications. Knowledge of the characteristics of the audiences for the information and how they might use it may dictate any of a variety of communications systems. Routine, public access to the data—consistent with privacy constraints—should be planned for and provided. This access can be facilitated with various electronic media, ranging from systems with structured analysis features suitable for general users to files of raw data for persons who can do special or more detailed analyses themselves. The advent of the Internet and easily used graphic and mapping techniques have enhanced the availability of readily understood information.

The primary users of surveillance information, however, are public health professionals and health-care providers. More and more health-care purchasers and consumers look for information on quality-of-care and surveillance information to enhance management of the health-care system. Information directed primarily to those individuals should include the analyses and interpretation of surveillance results, along with recommendations that stem from the surveillance data. Graphs and maps should be used liberally to facilitate rapid review and comprehension of the data. Communications media represent a valuable secondary audience that can be used to amplify the messages from surveillance information. The media play an important role in presenting and reinforcing health messages. Innovative methods for presenting information that capitalize on current audiovisual technology should be explored (*see* Chapter 7).

Evaluation of Surveillance Systems

Planning, like surveillance itself, is an iterative process requiring the regular reassessment of objectives and methods (*see* Chapter 8). The fundamental question to be answered in evaluation is whether the purposes of the surveillance system have been met. Did the system generate needed answers to problems? Was the information timely? Was it useful for planners, researchers, health-care providers, and public health professionals? How was the information used? Was it indeed worth the effort? Would those who participated in the system wish to (or be willing to) continue to participate? What could be done to enhance the attributes of the system (timeliness, simplicity, flexibility, acceptability, sensitivity, positive predictive value, and representativeness)?

Answers to these questions will direct subsequent efforts to revise the system. Changes might be minor (e.g., the addition of data elements to existing forms) or major (e.g., the need to obtain information from entirely different data sources). For example, a system to determine use of mammography might be based on administrative billing systems, yet problems with reports of multiple mammography examinations for the same individual might require the addition of unique patient identifiers or the addition of questions on mammography use from self-reports on health interview surveys. If access emerges as a critical factor in mammography use, then ongoing monitoring of the quantity and location of mammography facilities or monitoring for appropriate medical care coverage for mammography might be indicated.

Periodic rigorous evaluation assures that surveillance systems remain vibrant. Systems that assess problems whose only interest is historical should be discontinued or simplified to reduce the burden. Contemporary systems should take advantage of the emergence of new technology for information collection, analysis, and dissemination. They should capitalize on new information systems. For example, sentinel surveillance systems have become more flexible to allow the inclusion of an array of topics. Electronic medical records and standardized clinical databases all provide opportunities to obtain data that have been burdensome or difficult to acquire (*15*). These information sources often provide data in a more timely fashion and allow individuals to be tracked—an option that would be virtually impossible without such electronic systems.

INVOLVEMENT OF INTERESTED PARTIES
IN SURVEILLANCE

Virtually all surveillance systems involve networks of organizations and individuals at all levels of public health—federal, state, and local. Surveillance of notifiable disease (*see* Appendix 2A) relies on health-care providers, including clinicians, hospitals, and laboratories, to report to local health departments, which have the initial responsibility for responding to reports and amassing data. In many states, epidemiologists in the state health departments are responsible for surveillance and control of notifiable diseases in their states. In larger states, other organizational units (such as those dealing with sexually transmitted disease, immunization, or tuberculosis control) often have primary responsibility for surveillance and control of specific diseases or injuries. The state epidemiologist is responsible for the ongoing quality control, collection, analysis, interpretation, dissemination, and use of notifiable-disease data within that state (*see* Chapter 18). Data are subsequently forwarded to the national level, where they are again analyzed, interpreted, and disseminated.

Programs for injuries, chronic diseases, environmental exposures, risk behaviors, and disease determinants also have complex organizational structures and involve a wide array of external professional and voluntary interest groups whose needs must be addressed. Some basic surveillance information can be gleaned from such ongoing information systems as vital records, hospitalization programs, and registries. Although some of these conditions are part of state notifiable-disease lists, many require surveillance systems to be established in unique places (e.g., rehabilitation units and emergency medical services for spinal cord injuries or radiology centers for mammography). The support and interest of these groups of constituents are valuable in establishing the systems; these groups can provide key input regarding purposes of systems and users of systems, as well as assistance in developing the systems themselves.

The complex relationships among these organizational units and their constituents requires open communication to establish priorities and methods consistent with the needs and resources of each group. The conflicting desire for more detailed information must be balanced against the associated burden and cost, as well as against the utility of collecting extensive amounts of data. For example, electronic systems that may facilitate higher quality, more complete, and more timely data also involve the commitment of equipment, training, and changes in day-to-day activities that may permeate all levels of the system. One must understand the needs of each recipient group for the information and assess and assure their commitment to the system. It is also critical to be attentive to how components of the system can best be integrated into the day-to-day operation of the overall system.

The Council of State and Territorial Epidemiologists (CSTE) has the authority in the United States to recommend which health conditions should be notifiable. After this list has been agreed on by CSTE membership, it is then up to each state to determine whether and how the conditions should be made reportable. Although most states report all those conditions considered to be nationally notifiable, a wide range of additional conditions is reportable in only a few states (7). States may exercise their authority through regulations, boards of health, or legislative procedures. The diversity of these methods is described more fully in Chapters 10 and 18. Each of these mechanisms entails the involvement of groups with an array of medical, administrative, public health, and policy interests.

The success of surveillance depends heavily on the quality of the information entered into the system and on the value of the information to its intended users. A clear understanding of how policymakers, voluntary and professional groups, public health professionals, and others might use surveillance data is valuable in garnering the support of these audiences for the surveillance system.

Appendix 2A

*The National Notifiable Diseases Surveillance System in the United States**

PURPOSE

The National Notifiable Diseases Surveillance System (NNDSS) collects information on approximately 78 diseases and conditions that are notifiable at the federal level in the United States for the purpose of preventing and controlling those conditions (*16,17*). In 2009, CSTE approved, for the first time, a list of nationally notifiable conditions categorized by three notification timelines: *(1)* immediate, extremely urgent notification within 4 hours; *(2)* immediate, urgent notification within 24 hours; and *(3)* standard notification within 7 days. NNDSS conditions are primarily infectious. Other nationally notifiable conditions include environmental and occupational events and are notifiable to other surveillance systems.

LEGAL BASIS

Diseases, injuries, and other conditions are reportable to state and local health departments as indicated by relevant laws and regulations. The legal basis varies by state, as does the authority for determining which conditions are reportable. Some are legislatively mandated; others are declared reportable by the state health officer, state epidemiologist, or board of health (7).

CSTE determines which conditions should be nationally notifiable to the Centers for Disease Control and Prevention (CDC). Notifications sent from states

* The author thanks Dr Scott J. McNabb and Ruth A. Jajosky of CDC for their review and comment to Appendix 2A.

to CDC are sent voluntarily. U.S. State and Territorial Health Departments have agreed to notify CDC about public health emergencies of international concern involving human health, as outlined in the revised 2005 International Health Regulations (IHR) that went into effect in the United States on July 18, 2007. CDC analyzes these notifications based on a decision algorithm in Annex 2 of the revised IHR and determines whether further notification to the Department of Health and Human Services (DHHS) Secretary's Operations Center is appropriate. The DHHS has the lead role in carrying out the IHR.

REPORTING MECHANISM

Health-care providers, including laboratories, transmit reports of reportable conditions to their state or local health departments within specified time-frames.

DATA COLLECTION

Basic demographic information, date of illness onset or diagnosis, county and state of residence, and similar data are collected for all conditions. Health department personnel obtain additional information as needed on a case-by-case basis. Data are entered into electronic formats, usually at the state level. Data are edited for accuracy and validity.

DATA TRANSFER

The NNDSS is undergoing a transition in notification protocol from the National Electronic Telecommunciations System for Surveillance (NETSS) to the National Electronic Disease Surveillance System (NEDSS) (*18*). Data are sent to the appropriate state health department, which, in turn, forwards the information electronically and without personal identifiers to CDC through different mechanisms, including, but not limited to, the NETSS format and NEDSS format using PHIN Case Notification HL7 (version 2.5) messages.

ANALYSIS

Reports are reviewed on a case-by-case basis at the local level to determine the need for action on individual cases. More complete analysis by person, place, and time is performed at the state or local level to detect unusual patterns in reported conditions. Data are tabulated and graphed weekly by CDC and published. Maps with rates, by county, are prepared for selected conditions annually. Finalized data are included in the *Morbidity and Mortality Weekly Report (MMWR) Summary of Notifiable Diseases—United States.*

INTERPRETATION

On the basis of the analyses, an assessment of the characteristics of the conditions by person, place, and time are reviewed and additional investigations or actions are suggested.

DISSEMINATION

Data are disseminated through state and local newsletters and nationally through the *MMWR*. Reports include tables, graphs, and maps. National data are also available electronically. Information is transmitted directly to state and local health departments when necessary. The media often disseminate the information more widely.

USE

The data are used at the local level most directly for controlling conditions when direct action is possible and necessary. Such actions include therapy for patients, prophylaxis for contacts, initiation of research, program evaluation, and control of outbreaks.

At a state and national level, broader patterns of these conditions are assessed, such as historical trends and geographical clustering, and appropriate actions are initiated (e.g., outbreak investigations, control activities, or development of guidelines).

EVALUATION

The NNDSS is evaluated by CDC program offices that have prevention and control responsibilities for nationally notifiable conditions. Evaluations include assessments of completeness and timeliness as well as the usefulness of the data for monitoring and tracking trends. Annually, CSTE and CDC examine the reportable conditions for importance, reporting burden and preventability. CSTE also provides recommendations for the data to be collected and the data-handling systems. The frequency of reviews in the states varies. Evaluations have led to changes in the graphical presentation of information, the list of reportable conditions, the data to be collected, and the computer systems used in collection and analysis.

REFERENCES

1. U.S. Department of Health and Human Services. *Healthy People 2010*, 2nd ed. With Understanding and Improving Health and Objectives for Improving Health. 2 vols. Washington, DC: U.S. Government Printing Office; November 2000. http://www. healthypeople.gov/.

2. Centers for Disease Control and Prevention. Public Health Guidance for Community-Level Preparedness and Response to Severe Acute Respiratory Syndrome (SARS) Version 2. Supplement B: SARS Surveillance. May 3, 2005. http://www.cdc.gov/ncidod/sars/guidance/B/index.htm. Accessed March 3, 2010.

3. Centers for Disease Control and Prevention. Surveillance for illness and injury after hurricane Katrina—New Orleans, Louisiana, September 8–25, 2005. *MMWR* 2005; 54:1018–1021.

4. Centers for Disease Control and Prevention. Overview of Influenza Surveillance in the United States. http://www.cdc.gov/flu/weekly/pdf/overview.pdf. Accessed August 3, 2009.

5. Centers for Disease Control. Consensus set of health status indicators for the general assessment of community health status—United States. *MMWR* 1991;40:449–451.

6. America's Health Rankings—2009 Edition. United Health Foundation, Minnetonka, MN, 2009.

7. Chorba TL, Berkelman RL, Safford SK, Gibbs NP, Hull HF. Mandatory reporting of infectious diseases by clinicians. *JAMA* 1989;262:3018–3026.

8. Centers for Disease Control and Prevention. Case definitions for infectious conditions under public health surveillance. *MMWR* 1997;46(No. RR-10):1–55.

9. Centers for Disease Control and Prevention. Strategies to improve external cause-of-injury coding in state-based hospital discharge and emergency department data systems. Recommendations of the CDC Workgroup for Improvement of External Cause-of-Injury Coding. *MMWR* 2008;57(RR-1):1–15.

10. Teutsch SM, Herman WH, Dwyer DM, Lane JM. Mortality among diabetic patients using continuous subcutaneous insulin infusion pumps. *N Engl J Med* 1984;310:361–368.

11. Gostin LO, Lazzarini Z, Neslund VS, Osterholm MT. The public health information infrastructure: a national review of the law on health information privacy. *JAMA* 1996;275(24):1921–1927.

12. The Turning Point Public Health Statute Modernization Collaborative. The Turning Point Model State Public Health Act: A Tool for Assessing Public Health Laws. September 2003. http://www.turningpointprogram.org/Pages/pdfs/statute_mod/MSPHAfinal.pdf. Accessed July 31, 2009.

13. American Cancer Society. *Cancer Facts and Figures—2008*. Atlanta: American Cancer Society; 2008.

14. Lee LM, Gostin LO. Ethical collection, storage, and use of public health data: a proposal for a national privacy protection. *JAMA* 2009;302:82–84.

15. Ellwood PM. Outcomes management. A technology of patient experience. *N Engl J Med* 1988;318:1549–1556.

16. Roush SW, Birkhead GS, Koo D, Cobb AN, Fleming DW. Mandatory reporting of diseases and conditions by health-care providers and laboratories. *JAMA* 1999;282:164–170.

17. Koo D, Wetterhall SF. History and current status of the national notifiable diseases surveillance system. *J Public Health Manag Pract* 1996;2:4–10.

18. Centers for Disease Control and Prevention. Status of state electronic disease surveillance systems—United States, 2007. *MMWR* 2009;58:804–807.

3

Economic and Policy Justification for Public Health Surveillance

DAVID B. REIN

It's more fun to arrive at a conclusion than to justify it.

—Malcolm Forbes

> *In December 2007, I attended a session on funding allocations presented by members of the Centers for Disease Control and Prevention (CDC) and the Health Resources and Services Administration's (HRSA's) Ryan White HIV/AIDS Program. The HRSA speakers explained the increased importance of newer surveillance activities (such as name-based HIV reporting and annual matching of case reports to death certificate data) to annual funding allocations as directed by the U.S. Congress in 2007. In the question-and-answer period, the first few questions were mostly technical. Finally, someone cut to the chase and said something like this:*
>
> *"Without our data, HIV treatment programs like the Ryan White Program could not function. Every year we come to these surveillance workshops, and every year representatives from HRSA, or the CDC, or wherever talk to us about the importance of our surveillance data. Every year we get new requests for better data, or cleaner data, or more sophisticated data, but nobody ever offers us more funding to collect them. Why is it that if everyone agrees these data are essential, no one steps up to provide the funding to collect them?"*
>
> *The panelists had no answer for her but, as she noted, neither had anyone else in her 20-year surveillance career. She smiled, the joke had gone over well, and the audience, primarily surveillance specialists from across the country, were laughing and applauding. Before sitting, she stepped back to the microphone:*
>
> *"Don't blame CDC or HRSA; they're our friends in this. The truth is nobody knows how to put a value on what we do." With this statement, the questioner had underscored a core liability of the public health system. Although everyone in public health agrees that surveillance is essential, no one seems to know how to communicate that value in a way the public can easily understand.*

JUSTIFYING SURVEILLANCE

In the business world, building a business case often refers to understanding an up-front expenditure in terms of its future monetary benefits (*1*). An upgrade of a company's Web site can be justified in terms of expected future sales. In public health, the business case is often made in the form of a cost-effectiveness analysis in which the cost of a project or an intervention is presented in terms of the health benefits gained from the stakeholders' perspective. For example, a given evaluation might estimate a cost-per-year of life or quality-adjusted life year (QALY) gained compared with a less effective intervention. Since 2002, the U.S. government, through the mechanism of the Office of Management and Budget, has been encouraging federal agencies to demonstrate the independent impact of their programs on end-stage outcomes using methods ranging from randomized clinical trials to quasi-experimental designs (2). Programs are encouraged to evaluate their costs in terms of the incremental benefits they deliver, much in the way a business case analysis would evaluate a private investment decision or a cost-effectiveness analysis would evaluate the implementation of a new intervention.

Unfortunately, linking surveillance systems to outcomes in this way is often infeasible for a number of reasons. First, the public lacks the desire to finance the types of studies needed to reveal the incremental benefits of surveillance data in focusing or targeting effective programs. Second, because surveillance is in large part a method to track outcomes, more sophisticated (and presumably more expensive) systems are likely to capture more cases, confounding efforts to link the use of surveillance data to improvements in health outcomes. Third, in many instances, surveillance data can only result in health improvements when they are combined with other programmatic functions. Surveillance systems enable programmatic improvements when their information is used intelligently, and when there are effective interventions that can benefit from surveillance information. Fourth, in some instances surveillance systems are put in place to help prevent rare events, such as uncontrolled outbreaks of emergent infections. Although the preparedness the system provides in normal circumstances has value, this value is very difficult to quantify. For example, a surveillance system to detect emergent infections only results in concrete health benefits if a previously unknown infection emerges and is identified by the system and its spread is controlled.

Although surveillance data are vital to achieving public health goals, connecting surveillance directly to health outcomes is complicated by the reality that surveillance information can only improve public health in the presence of other programs and activities that put the information to use. Strong surveillance systems can support weak or limited programmatic interventions and vice versa. Further, no preventive interventions or treatments are currently available to treat many thousands of common and rare conditions. For some conditions, surveillance systems will likely need to be maintained for years simply to collect sufficient information to understand the etiology of the disease (3).

Still, while surveillance systems are difficult and in many cases impossible to link to end-stage health outcomes, they can and should be evaluated for quality, effectiveness, and efficiency, and a strong attempt should be made to articulate a rationale for their perpetuation. Other chapters in this text outline the quality standards that surveillance systems should fulfill and provide methods to evaluate the effectiveness of systems to collect data as intended (4). This chapter focuses on ways to justify a surveillance system, first by describing its specific uses and second by appealing to an economic public good or market failure rationale.

JUSTIFYING SURVEILLANCE IN TERMS OF ITS USES

The first step in justifying any surveillance system is to articulate its concrete uses in language that a wide audience can understand. Surprisingly, surveillance has not always played a central role in public health prevention efforts. As noted by Thacker and Berkelman (5), before 1950, the term *surveillance* was primarily used to refer to monitoring secondary cases of infection that resulted among the contacts of a patient with a serious infectious disease, such as smallpox. Langmuir (6) expanded the concept of surveillance to incorporate the monitoring of incidence, prevalence, and disease outcomes. Beginning in 1967, active surveillance was incorporated as an element of program operations when it was used as a strategic element of the World Health Organization's smallpox eradication effort (5). The success of this program in part led to the expanded use of surveillance in other areas of public health. The concept of surveillance has grown to incorporate a wide range of activities and health conditions. This growth created opportunities to enhance public health based on new information but also created new challenges in disseminating surveillance information and ensuring its efficacious use. The World Bank has outlined six general categories of uses for public health surveillance data (7):

1. *Identifying newly emergent health problems and infections and triggering initial health responses to clusters of symptomatic illness.* A good example of this is the role surveillance played in detecting early cases of severe acute respiratory syndrome (SARS). Detecting SARS early, and the subsequent contact tracing and quarantine that resulted from this detection, might have prevented a widespread global outbreak with potentially catastrophic consequences (8,9).
2. *Assessing the public health impact of problems and measuring temporal trends in disease burden.* Examples of this include the *Morbidity and Mortality Weekly Report* annual summary of notifiable diseases, which reports cumulative totals of notifiable disease data collected through the National Notifiable Disease Surveillance System (NNDSS) for use by federal agencies, state and local health departments, schools of medicine, the media, and other individuals interested in tracking annual trends of diseases as reported from the states (10).
3. *Identifying correlative risk factors for disease acquisition or progression.* In the early 1980s, researchers from CDC used extensive surveillance data (e.g., data collected from patients with hemophilia) to determine that the syndrome known as AIDS was caused by an infectious agent (later discovered as HIV) transmitted through blood and semen (11). These realizations led to early prevention campaigns that likely saved thousands—if not millions—of lives (12).
4. *Allocating resources for disease management, care, and control and targeting intervention or research investments.* The strongest current example of this is the use of HIV and AIDS case reports by HRSA to allocate Ryan White treatment funding to jurisdictions and states. However,

surveillance data are frequently used by Congress and other health policymakers to understand the relative burden of different diseases and to
prioritize the allocation of prevention and care resources.

5. *Evaluating the effectiveness and impact of interventions, policies, and
   public health strategies.* In the United States, the National Immunization
   Survey (a surveillance system of vaccine adoption rates) has been used
   to evaluate the effectiveness of federal programs to enhance vaccination
   (*13*). Similar studies have used sexually transmitted disease surveillance
   data to evaluate the impact of public prevention programs (*14*).

6. *Supporting research inquiries and scientific hypothesis generation.*
   Recently, the U.S. National Institute for Occupational Safety and Health
   sponsored an expansion of the National Mesothelioma Virtual Registry
   and Tissue Bank (*15*). Mesothelioma is a lethal and difficult-to-treat form
   of lung cancer caused by exposure to asbestos. The hope is that enhancing
   this registry system will allow scientists to develop new theories of the
   etiology of the disease that will lead to better therapy and treatment.

Surveillance needs to serve applied and programmatic purposes rather than
academic and/or purely scientific pursuits (*7,16*). Confusing a surveillance system with a research database can place the system at risk if those responsible for
populating the system think the burden and costs of collecting the system's data
exceed its programmatic benefits.

In her foundational discussions of the use of evaluation research, Carol Weiss
(*17*) outlined several principles regarding the utility of evaluation research that
are applicable to surveillance. She argued that evaluative results have both instrumental uses (the specific use of results to inform policy or programmatic action)
and enlightenment uses (uses of evaluation to understand issues and generate new
ideas and perspectives), and both forms of uses are highly valuable (*18*). Weiss
argued that the most useful results lead to feasible actions or directly challenge
assumptions about existing policies (*18*).

Articulating the uses of a surveillance system is essential to creating a credible
justification for it even when linking these uses to independent health impacts
is infeasible or impossible. However, simply stating that surveillance activities
cannot (in most cases) be feasibly justified using a business case, return on investment, or cost-effectiveness analysis does not in itself justify surveillance, much
less the government provision of the services. The next section attempts to justify
the government provision of public health surveillance by drawing on the economic literature on market failures and public goods.

A MARKET FAILURE ARGUMENT FOR GOVERNMENT SURVEILLANCE

Market failures refer to situations where the rational actions of individual consumers result in an inefficient level of production of a certain good or service by the
private market (*19*). Market failures are often used to justify government intervention to correct the inefficiency created by the failure or lack of incentives for private

market provisions. Market failures generally occur when the private costs of a good or service do not capture the good's total societal costs or benefits. Because the marginal costs and benefits to the buyer are not the same as the price of the good, free market transactions will not produce an optimal quantity of the good.

In terms of surveillance, the most important types of market failures are those that create positive or negative externalities. Externalities refer to costs or benefits that fall outside the scope of the market transaction and, therefore, are not considered when the price is set by the market. Positive externalities refer to situations where benefits to others are created by individual consumption of a good, and negative externalities refer to situations where individual consumption imposes additional costs on others. The free market will supply too little of a good that has positive externalities because most buyers will be unwilling to pay for benefits of others and too much of a good with negative externalities because most buyers will ignore costs of the good that are not contained in the price.

A good example of a positive externality in public health is herd immunity, the additional protection offered to non-vaccinated individuals that results from the partial or full interruption of transmission attributable to the vaccination of others. For example, influenza is spread primarily through children, but its negative impacts fall primarily on adults. Universal vaccination of children against influenza (when the vaccine is effective) has the potential to substantially reduce influenza morbidity across all age groups (20), and such a policy could be the most efficient way to reduce the societal burden of influenza. Despite these societal benefits, a free-market allocation of influenza vaccine would likely lead to greater vaccination use by adults than children because adults benefit more from vaccination than children (21). In this case, a public role in subsidizing childhood vaccination is supported by the large additional benefits that accrue across society—in other words, the positive externality of the policy.

Surveillance data have the potential to create positive externalities or prevent negative externalities through their various uses. Surveillance was used to detect SARS and prevent its spread, which resulted in the benefits of preventing a global SARS epidemic. Besides being large, what is important from a justification standpoint is that these benefits accrued to far more individuals than the initial individuals detected and their social contacts. The societal benefits of preventing a global SARS epidemic were so vast, dispersed, and unpredictable that no one individual or private firm could be expected to have sufficient market-driven incentives sufficient to create the surveillance system needed to detect the outbreak. This is particularly true when one considers that SARS was discovered in the absence of any previously identified threat.

Because of externalities, the free market cannot be relied on to provide the societal optimum quantity of surveillance needed to identify emergent infections, and therefore, government involvement is required to ensure the service is provided. Similar arguments can be made for other possible uses of surveillance. Such justifications should be articulated in the context of how the outcome would not be possible without the surveillance activity and how the benefits of the outcome accrue outside any single market transaction, so therefore the private market cannot be counted on to provide an optimal quantity of surveillance activities.

WHAT TYPE OF GOOD IS SURVEILLANCE?

Understanding how the characteristics of surveillance fit into a general economic framework of goods and services can also help us develop a policy justification for it. All goods and services can be thought of as falling somewhere along a continuum of rivalry and excludability properties (Table 3–1). Rival goods are those whose consumption, by definition, limits their consumption by others. A chocolate bar is a rival good in that once I eat it, none is left for anyone else to enjoy. In contrast, non-rival goods are those whose consumption or use by one person does not diminish their consumption or use by someone else. Radio broadcasts are non-rival because anyone within range can tune in to a station without diminishing the enjoyment of others. Excludability is a related property. Excludable goods are those for which a seller can easily restrict access based on payment. Tangible goods like commodities, industrial equipment, or consumer goods are examples of excludable goods. A non-excludable good is the opposite, one whose nature makes it impossible or extremely expensive for a seller to exclude people who do not pay from enjoying the good. A fish caught from a river is an example of a non-excludable good.

Non-rivalry and non-excludability complicate the ability of market forces to set a price that results in the economy producing an optimal quantity of a good where the marginal cost of the last unit provided is equal to its price. For non-rival items, this is because the marginal cost of an incremental use of an item is zero, and thus any fee charged for the good will result in a suboptimal and inefficient level of consumption of the good (22). The problem is roughly the opposite with non-excludability. Because there is no way to feasibly exclude people from using the good, there is also no way to ensure that people pay the marginal cost of producing that good. This is referred to as the free-rider problem. Anyone who has ever listened to public radio but ignored the pledge drive can understand the pernicious power of the incentive to free-ride.

Pure public goods, such as national defense or law enforcement, are both non-rival and non-excludable. Pure private goods such as clothing or automobiles are

Table 3–1 Public Health Examples of Types of Goods

	Non-rival	Rival
Non-excludability	Public goods – Herd immunity – Safe food supply – Disease eradication	Common goods – Public emergency room access – Public parks – Public bodies of water
Excludability	Toll goods* – Surveillance – Medical information – Public sanitation and sewage	Private goods – Prescription drugs – Bandages – Toothbrushes

* Toll goods refer to goods for which a fee can easily be charged for use but whose use (up to a point of overcapacity) does not limit its enjoyment by others.

both rival and easily excludable. In general, most economists would argue that a clear rationale exists for government involvement in the provision of pure public goods and that the government should try to avoid or limit its role in providing purely private goods.

Many aspects of the public health system can be thought of as pure public goods or nearly so. A safe and secure food supply, disease eradication, and herd immunity created through mass vaccination programs are each "goods" with non-excludable and non-rival properties. Government interventions in markets for goods that are non-excludable yet rival are also often justified, and failure of the government to intervene can result in what is known as the tragedy of the commons problem. The tragedy of the commons problem refers to goods such as public lands that are owned jointly by all and thus non-excludable but for which the actions of one person may have heavy consequences on the enjoyment of another. Because users do not incur the full costs of consuming these goods, each user has an incentive to use more than is optimal, which can lead to the destruction of the resource.

Goods that are non-rival yet excludable are a special case, and significant debate exists regarding whether the government should provide them and why. Satellite radio is a non-rival yet easily excludable good that is currently provided solely by the private market. In the past, many national roadways, which are somewhat non-rival (overlooking traffic congestion) yet easily excludable, were often provided by private toll companies, although increasingly roadways and especially national highways have been publicly financed and maintained by the federal government.

SURVEILLANCE IS AN EXAMPLE OF A NON-RIVAL YET EXCLUDABLE GOOD

Surveillance data are non-rival because once collected and disseminated in the form of reports or public use data sets, the incremental cost of new uses of the data are zero. However, surveillance data are also fairly easily excludable because the government or another producer of the data can easily restrict or charge a fee for access.

In the United States, a great deal of surveillance datasets are produced by the government and made freely accessible to the public (or provided in exchange for a nominal fee). Examples are the nationally notifiable disease reports published in CDC's *MMWR* and the Behavioral Risk Factor Surveillance System, which provides annual state-level estimates of a range of conditions from alcohol consumption to women's health.

Still, even in the United States, not all surveillance data are collected by the government. Several private companies have created businesses out of compiling specific information from complex administrative data sources, cleaning these data to facilitate more potential uses, and then selling access for a fee. For example, the MarketScan Disease Profiler data for a fee offers to "quickly project the estimated prevalence of a treated condition or diagnosis among patients actively engaged in the U.S. healthcare system and covered by employer-sponsored insurance (*23*)." IMS Health offers retail pharmacy sales data for six countries.

Although these systems might not strictly meet the definition of a surveillance system, neither do many publicly funded health information systems, and the new systems have rushed in and addressed a void of information that the government previously lacked the will, foresight, or ability to fill. Why then should the government finance and build surveillance systems, when several companies have demonstrated that the private market can produce its own competing systems?

PUBLIC GOOD AND MARKET FAILURE ARGUMENTS IN SUPPORT OF PUBLIC HEALTH SURVEILLANCE

The concepts of public goods and market failures suggest at least two arguments in favor of a government role in surveillance. The strongest argument is that because surveillance data are non-rival, any price charged for them will lead to an economically inefficient allocation. This is simply a formal way of stating that the public derives the most good from surveillance data when they are offered freely because the data result in greater benefits at no additional cost. This is because the marginal cost of providing additional access to the information is zero (or very nearly so) in relation to the costs of compiling the data. Therefore, assuming a need for the data exists, any price charged for them will exclude at least some of the data's positive possible uses. In fact, many of the possible uses of surveillance data are unknown until after they are collected and scientists have an opportunity to use them and draw conclusions. For example, existing and publicly available sources of surveillance data such as the NNDSS data combined with other sources, have been used and reused over the past 10 years to model and understand historical trends in hepatitis A, B, and C and, based on this understanding, to alter federal vaccination, screening, and treatment recommendations in a way that enhances global health (*24–26*). Countless graduate school dissertations would never have been written without the benefit of freely available, government-provided surveillance data.

Second, surveillance is an essential ingredient in the prevention and control of diseases that results in a wide range of positive societal externalities. Preventing the spread of infectious diseases creates positive externalities in two ways. First, responsible management of one's own disease once infected can prevent the spread of disease to others. Unfortunately, individuals have few incentives outside altruism to consider these benefits in their actions, as evidenced by Andrew Speaker, the U.S. citizen who traveled internationally while infected with drug-resistant tuberculosis (*27*). Well funded surveillance systems maintained by public entities can enhance the likelihood that individual infectious cases are detected before infection is spread to others. Second, individual actions to prevent infection such as getting yourself or your children vaccinated reduce the probabilities of others becoming infected through herd immunity (*28*).

Second, controlling chronic diseases likely reduces externalities on others through the reductions of shared health-care costs borne through insurance premiums to fund either national or privatized insurance (*29*). Enhancing overall public health can lead to substantial improvements in prosperity and economic development both because healthy individuals tend to be more productive and also because, as life expectancy increases, individuals have greater incentives to invest in long-term projects that result in societal benefits (*30*). Surveillance is strongly justified through externality arguments to the extent that the efficacy of disease control and prevention depends on or are enhanced by surveillance data.

PUBLIC AUTHORITY ARGUMENTS FOR GOVERNMENT INVOLVEMENT IN SURVEILLANCE

Although government financing of surveillance can be justified using the arguments above, these arguments do little to justify the government production of surveillance data. In theory and in practice, surveillance data can be collected by private firms through direct contracting or through cooperative agreements with federal agencies, and in many cases these business arrangements are likely to lead to data of high quality and value to the public. For example, in the United States, private-sector contractors currently compile data for the Pregnancy Risk Assessment Monitoring System and the National Immunization Survey among others.

Although private or public entities are often on equivalent footing to produce surveillance, only the government has the legal authority to compel many of the types of reporting that make surveillance possible. In the United States, the Council of State and Territorial Epidemiologists recommends which diseases should be reportable to public health departments and then, in turn, which of those data should be reported to CDC. State legislatures then act to require the collection and reporting of such data at the state level. In instances where surveillance data are deemed to be absolutely necessary to protect the public's health, only the government has the power to compel disease reporting. Further, the use of government power to compel the reporting of certain types of data can reduce substantially the transaction costs of collecting those data (*31*).

CRITIQUES OF GOVERNMENT INTERVENTION AND OTHER NON-ECONOMIC JUSTIFICATIONS

Readers should be aware that government intervention in any function often is criticized even in situations of public goods and when the private provision results in market failures. Public choice theorists argue that government policy failures are often worse and more costly than the market failures they were designed to address. To these theorists, the greater the cost of a government intervention, the greater the degree of public support should be required to support it, with supermajorities required to support the expansion of government programs (*32*). Public choice theorists' solution to government overreach is to keep as much activity centered in the private sector as possible and to contract out or sell government functions and assets to private entities in an attempt to increase efficiency.

In contrast, public value theorists reject the idea that government activities can only be justified using economic arguments of market failure and externalities. Bozeman (33) argues that economic approaches only assess the "private value of public things" and many activities of government forward inherently social goods such as societal equity and justice. Okun (34) argued that economic efficiency and social equality were two competing values and neither had primacy over the other. American history is full of examples of the continual renegotiated trade-off of equity and efficiency, and losses of market efficiency are easily justifiable if they can be demonstrated to lead to concomitant and worthwhile increases in social equity.

Finally, behavioral economists argue that contrary to classical economic theory, private markets often operate inefficiently and inequitably because private entities use a variety of mechanisms to hoard benefits and resources or because players in a private market often behave irrationally (35). Because of this, government involvement in markets and service delivery might be both desirable to forward the interests of the public as well as more efficient than allowing the private markets to operate independently.

CONCLUSIONS

This chapter discussed ways in which surveillance can be thought of as a special type of public good. Surveillance information is non-rival, which means that once it is produced it can be used freely by all without diminishing its value to any individual user. It follows then that one of the simplest ways to increase the value of a surveillance system is to broaden its uses, by making its data available to the widest audience possible. At its core, surveillance is intended to be used with other policies and interventions to enhance public health outcomes. Many aspects of improved public health, such as protection from infectious diseases or a more prosperous and productive society from reduced levels of morbidity and mortality, are pure public goods that result in substantial positive externalities. Surveillance can be justified using an externality argument to the extent that surveillance activities are essential to enhancing public health.

Surveillance systems have multiple primary, secondary, and tertiary uses and users. A robust assessment of a system's value will attempt to capture at least as many legitimate benefits as possible. Ultimately, it is often impossible to link surveillance data to independent and isolated improvements in public health, because surveillance data are a necessary but insufficient input used to achieve public health. When justifying a surveillance system, public health practitioners should accept that many of the system's costs and benefits will be inherently uncertain. Articulating the possible range of values and discussing the nature and causes of this uncertainty is a fundamental component of justifying the system and can help to explain what uses and factors are driving a system's value.

REFERENCES

1. Bourne A. Making the business case for restructuring. *People Manag* 2008;14(25):41.
2. Office of Management and Budget. What constitutes strong evidence of a program's effectiveness? http://www.whitehouse.gov/omb/assets/omb/part/2004_program_eval.pdf. Accessed February 13, 2009.
3. U.S. General Accounting Office. Global health: Challenges in improving infectious disease surveillance systems. Washington, DC: U.S. General Accounting Office; 2001. GAO-01-722. http://www.gao.gov/new.items/d01722.pdf 2001. Accessed February 12, 2009.
4. Groseclose S. Evaluation of public health surveillance systems. In: Lee LM, St. Louis ME, Thacker SB, ed. *Principles and Practice of Public Health Surveillance*, 3rd ed. New York, NY: Oxford University Press; 2009.
5. Thacker S, Berkelman R. History of public health surveillance. In: Halperin W, Baker E, eds. *Public Health Surveillance*. New York, NY: Van Nostrand Reinhold; 1992: 1–12.
6. Langmuir A. The surveillance of communicable diseases of national importance. *N Engl J Med* 1963;268:182–192.
7. Garcia-Abreu A, Halperin W, Danel I. *Public Health Surveillance Toolkit: A Guide for Busy Task Managers*. Washington, DC: The World Bank; 2002.
8. Krumkamp R, Duerr HP, Reintjes R, Ahmad A, Kassen A, Eichner M. Impact of public health interventions in controlling the spread of SARS: Modelling of intervention scenarios. *Int J Hyg Environ Health* 2009;212(1):67–75.
9. Lee SH. The SARS epidemic in Hong Kong—a human calamity in the 21st century. *Methods Inf Med* 2005;44(2):293–298.
10. McNabb SJ, Jajosky RA, Hall-Baker PA, et al. Summary of notifiable diseases— United States, 2006. *MMWR* 2008;55(53):1–92.
11. Leads from the MMWR. Surveillance of hemophilia-associated acquired immunodeficiency syndrome. *JAMA* 1986;256(23):3205–3206.
12. Holtgrave DR. Estimating the effectiveness and efficiency of US HIV prevention efforts using scenario and cost-effectiveness analysis. *AIDS* 2002;16(17):2347–2349.
13. Rein DB, Honeycutt AA, Rojas-Smith L, Hersey JC. Impact of the CDC's section 317 immunization grants program funding on childhood vaccination coverage. *Am J Public Health* 2006;96(9):1548–1553.
14. Chesson HW. Estimated effectiveness and cost-effectiveness of federally funded prevention efforts on gonorrhea rates in the United States, 1971–2003, under various assumptions about the impact of prevention funding. *Sex Transm Dis* 2006;33(10 suppl):S140–S144.
15. Amin W, Parwani AV, Schmandt L, et al. National Mesothelioma Virtual Bank: A standard based biospecimen and clinical data resource to enhance translational research. *BMC Cancer* 2008;8:236. doi 10.1186/1471-2407-8-236.
16. Thacker S, Berkelman R. Public health surveillance in the United States. *Epidemiol Rev* 1988;10:164–190.
17. Weiss C. *Evaluation: Methods for Studying Programs and Policies,* 2nd ed. Upper Saddle River, NJ: Prentice Hall; 1998.
18. Shaddish WJ, Cook T, Leviton L, Carol H. Weiss: Linking evaluation to policy research. In: *Foundations of Program Evaluation: Theories of Practice*. Newbury Park, CA: Sage Publications; 1995:179–224.
19. Bator FM. The anatomy of market failure. *Quarterly J Econ* 1958;72(3):351–379.

20. Piedra PA, Gaglani MJ, Kozinetz CA, et al. Herd immunity in adults against influenza-related illnesses with use of the trivalent-live attenuated influenza vaccine (CAIV-T) in children. *Vaccine* 2005;23(13):1540–1548.

21. Galvani AP, Reluga TC, Chapman GB. Long-standing influenza vaccination policy is in accord with individual self-interest but not with the utilitarian optimum. *Proc Natl Acad Sci* 2007;104(13):5692–5697.

22. Musgrave RA, Musgrave PB. *Public Finance in Theory and Practice*, 4th ed. New York, NY: McGraw-Hill; 1984.

23. Adamson DM, Chang S, Hansen LG. Health research data for the real world: The MarketScan databases; 2008. http://pharma.thomsonhealthcare.com/uploadedFiles/docs/2008HealthResearchDatafortheRealWorldThe%20MarketScanDatabases(1).pdf. Accessed March 3, 2009.

24. Armstrong GL, Bell BP. Hepatitis A virus infections in the United States: model-based estimates and implications for childhood immunization. *Pediatrics* 2002;109(5):839–845.

25. Armstrong GL, Mast EE, Wojczynski M, Margolis HS. Childhood hepatitis B virus infections in the United States before hepatitis B immunization. *Pediatrics* 2001;108(5):1123–1128.

26. Armstrong GL, Wasley A, Simard EP, McQuillan GM, Kuhnert WL, Alter MJ. The prevalence of hepatitis C virus infection in the United States, 1999 through 2002. *Ann Intern Med* 2006;144(10):705–714.

27. Fidler DP, Gostin LO, Markel H. Through the quarantine looking glass: drug-resistant tuberculosis and public health governance, law, and ethics. *J Law Med Ethics* 2007;35(4):616–628.

28. Gersovitz M, Hammer JS. *The Economic Control of Infectious Diseases.* Policy Research Working Paper Series 2607. Geneva, Switzerland: The World Bank; 2001.

29. Abegunde DO, Mathers CD, Adam T, Ortegon M, Strong K. The burden and costs of chronic diseases in low-income and middle-income countries. *Lancet* 2007;370(9603):1929–1938.

30. Finlay JE. *The Role of Health in Economic Development.* Program on the global demography of aging working paper. Cambridge, MA: Harvard University; 2007.

31. Williamson O. Why law, economics, and organization? *Ann Rev Law Social Sci* 2005;1:369–396.

32. Buchanan JM, Tullock G. *The Calculus of Consent, Logical Foundations of Constitutional Democracy.* Ann Arbor, MI: University of Michigan Press; 1962.

33. Bozeman B. Public-value failure: When efficient markets may not do. *Pub Admin Rev* 2002;62(2):145–161.

34. Okun A. *Equality and Efficiency, The Big Tradeoff.* Washington, DC: The Brookings Institution; 1975.

35. Shiller RJ. From efficient markets theory to behavioral finance. *J Econ Perspect* 2003;17(1):83–104.

4

Collecting Public Health Surveillance Data

Creating a Surveillance System

M. KATHLEEN GLYNN AND LORRAINE C. BACKER

If you don't know where you are going, any road will get you there.
—Lewis Carroll

Surveillance systems are created to address a need for specific information, such as the incidence or prevalence of a disease, the association between disease and a specific exposure, or the effectiveness of a public health intervention. Creation of a new surveillance system might be considered when existing systems cannot answer a specific surveillance question or cannot address the new information need. A new system might be necessary when critical (e.g., time-sensitive) public health questions need to be answered, other accessible health information systems do not hold data adequate to answer the specific question, or the question needs more than a one-time answer.

In 1996, Thacker and Stroup laid out a vision for the development of a comprehensive public health surveillance system by the year 2000; this system would comprise a network of interoperable health information systems linked electronically, capturing data from many sources (*1*). Although significant progress has been made, we are still far from having such an integrated system. The development of new surveillance systems must consider data collection needs as well as the mechanism and information technology framework required to support the new system.

Considerations for planning a surveillance system were outlined in Chapter 2. In this chapter, we assume the decision has been made to create a new surveillance system, and we address the implementation of this decision. Creation of a new surveillance system should focus on four basic tenets: incorporating common data elements, maximizing appropriate timeliness of data collection, ensuring accessibility to appropriate partners, and establishing flexibility for future enhancement (*1*). Another critical component of surveillance is data protection to ensure that personal confidentiality and privacy are protected. A clear purpose of the surveillance system must be established and consistent with public health surveillance principles.

It is critical to remember that disease reporting and monitoring are not the full complement of surveillance-related public health actions. Using surveillance data to inform and direct public health actions, and to evaluate effectiveness of these actions, are absolute requirements of any surveillance system. New system design can be optimized by examining the features of well-functioning surveillance systems and incorporating standards intended to enhance interoperability and data sharing capacity. For example, the specific public health areas of infection control (2), injury (3,4), chronic disease (5), stroke (6), and syndromes suggestive of bioterrorism (7) are just a sample of those that have developed guidelines to promote commonality across related surveillance activities.

This chapter outlines the process of creating a new surveillance system and discusses issues critical to system implementation. As a practical example of how these steps are applied, we discuss the development and implementation of the Harmful Algal Bloom-related Illness Surveillance System (HABISS) by the Centers for Disease Control and Prevention (CDC) (Box 4–1).

Box 4–1 Creating a New Surveillance System—Development and Characteristics of the Harmful Algal Bloom-Related Illness Surveillance System (HABISS), United States, 1997–2009

Public Health Need Requiring a New Surveillance System
The need for surveillance to assess the public health impacts of harmful algal blooms (HABs) was first identified in 1997 following reports of human illnesses purportedly associated with exposure to the newly identified phytoplankton, *Pfiesteria piscicida* in laboratory personnel working with the organism in open aquaria (8) and Maryland waterman occupationally exposed to the Chesapeake Bay and its tributaries (9). No existing surveillance or other health information system could clarify the relationship between exposure and illness. In response, CDC created the Harmful Algal Bloom-Related Illness Surveillance System (HABISS).

Statement of the Problem
The purpose of HABISS is to define and reduce the public health impact of HABs (10,11). The goals of the system are to identify HAB-related illness cases, mitigate exposure risks, identify outbreaks, prevent further cases, and link health and environmental data.

Case Definitions
Few applicable case definitions existed. CDC worked with public health partners and stakeholders to develop case definitions for illnesses in humans and animals associated with the known HABs. These definitions were also disseminated in Poisindex Managements, the reference used by a key data source, Poison Information Centers. CDC also identified descriptive criteria for harmful algal blooms.

Unit of Surveillance
The original unit of surveillance was a case of disease in a person. As the system evolved, cases of disease in an animal were added (because animal deaths were often the first indication of a toxic HAB in the local environment) and the occurrence of algal blooms was added (to allow prediction of future blooms and thus proactively protect health.)

(continued)

Duration of Data Collection

HABISS is an ongoing surveillance system with continuous data collection. Because mounting evidence indicates that HABs are increasing in duration, frequency, and geographic extent (*12*), HABISS data collection will continue into the future.

Timeliness

CDC's public health partners wanted HABISS to provide information to support timely local public health decision making, such as posting or closing beaches because of the presence of current HAB-related health hazards. Timeliness of reporting depends on the communication systems developed within each state and ranges from less than a day to several weeks. In addition, CDC maintains an informal network for rapid information sharing among HABISS partners. CDC plans to create an automatic email messaging system to alert relevant entities when illness cases or specific environmental data are entered into HABISS.

Data Elements

One of the goals of HABISS is to support public health actions and generate research hypotheses about the impact of HABs, ideally without creating an excessive burden on reporting agencies. HABISS requires all users to input date of report and state identification code. HABISS prompts users to report specified data elements for a suspected illness in a human or animal, including (*1*) point of contact with the system, (*2*) case identifying information and demographics, (*3*) environmental and exposure information, and (*4*) medical information or specified data elements characterizing algal blooms, including (*1*) GIS coordinates of the relevant water body, (*2*) water quality criteria, (*3*) HAB species, and (*4*) toxin analyses.

Data Sources

Data for HABISS are predominantly input directly into HABISS during telephone interviews with a primary physician, an emergency room physician, or an ill individual. Other data are abstracted from daily searches of the National Poisonings Data System. Foodborne illnesses data might be abstracted from emergency room records or state-based foodborne disease outbreak records. Data describing HABs might be abstracted from routine water quality-monitoring efforts.

Data Collection

Data collection for HABISS occurs in standardized format and might include a telephone interview with the reporting individual as well as data abstraction from the various sources described above. Database entry is modular, units are specified, and ranges are specified for results such as laboratory tests or toxin concentrations. Data are directly input into CDC system and are centrally stored at CDC.

Data Access

HABISS operates on CDC's secure platform, the Rapid Data Collector (RDC) and is protected by approved access and password. Access is limited to CDC HABISS staff and State partners with digital certificates. Conditions of sharing data outside of the contributing states have not yet been determined. Currently, the data are available to outside researchers only in a planned summary published in CDC's *Morbidity and Mortality Weekly Report.*

Data Quality

Procedures include extensive training for persons entering data into HABISS and an extensive data dictionary. CDC provides ongoing feedback and has modified the application to improve data quality.

(continued)

Standardized Vocabularies

Ongoing standardization of HABISS includes mapping vocabulary to CDC's Event Anomaly Reporting System (EARS), using standardize nomenclature of medicine (SNOMED), and logical observation identifiers names and codes (LOINC); matching marine animal health vocabulary with the data base of the National Oceanic and Atmospheric Marine Mammal Stranding Program; and working with veterinarians to ensure that animal health data are collected using the standardized vocabularies. HABISS will use messaging consistent with the Public Health Information Network (PHIN) standards.

Confidentiality

HABISS protects data confidentiality by requiring all users to have electronic certificates. The system is periodically reviewed for data integrity and security.

Reports

HABISS data collection began with four states in 2007 and expanded to 12 in 2008. Currently, there are over 500 bloom reports, over 50 human disease cases and over 20 animal cases in the data base.

STATEMENT OF THE PROBLEM: WHAT IS (ARE) THE INTENDED USE(S) OF THE SURVEILLANCE DATA?

> *The reason for collecting, analyzing, and disseminating information on a disease is to control that disease. Collection and analysis should not be allowed to consume resources if action does not follow.*
>
> —WH Foege (*13*)

Surveillance systems can be designed to monitor many different determinants of health. The oldest monitor cases of infectious diseases (*14*), but increasingly systems monitor other events, particularly indicators of overall population health. Public health practitioners must define the characteristics of the condition or behavior under surveillance. They must also define the purpose of the system, such as monitoring ongoing occurrence of an endemic disease or condition; detecting epidemics of diseases that routinely occur at low levels; identifying the emergence of new conditions; monitoring health outcomes from exposures to environmental or occupational hazards; monitoring the presence of genetic anomalies; recording certain health risk or health protection behaviors; or tracking uptake of health interventions to control disease or promote health, such as childhood vaccinations (*15*) or mammography in women (*16*). Finally, any system should support the main areas of surveillance data use: detection (e.g., of newly emerging health problems); periodic data dissemination (e.g., for assessing implemented control activities); archival information storage (e.g., to document the evolving health status of a population) (*17*); and application in public health protection.

The identified goals of the surveillance system will inform its design. The unit of surveillance, sources of data, and planned analyses will be different if the goal, for example, is to identify cases of a rare disease, detect outbreaks of diseases that are epidemic-prone, or monitor the effect of an intervention to reduce a health risk behavior. Most systems will have goals that include improving the ability to detect cases and outbreaks, informing design of targeted intervention and control measures, and evaluating interventions (*18*). Systems should have the capacity to identify unusual patterns that could indicate changes or the emergence of new events (*19,20*).

CASE DEFINITION

For any surveillance system, case definitions must be established and disseminated. Case definitions should include the unit of surveillance along with specific and achievable diagnostic or other characterizing parameters. The case definition must also define whether multiple occurrences of a condition or exposure can occur in an individual and, if so, what the criteria are for determining a new case. For example, over a lifetime, one person can have multiple unrelated cases of salmonellosis; one case of HIV infection; varying levels of lead exposure; or multiple cancers. Public health surveillance case definitions for conditions reported through the U.S. National Notifiable Diseases Surveillance System (NNDSS) have specific structure and requirements determined by the Council of State and Territorial Epidemiologists (CSTE) (*21*), and this template could be applied to new surveillance systems. For example, the infectious disease botulism is listed in the NNDSS; and the clinical description, laboratory criteria for diagnosis, and case classification are clearly specified (*22*). By contrast, case definitions for ciguatera fish poisoning vary by state, making it difficult to accurately assess national or international disease incidence.

In this template, case reporting should include the criteria to be used by both humans (based on clinical judgment and clinical diagnosis) and machines (using computerized algorithms that operate in electronic health record and health information systems). In addition, the "human-based" component should describe, as appropriate, the clinical presentation, laboratory evidence, and criteria for epidemiologic linkage.

DEFINING THE UNIT(S) OF SURVEILLANCE

Perhaps the most common unit of public health surveillance is a case of disease in an individual. However, the unit of surveillance could be a test result, exposure to an environmental factor, the practice of certain behaviors, the combination of specific clinical signs and symptoms, or the presence of a certain genetic marker or other bio-indicator. Alternatively, the unit of surveillance could be something other than the individual level, such as the number of disease clusters or outbreaks.

Conducting surveillance for occurrence of a disease alone might not provide the most useful information to direct or measure the success of public health interventions, particularly when infection or exposure substantially predates the observable health outcome (*23*). For diseases where diagnosis and treatment play a minimal role in breaking the overall population transmission cycle, a surveillance system should be expanded beyond simple case reporting. In such circumstances, additional units of surveillance to assess the effectiveness of public health interventions might focus on behaviors (to predict the future disease incidence or morbidity based on the prevalence of certain behavioral practices) or the environment (to predict the future disease incidence or morbidity based on the environmental presence or level of certain factors). Behavioral surveillance of sexual practices or the use of insecticide-treated nets might be useful in designing and monitoring population level interventions for HIV (*24*) and malaria (*25*), respectively. Similarly, monitoring vector populations as a component of malaria surveillance (*25*) or community lead paint levels as a component of lead level surveillance (*26*) would provide data to direct public health responses.

POPULATION UNDER SURVEILLANCE

Information collected in a surveillance system is directly interpretable and applicable only to the population represented by the group under surveillance. Thus, the next critical decision for creating a surveillance system is to identify the population under surveillance. For many public health surveillance systems in the United States, the most common population under surveillance is the U.S. population, because any conclusions drawn from surveillance are intended to be applicable to the entire population.

However, one must assess whether conducting surveillance in the entire population is necessary to make valid statements about a given condition. For feasibility, economy, convenience, and as supported by scientific plausibility, a variety of population subsets can be considered for specific surveillance efforts. These subsets can be those most representative of the population as a whole, most likely to identify the condition of interest, or most convenient from which to collect data. In some instances, conditions or exposures might be limited to, more likely to occur among, or of greater interest when occurring among persons in a certain population. Examples include the incidence of sexually transmitted diseases or unintended pregnancy among adolescents (*27*), the occurrence of specific behaviors and outcomes among pregnant women (*28*), or the occurrence of specific diseases among workers in specific occupations. Surveillance for diseases resulting from specific exposures might only be relevant in geographically limited areas because of environmental conditions, population density, or other factors. For some conditions, to ensure completeness of reporting, special efforts are taken to ascertain all cases. In these situations, facilities or locations preferentially providing care for affected populations should be identified as targets for surveillance.

If the decision is made that surveillance within a population subset will adequately fulfill the surveillance objectives, then varying methods to identify the subset can be used. Surveillance can be limited to the entire population residing in a specific geographic area that possesses the general demographic characteristics of the population as a whole. For example, in one system, laboratory-based surveillance for foodborne pathogens is conducted among all residents in a defined geographical (catchment) area (29). Another alternative strategy is sentinel surveillance, where a specific set of health-care providers, hospitals, laboratories, or other potential reporting sources agree to report the conditions under surveillance. These types of sentinel systems can be targeted at high population areas, areas where occurrence of exposures or risk factors is highest, or at hospitals or health-care providers most able to provide timely and accurate data. Some surveillance in the United States is conducted on limited populations because there is ongoing access to specific data only for that particular population, such as members and families of members of the uniformed services (30) or recipients of health care provided by a particular care provider or insurance agency (31).

Formal statistical sampling methods can be implemented to allow extrapolation of results to the entire population from which the sample is taken. Various methods can be used, such as the venue-based time–space sampling and respondent-driven sampling of the National HIV Behavioral Surveillance System (24). The National Youth Risk Behavior Survey, which serves as the major data source for the National Youth Risk Behavior Surveillance (YRBS), implemented a three-stage cluster sample design to generate a nationally representative sample of students in grades 9 through 12 who attend public and private schools (27). Statistical sampling methods might also be used to ensure adequate capture of persons with the conditions under surveillance who are part of hard-to-reach populations or who are underrepresented in the general population (32). Table 4–1 shows examples of surveillance systems that are conducted over a variety of population subsets, including use of sampling.

DURATION OF DATA COLLECTION

Most surveillance systems are implemented with an indefinite duration. Periodic assessment should be incorporated into system evaluation to determine whether surveillance should continue. A surveillance system that routinely collects data with a set frequency could also be modified or enhanced for a set period in response to a critical public health need—such as identifying cases of illness during a known outbreak or for an uncommon condition after a toxin release; conducting syndromic surveillance during a high profile event; or conducting active surveillance for cases in response to identification of a rare but epidemic-prone disease. If a known seasonality occurs for a given condition, event, or behavior, it is possible to vary the frequency of surveillance intensity by season. For example, influenza surveillance data collected by CDC are updated and analyzed weekly during the influenza season (from October through May), with lower levels of reporting at other times (33).

Table 4–1 Examples of Public Health Surveillance Systems Focusing on Different Population Subsets, United States, 2009

	Condition under surveillance	Subset or sampling strategy
National HIV Behavioral Surveillance System (*24*)	Behavioral risks for HIV	1) Metropolitan areas with the highest estimated prevalence of persons living with AIDS, then 2) Venue-based or respondent driven
Youth Risk Behavioral Surveillance (*27*)	Priority health-risk behaviors among youth and young adults	Three-stage cluster sample designed to produce a nationally representative sample of students in grades 9–12 who attend public and private schools
National Violent Death Reporting System (*34*)	Death resulting from either the intentional use of physical force or power against oneself, another person, or a group or community, or the unintentional use of a firearm	Seventeen states funded to conduct state-based active surveillance
Behavioral Risk Factor Surveillance System (*35*)	Health-risk behaviors and use of preventive health services related to the leading causes of death and disability in the United States	1) Noninstitutionalized U.S. population aged >18 years 2) Within US states and territories, select metropolitan areas and counties that reported data for at least 500 respondents or a minimum sample size of 19 per weighting class
Surveillance for World Trade Center Disaster Health Effects Among Survivors of Collapsed and Damaged Buildings (*36*)	Mental and physical health	Adult survivors (aged >18 years at the time of interview and were office workers and visitors) who were present between the time of the first airplane impact and noon on September 11, 2001 in any one of the 38 primarily nonresidential buildings or structures that were damaged or that collapsed as a result of the September 11 attack, excluding those who were involved in rescue and recovery.
Metropolitan Atlanta Developmental Disabilities Surveillance Program (*37*)	Mental retardation, cerebral palsy, hearing loss, vision impairment, and autism spectrum disorders	Active surveillance methods to ascertain cases of the five select disabilities in the five-county Atlanta metropolitan area conducted in 2-year intervals a multiple source ascertainment methodology

(continued)

51

Table 4–1 (*continued*)

	Condition under surveillance	Subset or sampling strategy
Foodborne Diseases Active Surveillance Network (FoodNet) (*29*)	Laboratory-confirmed infections of common foodborne pathogens	Residents of defined cachment areas in 10 funded states
HABISS (*see* Box 4.1)	Cases of illness in animals and persons associated with exposure to harmful algal blooms (HABs); occurrence of HABs	Active surveillance in 12 states that are either supported by a CDC-sponsored cooperative agreement or with a specific public health interest in HABs Active surveillance of sentinel animal events (e.g., HAB-related pet dog or wild animal deaths)

TIMELINESS AND FREQUENCY OF DATA COLLECTION

Timeliness and frequency of data collection are complementary characteristics. Effective public health responses depend on the ability of surveillance systems to provide reliable and timely information to support action (*38*). To determine the timeliness required by a new surveillance system, one must determine how rapidly the information will be used for public health action. Although there is an increasing demand for real-time reporting, it is only reasonable to expect the implemented timeliness for reporting to be supported by a concordant timeliness of review, analysis, or response.

The goal of the surveillance system will inform the required timeliness; for example, identification of outbreaks or potential bioterrorism events requires immediate reporting, usually through a direct phone call to the health department. By contrast, surveillance systems used to monitor chronic diseases or the effect of population-level interventions can function effectively with less timely reporting.

Timely reporting often needs to strike a balance between reporting a confirmed case and more rapid reporting of a preliminary or potential case. Complete reports will be less timely and thus might miss a critical window for public health action. Alternatively, timelier but less complete reports might ultimately turn out to be "false alarms" that unnecessarily consume scarce resources. One way to maximize timeliness, accuracy, and completeness is to allow quick reporting of preliminary data, while supporting later routine submission of more complete, updated surveillance reports. However, this requires that the system establishes procedures to collect and manage accurately both initial and subsequent updated reports.

The required timeliness varies based on the level at which the reporting occurs. More rapid reporting is usually needed at the local level, where immediate public health action occurs to investigate and control disease. For many notifiable diseases, routinely scheduled (e.g., weekly or monthly) reporting to state or federal levels is adequate, even when more timely reporting is required at the local level.

Cases of disease that might be associated with a large-scale event, are associated with travel on common carriers, potentially indicate bioterrorism, or require rapid implementation of control measures require timelier reporting from local to state or federal levels to determine whether a geographically dispersed exposure might have occurred and a wider-scale response is necessary. Additionally, certain diseases are included among the international health reporting regulations and require timely international reporting (*39*).

Consideration of the frequency of data collection is an important step for creating a surveillance system and is closely related to timeliness. Reporting can be structured on a scheduled basis (e.g., weekly, indicating the presence or absence of cases) or in real time (e.g., immediately, but only when the condition under surveillance is identified). Contributing parameters to the frequency of surveillance include whether the data are collected actively (surveillance staff conduct specific and structured outreach to collect surveillance data) or passively (sources report based on expectations or requirements). The availability of data can determine the frequency of data collection. If a main data source for a surveillance system is a survey or vital statistics registry, then the frequency of the survey or release of the vital statistic data set determines the frequency of data collection from these sources and might drive the frequency of collection of any other contributing source.

REQUIRED DATA ELEMENTS

"If we confuse surveillance with research we may be motivated to collect large amounts of detailed data on each case. The burden of this approach is too great for the resources available for surveillance and usually leads to failure."
—A. Garcia-Abreu, World Bank (*40*)

What data are necessary to adequately conduct the surveillance? Public health surveillance is not intended to answer all possible questions about a disease or condition under surveillance. Rather, it should provide answers required to support public health practice, especially to implement or inform prevention or control measures. However, surveillance data should be adequate to generate hypotheses for targeted research.

To maximally protect personal privacy while informing and protecting public health, all efforts should be made to identify the minimum number of and simplest data elements to understand the current or realistically potential disease situation and to minimize the collection and maintenance of personally identifiable information. This serves two important purposes. First, it minimizes the burden on reporters and resources required to collect, validate, and evaluate the data, resulting in a higher probability of establishing and maintaining a successful and accurate surveillance system. Second, it limits the chance that personal information is vulnerable to a breach or other violation of confidentiality.

Once data elements are identified for collection, sources and mechanisms for their collection must be identified. Surveillance programs need to ensure that they have legal authority to collect the data and that there are mechanisms in place to access and collect the data required to support the surveillance. New local, state, or federal regulations might need to be enacted or existing ones enforced or data sharing agreements established. The medium and mechanism of data collection and storage should be reviewed to ensure they are consistent with statutory or legal requirements and controls.

SOURCES OF DATA

Historically, three sources of public health surveillance data have been described: individuals, health-care providers, and other entities. Currently, we recognize that although data originate from individuals, they can exist and are accessed in a variety of formats and media. With the increasing amount of electronic collection and storage of health information, the myriad of sources within "other entities" is now a greater focus of discussion.

Electronic Data Sources

Public health continues to recognize that data should be collected once and then reused by others to benefit the needs of public health and the primary data collectors (*41*). Effective and efficient use of electronic data from existing data stores for public health surveillance depends on the widespread use of standardized vocabularies and messaging standards and requires a complete understanding of how and for what purpose the data were originally created or collected. With varying degrees of availability, quality, comprehensiveness, timeliness, and feasibility, primary sources of electronic data for public health surveillance include laboratory data systems, electronic health records, administrative data systems, other traditional health information systems, and nontraditional data sources. Each of these sources is described briefly below.

Electronic Laboratory Information Management Systems

Because public health laboratories faced mandatory reporting of an increasing volume of tests and results for public health surveillance, they were one of the original foci of electronic data management in the health-care setting. Standardized vocabulary (data coding) and messaging (exporting data to another electronic data system, such as a surveillance system) have been more widely investigated and implemented for electronic laboratory reporting (ELR) to surveillance systems than for other data sources.

ELR generally provides more complete and timely notification of reportable events than case reporting from providers and might be useful for conditions requiring immediate public health response or that might indicate an urgent event. Most laboratories, however, cannot provide the same amount of case data as available from clinical data sources, and they might not be able to provide the information needed to determine whether the report represents a true case (*42,43*). ELR includes laboratory reports that are repeat, follow-up, or confirmatory tests for a known case or negative results ruling out a case and, therefore, generally require more follow-up activity by the surveillance program to investigate and verify than traditional case reports (*42*). Given the effort required to follow-up on the high volume of laboratory reports, every effort should be taken to maximize the probability that incoming reports to the surveillance system represent true cases (*42*). In addition, the volume of reports, and the desire to automatically import them into a surveillance system, will require detailed matching algorithms and procedures to ensure accuracy of matching to existing cases in the system and ultimately of case counts.

Electronic Health Records

For effective and efficient health-care provision, management of complex clinical data, and standardized insurance billing, electronic health records (EHRs) are seen as the inevitable future of clinical care patient records. Criteria have been established at the national level, ensuring that all EHR systems meet standards for functionality, security, reliability, and interoperability. A well-designed, fully implemented EHR system might be capable of providing all the information required for a complete surveillance report. Currently, however, it is more likely that all reporting needs will not be met by this source, and this creates some specific potential limitations. Initial implementation of EHRs incorporated propriety data coding that would not easily support routine data transmission to public health surveillance systems (*44*). Because of the expense of EHR systems, and the complexity of implementation in any health-care setting, EHRs are not in as widespread use as predicted (*45–47*). EHRs are primarily for clinical purposes and tend to have limited data on psychosocial, behavioral, and environmental elements (*48*), which are critical elements in some surveillance systems.

EHRs are designed to store data in a standard, predominantly coded, manner. Even EHRs that include a robust use of standard codes for data entry and storage will still support some free text entry options. Any data collection from such systems will need to consider accepting data exports or "messages" containing these codes and data stored as free text (*49,50*). The use of clinical data from EHRs for surveillance would be greatly facilitated by reliable and automated methods for identifying cases from clinical records (*21,45*).

Administrative Data Systems

Administrative data systems are those that have been created and exist within the health-care setting for reasons other than for clinical care. The most common administrative data systems are discharge databases created to facilitate billing for clinical services. As a result of the U.S. government-implemented data standards (*51,52*), these systems tend to be the most standardized of the electronic data sources, and their data can be collected and used relatively easily for surveillance systems. However, these systems are not intended to describe accurately the clinical condition of the patient but to reflect services provided for the patient. Some assessments of these data have identified errors that affect their ability to serve as sources of accurate surveillance data (*53,54*).

Additional Health Information Systems

Many surveillance systems depend on routine data collection from other health information systems—especially from vital registries and ongoing surveys—to provide adjunct, complementary, or even their primary source of data. For example, surveillance for mortality resulting from a specific cause, such as mortality from cardiovascular disease, could be exclusively based on reported death certificates—either from deaths reported to a county or state vital registry system or from the national all-causes death certificate database compiled by the National Center for Health Statistics. Alternately, these reports could also be combined with cardiac disease case data from specific surveillance systems. Many other condition-specific surveillance systems use data collected in the Behavioral Risk Factor Surveillance System (35) or the National Health Information Survey (55).

Non-Traditional Electronic Data Sources

As new surveillance systems are created for an increasingly diverse set of conditions, and as more data are collected, stored, and potentially available electronically, surveillance professionals should consider nontraditional data sources as components of new surveillance systems. These can include, for example, information on sales of drugs and biologics (56,57) or increases in school absenteeism (58) that might serve as early warning of an outbreak or a bioterrorism attack. Other alternative data sources used for similar purposes include pharmacy databases and those that monitor call-in centers, such as poison control centers (59) or nurse advice hotlines (60), surveillance data collected on animal populations (wildlife, livestock, or companion animals) (61,62), or listservs that report emerging issues (e.g., Promed).

Nonelectronic Data Sources

Virtually all surveillance data gathered from electronic sources ultimately originate from a person—frequently an affected individual or a health-care provider. The data can be collected directly from the affected person (e.g., through interview or survey) or from the health-care providers who gather information through medical encounters. The most common paper sources include case reporting cards (morbidity cards) and case investigation forms. Morbidity cards generally include only basic information: the case of disease or event being reported, a date of onset or diagnosis of the disease or event, limited patient demographics, and, for some diseases, the specific test results conducted to diagnose the case. Morbidity cards can be telephoned, mailed, or faxed to the surveillance program. Surveillance for other reportable conditions might require completion of a more detailed case investigation form that includes information on specific risk factors, vaccination or other disease prevention methods, more detailed clinical information, and names or contact information for other potentially exposed persons. Case investigation forms can be completed by health-care providers, by public health surveillance staff interviewing health-care providers, or through chart abstraction from information collected in patient histories. Increasingly, surveillance programs are migrating these nonelectronic forms into electronic reporting mechanisms.

ELECTRONIC DATA STORAGE AND SHARING

In addition to assessments of data sources, public health practitioners must determine the technical specifics of how data will be collected and compiled over time. Some details (e.g., data format and availability) are determined by the data source. Practitioners might also have to determine whether surveillance records will be entered as a single case report, representing a single person, or collected as separate reports from multiple sources and then compiled into a "virtual single case report" representing a single person. Creators must determine whether a new surveillance software application will be deployed or whether participants will be provided data element definitions and collection procedures and then allowed to develop their own software systems to collect, store, and transmit the data. Creators must decide how data transmission between local, state, and federal surveillance systems will occur—including messaging standards, error checks, and feedback between reporting entities. If a system uses electronic data from other sources, then procedures must be in place for routine reporting from those systems or routine access by surveillance staff to those systems.

PROCEDURES FOR DATA ACCESS

When personally identifying or other sensitive information is collected, the degree to which and at which jurisdictional level (e.g., local, state, or federal) that information is maintained must be considered when establishing data access and security procedures. Data elements are often collected locally but not reported to higher or next levels of the surveillance system. A variety and combination of data collection, storage, and access options can be considered in consultation with information technology and security advisors, depending on the data sources, timeliness, and other attributes being established in the surveillance system.

Data can be decentralized, centralized, or range across the two. Most public health surveillance systems are hybrids. For example, data collection occurs at the local level, individual but limited case data are forwarded to the central level, and all data are collected under standards and procedures agreed on at the local and central level. In a typical hybrid surveillance system, data are collected and managed locally but are also compiled and managed centrally. Local users have access to their own data but not to centrally managed data, and vice versa. Variations on these outlined models are almost unlimited; the key point here is that each of these issues must be addressed, clearly documented in detail, and agreed on between the central and local levels (frequently representing multiple tiers) before the system is implemented. For each of these kinds of systems, data sharing protocols must clearly outline who owns the data and has permission to change any data and how updates or corrections are accomplished.

Surveillance practitioners must also address broader data access issues. Provisions should be made for access to surveillance data for a variety of purposes and to a variety of users, each with appropriate controls to protect data integrity and confidentiality. For example, some systems allow controlled access to selected data for those with specific research needs. Other systems have created de-identified datasets or public use data sets in which data are modified such that individual cases cannot be directly or indirectly identified.

Issues of ethics are covered in more detail in Chapter 9, but creators of surveillance systems must also consider issues of data ownership. Criteria should be created that specify which entities can abstract, analyze, and generate reports from the data. In addition to ownership issues, creators of surveillance systems should consider whether external parties might attempt to gain access to surveillance data for other than public health purposes. Public health practitioners must determine what protections are in place at the local level and how these protections translate to the compilation or storage of data at the various jurisdictional levels. Rules, regulations, mandates, or other data access protection or provisions, including required disclosures, vary by jurisdiction (*63,64*). The potential for external access reinforces the goal of collecting only those data truly required for surveillance purposes.

DATA QUALITY

> *"The importance of the weekly Bills of Mortality to Graunt reminds us that epidemiology is largely dependent on the availability of good records...We could get along fine today, if we had to, with low-tech methods, but not without the existence of systematic records."*
>
> —K.J. Rothman (*65*)

Appropriate use of data (covered in greater detail in Chapters 6 and 7) and conclusions that can be drawn from surveillance data will depend on the quality of data collected. The data quality of the surveillance system as a whole depends on the compilation of the quality of all of the sources. For electronically derived data, data quality in the surveillance system will depend on the underlying accuracy of the data that were entered into the source system and the accuracy of mapping the source data to the data fields in the surveillance system. For data collected from nonelectronic sources, data quality will depend on the accuracy of the original data collection and surveillance form completion and the accuracy of data entry from those forms into the surveillance system.

For all incoming data, procedures must be established to ensure the highest quality, including accurate data entry or importation. Procedures should address clear instructions for form completion (if applicable), definitions of data elements, a detailed understanding of any data elements derived from electronic data sources, and accurate mapping of data elements from electronic data sources to data fields in the surveillance system. If electronic records or data to be placed within records are automatically loaded into the surveillance system, then detailed matching algorithms for de-duplication, linking data to existing records, or importing new records must be defined, validated, and periodically reassessed. Any software designed for a surveillance system should have available documentation and built in data checks, such as automated validation steps (e.g., acceptable ranges and values). Finally, feedback to reporting sources regarding common errors might be a useful tool in attaining and maintaining data quality. These procedures must be accompanied by ongoing assessment of data quality as part of the routine surveillance system evaluation procedures.

Standardized Vocabularies

If a surveillance system is intended to have the capacity to export data to another electronic system, or to merge, match, or accept data from another source, then standardized vocabularies are a critical way to ensure data quality (41). Implementation of data standards through the use of predetermined vocabularies increases the accuracy of data entry and use and simplifies the ability to merge and map collected precoded data (66,67).

In support of these needs, the U.S. Government has implemented regulations regarding health information standards. These were predominantly established through the Health Insurance Portability and Accountability Act (HIPAA) (51,52). HIPAA established electronic data interchange standards and required every provider doing business electronically to use the same health-care transactions, code sets, and identifiers (68). Standard vocabulary code sets use specific codes to identify the diagnosis and clinical procedures on claims and encounter forms; standard message structures support transmission of data.

These same standards are key components for implementation in surveillance systems because (1) there is wide investment in their advancement and disseminated use, (2) health information systems are major data sources for many public health surveillance systems, and (3) limited surveillance resources can be used best by adopting standards already in use by broader health information communities. To facilitate the development of standard public health messages, CDC laid out a conceptual data model for common data collected in public health surveillance (69). Use of these data standards in establishing surveillance systems should minimize the degree of error and time investment associated with recoding or mapping of data from other data sources. Additional discussion of standardized vocabularies and the standardized messaging can be found in Chapter 5.

UNIVERSAL HEALTH IDENTIFIERS

In creating a new system, one might need to link data from an individual person-case across multiple data sources and over time (45,70). A key data element that could facilitate this linkage is a universal health identifier. The requirement for such a health identifier was included for implementation within the standards outlined by HIPAA, but the actual implementation was subsequently halted in 2006 (*52*). The lack of a universal unique health identifier continues to pose a challenge to both health information and public health surveillance systems.

CONFIDENTIALITY AND SECURITY OF HEALTH INFORMATION

With respect to data collection using universal health identifiers, or at times even to conducting surveillance *per se*, there has always been a tension between private rights and public good and a need to balance between having adequate data to inform public health practice and the ability to protect confidentiality of personal health information (*see* earlier discussion of data elements) (*71*). The collection of detailed and sensitive data frequently included in surveillance systems is supported by legal authority at the state (or occasionally local) level; however, these data are almost always collected without the specific consent of the individual. Thus, success of public health surveillance requires public trust. Public health entities need to demonstrate that data collection and storage is done with the greatest possible care so as not to risk the loss confidentiality and that data will be used only for public health good. A surveillance system design that specifically states its intent to minimize the risk of inadvertent disclosure will almost certainly elicit greater participation by data providers and will thus improve its feasibility, accuracy, and representativeness (*72*). There must be clearly defined legal protections at all levels of the public health system that prohibit the release of data and the specifics of these ethical and legal issues are outlined at length in Chapters 9 and 10.

CONCLUSIONS

An effective surveillance system requires substantial investment of effort before a single report is collected—careful and thoughtful design will ensure that each of the major goals of surveillance can be met once the data are collected. Once the key characteristics of a new surveillance system have been outlined, it is an optimal time to assess whether there are opportunities to build in components that will support required analyses, ensure appropriate dissemination for public health action, and allow system evaluation. Creators must determine if the system as designed will support ongoing assessment of whether the goals and objectives are being met and whether it should be continued. The specifics of these components (analysis, dissemination, and evaluation) are covered in detail in later chapters. The ability of a surveillance system to meet these needs, however, is critically dependent on system design.

Developments in surveillance as a part of public health practice are clearly moving us toward the goal of an integrated and interoperable network of health information systems, where new surveillance systems need not be created entirely anew. Persons initiating surveillance for a new condition truly have the opportunity to build a new system that takes full advantage of data existing in other health information systems while still achieving the public health goals. Regardless of how a new system is designed, however, experience has demonstrated that new surveillance systems should be flexible, and thus adaptable, to changing public health needs and goals. Even more importantly, new surveillance systems should collect accurate high-quality data to maintain for the future the critical historical role surveillance has played in protecting and promoting public health.

REFERENCES

1. Thacker SB, Stroup DF. The future of national public health surveillance in the United States. *J Public Health Manag Pract* 1996;2(4):1–3.
2. Lee TB, Baker OG, Lee, JT, Scheckler WE, Steele L, Laxton CE. Recommended practices for surveillance. *Am J Infect Control* 1998;26(3):277–288.
3. Pollock DA, Adams DL, Bernardo LM, et al. Data elements for emergency departments systems, release 1.0 (DEEDS): a summary report. *Ann Emerg Med* 1998;31(2):264–273.
4. Horan JM, Mallonee S. Injury surveillance. *Epidemiologic Rev* 2003;25:24–42.
5. Centers for Disease Control and Prevention. Indicators for chronic disease surveillance. *MMWR Recomm Rep* 2004;53(RR-11):1–114.
6. Goff DC Jr, Brass L, Braun LT, *et al*. Essential features of a surveillance system to support the prevention and management of heart disease and stroke. *Circulation* 2007;115(1):127–155.
7. Mandl KD, Overhage JM, Wagner MM, *et al*. Implementing syndromic surveillance: a practical guide informed by the early experience. *J Am Med Inform Assoc*, 2004;11(2):141–150.
8. Glasgow HB Jr, Burkholder JM, Schmechel DE, Tester PA, Rublee PA. Insidious effects of a toxic estuarine dinoflagellate on fish survival and human health. *J Toxicol Environ Health* 1995;46(4):501–522.
9. Grattan L M, Oldach D, Perl TM, *et al*. Learning and memory difficulties after environmental exposure to waterways containing toxin-producing *Pfiesteria* or *Pfiesteria*-like dinoflagellates. *Lancet* 1998;352:532–549.
10. Centers for Disease Control and Prevention. Notice to readers: Results of the public health response to *Pfiesteria* workshop—Atlanta, GA, September 29–30, 1997. *MMWR* 1997;46(40):951–952.
11. Centers for Disease Control and Prevention. Notice to readers: Possible estuary-associated syndrome. *MMWR* 1999;48(18):381.
12. Glibert PM, Anderson DM, Gentien PG, Graneli E, Sellner KG. The global complex phenomona of harmful algal blooms. *Oceanograph* 2005;18(20):136–147.
13. Foege WH, Hogan RC, Newton LH. Surveillance projects for selected diseases. *Int J Epidemiol* 1976;1:29–37.
14. Declich S, Carter AO. Public health surveillance: historical origins, methods and evaluation. *Bull World Health Organ* 1994;72(2):285–304.
15. McDonald L, Yiannakoulias N, Svenson L. A Novel Application of Surveillance Algorithms in Childhood Immunization Program Monitoring. *Adv Dis Surv* 2007; 4:178.
16. Centers for Disease Control and Prevention. Use of mammograms among women aged >40 years—United States, 2000–2005. *MMWR* 2007;56(3):49–51.

17. Thacker SB, Stroup DF. Future directions for comprehensive public health surveillance and health information systems in the United States. *Am J Epidemiol* 1994;140(5):383–397.
18. Hopkins RS. Design and operation of state and local infectious disease surveillance systems. *J Public Health Manag Pract* 2005;11(3):184–190.
19. Spitalny KC. Learning to design new systems: communicable disease surveillance. *J Public Health Manag Pract* 1996;2(4):40–41.
20. Dato V, Wagner MM, Fapohunda A. How outbreaks of infectious disease are detected: a review of surveillance systems and outbreaks. *Public Health Rep* 2004;119(5): 464–471.
21. Council of State and Territorial Epidemiologists. Template for placing diseases or conditions under national surveillance, 2008. http://www.cste.org/PS/2008pdfs/ PSTemplateNNDSS2008V7final.doc. Accessed February 24, 2009.
22. Centers for Disease Control and Prevention. Case definitions for infectious conditions under public health surveillance. *MMWR Recomm Rep* 1997;46(RR-10):1–55.
23. Ritz B, Tager I, Balmes J. Can lessons from public health disease surveillance be applied to environmental public health tracking? *Env Health Perspect* 2005;113(3):243–249.
24. Gallagher KM, Sullivan PS, Lansky A, Onorato IM. Behavioral surveillance among people at risk for HIV infection in the US: the National HIV Behavioral Surveillance System. *Public Health Rep* 2007;122(Suppl 1):32–38.
25. Breman JG, Holloway CN. Malaria surveillance counts. *Am J Trop Med Hyg* 2007;77(6 Suppl):36–47.
26. Jacobs DE, Nevin R. Validation of a 20-year forecast of US childhood lead poisoning: Updated prospects for 2010. *Environ Res* 2006;102(3):352–364.
27. Centers for Disease Control and Prevention. Youth risk behavior surveillance— United States, 2007. *MMWR Surveill Summ* 2008;57(SS-4):1–131.
28. Centers for Disease Control and Prevention. Surveillance for selected maternal behaviors and experiences before, during, and after pregnancy. *MMWR Surveill Summ* 2003;52(SS-11):1–15.
29. Centers for Disease Control and Prevention. Preliminary FoodNet data on the incidence of infection with pathogens transmitted commonly through food—10 states, 2007. *MMWR* 2008;57(14):366–370.
30. Rubertone MV, Brundage JF. The Defense Medical Surveillance System and the Department of Defense serum repository: glimpses of the future of public health surveillance. *Am J Pub Health* 2002;92(12):1900–1904.
31. Nelson JC, Jackson M, Yua O, *et al.* Impact of the introduction of pneumococcal conjugate vaccine on rates of community acquired pneumonia in children and adults. *Vaccine* 2008;26:4947–4954.
32. Faugier J, Sargeant M. Sampling hard to reach populations. *J Adv Nursing* 1997;26(4):790–797.
33. Centers for Disease Control and Prevention. Influenza activity—United States and worldwide, 2007–08 season. *MMWR* 2008;57(25):692–697.
34. Butchart A. The National Violent Death Reporting System: a new gold standard for the surveillance of violence related deaths? *Inj Prev* 2006;12(Suppl 2):ii63–ii64.
35. Centers for Disease Control and Prevention. Surveillance of certain health behaviors and conditions among states and selected local areas—Behavioral Risk Factor Surveillance System (BRFSS), United States, 2006. *MMWR Surveill Summ* 2008;57(SS-7):1–188.

36. Centers for Disease Control and Prevention. Surveillance for World Trade Center disaster health effects among survivors of collapsed and damaged buildings. *MMWR Surveill Summ* 2006;55(SS-2):1–18.

37. Centers for Disease Control and Prevention. Prevalence of four developmental disabilities among children aged 8 years—Metropolitan Atlanta Developmental Disabilities Surveillance Program, 1996 and 2000. *MMWR Surveill Summ* 2006;55(SS-1):1–9.

38. Thacker SB. Surveillance. In: Gregg MB, ed. *Field Epidemiology*. New York: Oxford University Press; 2002:16–32.

39. World Health Organization. *International Health Regulations (2005)*, 2nd ed. 2008. Geneva: World Health Organization; 2008.

40. Garcia-Abreu A, Halperin WE, Danel I. *Public Health Surveillance Toolkit*. Washington, DC: The World Bank. 2002.

41. Chute CG, Koo D. Public health, data standards, and vocabulary: crucial infrastructure for reliable public health surveillance. *J Public Health Manag Pract* 2002;8(3):11–17.

42. Overhage JM, Grannis S, McDonald CJ. A comparison of the completeness and timeliness of automated electronic laboratory reporting and spontaneous reporting of notifiable conditions. *Am J Pub Health* 2008;98(2):344–350.

43. Centers for Disease Control and Prevention. Automated detection and reporting of notifiable diseases using electronic medical records versus passive surveillance—Massachusetts, June 2006–July 2007. *MMWR* 2008;57(14):373–376.

44. Erstad TL. Analyzing computer based patient records: a review of the literature. *J Healthcare Inform Manag* 2003;17(4):51–57.

45. Kukafka R, Ancker JS, Chan C, Chelico J, Khan S. Redesigning electronic health record systems to support public health. *J Biomed Inform* 2007;40(4):398–409.

46. Simon SR, McCarthy ML, Kaushal R, et al. Electronic health records: which practices have them, and how are clinicians using them? *J Eval Clin Prac* 2008;14:43–47.

47. Ford EW, Menachemi N, Phillips MT. Predicting the adoption of electronic health records by physicians: when will health care be paperless? *J Am Med Inform Assoc* 2006;13:106–112.

48. Mayo NE, Poissant L, Ahmed S, *et al*. Incorporating the International Classification of Functioning, Disability. and Health (ICF) into an electronic health record to create indicators of function: proof of concept using the SF-12. *J Am Med Inform Assoc* 2004;11:514–522.

49. Shapiro AR. Taming variability in free text: application to health surveillance. *MMWR* 2004;53(Suppl):95–100.

50. Meystre SM, Savova GK, Kipper-Schuler KC, Hurdle JF. Extracting information from textual documents in the electronic health record: a review of recent research. *Yearb Med Inform* 2008;128–144.

51. Health Insurance Portability and Accountability Act of 1996. Pub. L. No. 104–191, 110 Stat 1936 (1996).

52. U.S. Department of Health and Human Services Office for Civil Rights. *HIPAA Administrative Simplification Regulation Text*, Regulation Text 45 CFR Parts 160, 162, and 164 (Unofficial Version, as amended through February 16, 2006), 2006. US Department of Health and Human Services: Washington, D.C.

53. Peabody JW, Luck J, Jain S, Bertenthal D, Glassman P. Assessing the accuracy of administrative data in health information systems. *Med Care* 2004;42(11):1066–1072.

54. Campbell SE, Campbell MK, Grimshaw JM, Walker AE. A systematic review of discharge coding accuracy. *J Public Health Med* 2001;23(3):205–211.

55. Centers for Disease Control and Prevention. *National Health Interview Survey (NHIS).* http://www.cdc.gov/nchs/nhis.htm. Accessed November 21, 2008.
56. Popovich ML, Henderson JM, Stinn J. Information technology in the age of emergency public health response. The framework for an integrated disease surveillance system for rapid detection, tracking, and managing of public health threats. *IEEE Eng Med Biol Mag* 2002;21(5):48–55.
57. Wagner MM, Robinson JM, Tsui FC, Espino JU, Hogan WR. Design of a national retail data monitor for public health surveillance. *J Am Med Inform Assoc* 2003;10(5):409–418.
58. Mook P, Joseph C, Gates P, Phin N. Pilot scheme for monitoring sickness absence in schools during the 2006/07 winter in England: can these data be used as a proxy for influenza activity? *Eurosurv* 2007;12(12):E11–E12.
59. Lober, W.B., Karras BT, Wagner MM, *et al.* Roundtable on bioterrorism detection: information system-based surveillance. *J Am Med Inform Assoc* 2002;9(2):105–115.
60. Henry JV, Magruder S, Snyder M. Comparison of office visit and nurse advice hotline data for syndromic surveillance—Baltimore-Washington, D.C., metropolitan area, 2002. *MMWR* 2004;53(Suppl):112–116.
61. Lynn T, Marano N, Treadwell T, Bokma B. Linking human and animal health surveillance for emerging diseases in the United States: achievements and challenges. *Ann N Y Acad Sci* 2006;1081:108–111.
62. Glickman LT, Moore GE, Glickman NW, Caldanaro LJ, Aucoin D, Lewis HB. Purdue University-Banfield National Companion Animal Surveillance Program for emerging and zoonotic diseases. *Vector Borne Zoonotic Dis* 2006;6(1):14–23.
63. Gostin LO, Lazzarini Z, Neslund VS, Osterholm MT. The public health information infrastructure. A national review of the law on health information privacy. *JAMA* 1996;275(24):1921–1927.
64. Ouellette A, Reider J. Practical, state, and federal limits on the scope of compelled disclosure of health records. *Am J Bioethics* 2007;7(3):46–48.
65. Rothman KJ. Lessons from John Graunt. *Lancet* 2006;347:37–39.
66. McDonald CJ, Schadow G, Suico J, Overhage JM. Data standards in health care. *Ann Emerg Med* 2001;38(3):303–311.
67. Hammond WE. The making and adoption of health data standards. *Health Aff. (Millwood.),* 2005;24(5):1205–1213.
68. McDonald CJ, Overhage JM, Dexter P, Takesue BY, Dwyer DM. A framework for capturing clinical data sets from computerized sources. *Ann Intern Med* 1997;127:675–682.
69. Centers for Disease Control and Prevention. *Public Health Conceptual Data Model.* Atlanta: US Department of Health and Human Services 2000.
70. Yasnoff WA, Overhage JM, Humphreys BL, LaVenture M. A national agenda for public health informatics: summarized recommendations from the 2001 AMIA Spring Congress. *J Am Med Inform Assoc* 2001;8(6):535–545.
71. Bayer R, Fairchild AL. The limits of privacy: surveillance and the control of disease. *Health Care Anal* 2002;10:19–35.
72. Lazarus R, Yih K, Platt R. Distributed data processing for public health surveillance. *BMC Public Health* 2006;6. (doi:10.1186/1471-2458-6-235).

5

Informatics and the Management of Surveillance Data

RAMESH S. KRISHNAMURTHY AND
MICHAEL E. ST. LOUIS

If you want to travel fast, travel alone. If you want to travel far, travel together.

—African proverb

Without effective data management, even the best surveillance system will fail to yield timely and useful information. The volume of accessible digital information that now can be captured electronically for the purpose of surveillance easily can overwhelm traditional data management capabilities, so that data management is now routinely the Achilles' heel of surveillance. In 2009, the multiple information streams related to the outbreak of novel Influenza H1N1 threatened to overwhelm the ability of health officials to manage the information in Mexico City, New York City, and at both the U.S. Centers for Disease Control and Prevention (CDC) and the World Health Organization (WHO). If the new digital era ahead is to yield a great breakthrough for public health surveillance as many have prophesied, data management for surveillance needs to be elevated in priority and to become grounded in the emerging discipline of public health informatics.

At the broadest level, the process of surveillance data management can be broken down into three main categories: data capture (commonly referred to as data collection); data processing and storage; and data analysis and reporting. Frequently, data management and statistical analysis are overseen by single management unit to coordinate the collection and analysis functions of data management. The collection of public health data is addressed in Chapter 4 and the analysis and interpretation are described in Chapter 6.

Traditionally, surveillance data have been managed primarily using paper-based processes. Data capture forms are designed using word processors and are printed on paper to collect data and later stored for data management and record-keeping purposes. In industrialized countries, surveillance data from paper forms typically are entered routinely into electronic databases, with variable requirements for timeliness and quality of data transcription. In resource-limited environments, this practice of paper-based data capture and management often continues beyond the primary registration of a surveillance case report (*1,2*). Statistics such as aggregate numbers of cases seen during a reporting period may be tallied by hand, and the resulting summary statistics either entered into an electronic database or hand-written onto another form for submission to a higher level in the surveillance reporting chain. Paper-based systems are often too slow for analysis to guide urgent action and difficult to maintain, and the archival properties of paper tend toward deterioration and data loss if they are not protected.

In the recent years, surveillance data are increasingly collected using electronic devices at the point of origin of data, thereby eliminating the need for conventional paper-based data collection effort. A well-designed electronic information system allows: a streamlined data entry process or the direct digital capture of laboratory test results or clinical diagnoses; efficient data merge capabilities from multiple data sources; automated data quality checks; rapid search, retrieval, and visualization capabilities; and early warning alerts for potential disease threats and outbreaks (*3–6*). In light of the evolution of surveillance systems and health informatics even in low infrastructure settings (*7,8*), this chapter emphasizes the design and performance of electronic information systems instead of paper-based systems for public health surveillance.

In recent years, surveillance data management increasingly has been incorporated into the broader framework of the scientific discipline of public health informatics (*9*). The rapid expansion of information and communication technologies (ICT) and the growth of public health informatics have each contributed to blurring the demarcation among data collection, data management, and—to some extent—preliminary data analysis, throughout an integrated and interoperable environment. Future advances in informatics will likely have major impact across the subject matter of essentially every chapter contained in this text. Therefore, we will briefly introduce the discipline, concepts, and terminology of public health informatics as it applies to management of surveillance data.

PUBLIC HEALTH INFORMATICS AND ITS APPLICATION TO SURVEILLANCE

Public health informatics is an interdisciplinary science that focuses on the systematic use of information theories and of ICT to enhance the performance of individuals, groups, and organizations in public health practice (*10–12*). Epidemiologists use scientific disciplines such as microbiology, toxicology, ecology, and statistics to understand and monitor a disease or other public health concern in a population. Correspondingly, informaticians use disciplines such as information science, computer science, communications theory, psychology, neuroscience, and systems engineering to understand and address the information requirements of an organization. One such example—the topic of this chapter—would be application of those disciplines and the tools of informatics to the requirements of a public health department or agency for managing public health surveillance data. Although sophisticated, appropriate use of information technology (IT) is a critical dimension of health informatics, informatics is not synonymous with IT.

Concepts and Terminology of Informatics: An Introduction for Public Health Surveillance Practitioners

Table 5–1 introduces some basic terms, concepts, and tools of informatics, along with a description of how these concepts apply to surveillance information systems. The use of this terminology can be off-putting at first to public health professionals. Indeed, many public health and surveillance experts respond negatively to the application of terms such as *business process* or *business steward* (Table 5–1) to their public health work or their own role as a subject matter expert in public health. However, this language—adapted from engineering disciplines and systems analysis—simply reflects the agnostic posture of a systems engineer or informatician to the different specialized knowledge and expertise domains with which they need to interact. Within that engineering world, the entirety of public health can be considered as a business process, under which public health surveillance can be viewed as a subsidiary business process. Likewise, data management for public health surveillance can be viewed and described as a subsidiary process of public health surveillance. This chapter focuses on the business process of data management for public health surveillance.

For many surveillance professionals, the term *scoping document* seems an unnecessary and annoying term of jargon. Nonetheless, it denotes something that everyone in public health can value: the tangible output of a process that bridges between different expertise domains to translate the expectations of an epidemiologist (interested in improving surveillance) into a set of instructions that both the epidemiologist and the informatician can understand, agree on, and implement. The advantage of allowing the infiltration of such informatics language into public health is that it helps prepare public health for the larger scale importation of new skills, technologies, and expertise domains into public health surveillance. Similarly, "mapping of the stakeholders" in a surveillance system (Table 5–1) through a structured process seems an obvious step, and other terms might be commonly used in public health for this activity. However, once the terminology is adopted by all, it can facilitate the collaboration across fields about the importance of identifying all stakeholders in a surveillance operation, identifying the key locus of contribution of each, and articulating their interests and critical concerns. Moreover, a stakeholder-mapping exercise provides an opportunity to document ownership and stewardship of data (*13,14*). Mapping the understandings regarding data ownership; stewardship responsibilities; and access to which parts of the data for what purposes is essential to prevent misunderstanding and conflict among the stakeholders.

To an informatician, a "functional requirement" is a basic procedure or building block of any business process. It needs to be described systematically to allow the elements of the procedure to be translated into terminology or depicted in diagrams that can be modeled for the eventual purpose of electronic data processing. Once functional requirements are listed and described, a "requirements analysis" can be undertaken that arrays the different functional requirements being expressed and establishes a context in which conflicts or complexities can be identified and addressed. Upon completion of the requirements analysis, detailed "requirements specifications" can be generated for the new or modified systems. This provides the type of detailed instructions that can ultimately be translated into computer software code. "Use cases" will likely be developed along the way that reflect typical, important examples of the operation of the surveillance "business," such as the detection, reporting, and data capture for a case of one specific reportable event or condition. Once the informatician's understanding of what the experts in surveillance and other public health disciplines actually want to happen, the surveillance information system will be tested repeatedly by considering the response of the system to a set of these core use cases. One important byproduct of this process will be a summary "statement of methods for capture of surveillance data," which needs to be both technically sufficient to meet surveillance needs and to achieve concurrence of stakeholders for legal and policy considerations. This seemingly technical issue is actually sensitive and important: This is the critical documentation for how a government is authorized to gather health-related data about their citizens for the express purpose of protecting health. In fact, this seemingly arcane, technical issue is at the heart of the debate about the proper role of public health surveillance in modern society (*15,16*).

The concepts from the field of systems analysis typically are represented in abstract diagrams such as Figure 5–1. The re-engineering of any process (such as a component of a surveillance system) can be formalized as the application of a standardized set of steps to be applied to the process *input* and intended to result in an improved process *output*. These design steps typically involve a requirement analysis, functional analysis, design, and implementation. Feedback loops are defined at each stage to assure that every step in the design process continues to be guided by the needs of the stakeholders as expressed in the requirements document.

Another group of concepts listed in Table 5–1 comes from the field of "standards." Understanding the application and implications of standards to the

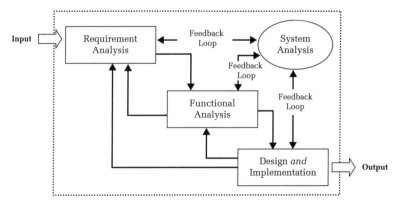

Figure 5–1 Typical engineering approach to design and implement a surveillance information system.

Table 5–1 Concepts and Terminology From the Field of Informatics Relevant to Data Management for Public Health Surveillance*

Informatics term or tool	Description for relevance of the term to data management for surveillance
Business process	A collection of related, structured activities or tasks that produce a specific service or product (serve a particular goal) for a particular customer or customers. For example, county-level reporting of *Neisseria meningitidis* infections in Fulton County, Georgia; National Notifiable Disease Surveillance in the United States; and U.S. Biosurveillance (*see* Chapter 14) are partly overlapping but distinguishable business processes at very different levels of complexity and aggregation.
Business steward or owner	Subject matter expert who has decision-making responsibility and authority for the business process in question.
Scope Document or Scoping Document	Output produced by an informatics practitioner when translating the objectives of a business steward into a set of statements, deliverable products, expected costs, time-frames, and other key parameters that allow the business steward and the informatics practitioner to achieve a deep consensus on mutual expectations for a data or informatics initiative or activity.
Stakeholder analysis or mapping	A process where all the individuals or groups that are likely to be affected by the activities of a business process (such as surveillance data management) or process improvement are identified and then characterized according to how much they can affect the project and how much the project can affect them.
Map of data ownership, stewardship, and access	Written document that describes who (i.e., which agency or entity) owns which component of surveillance data, who has rights to use which elements of the data and for what purpose, and who is responsible for maintaining the property protections and rights to the data.
Functional requirement	A functional requirement defines the function of a software system (http://en.wikipedia.org/wiki/Software_system) or its component. A function is described as a set of inputs, behaviors, and outputs. Functional requirements might specify calculations, technical details, data manipulation and processing, and other specific functionality that define *what* a system is supposed to accomplish.
Statement of methods of data capture	Description of all modes of data acquisition, input, or capture format: original data collection using paper forms; original data collection using electronic (machine readable) input devices (desktop/laptop computers, personal digital assistants (PDAs), smart phones, and other related formats); and extraction of primary data from existing systems.
Data dictionary	A centralized repository of information about data such as name, meaning, relationships to other data, origin, usage, format, possible values, etc.

(continued)

Table 5–1 (*continued*)

Informatics term or tool	Description for relevance of the term to data management for surveillance
Standards	A technical standard is an established norm or requirement. Usually it is reflected in a formal document that establishes uniform engineering or technical criteria, methods, processes, and practices. Most voluntary standards are offered for use by people, professional societies, regulators, or industry. When a published standard achieves widespread acceptance and dominance, it can become a broader de facto standard for an industry. This has happened with the modem protocol developed by Hayes, Apple's TrueType font standard, and the PCL protocol used by Hewlett-Packard in the computer printers they produced.
Interoperability	Ability of two or more systems or components to exchange information and to use the information that has been exchanged. This generally occurs in through mutual agreement to adopt published standards.
Syntactic interoperability	If two or more systems are capable of communicating and exchanging data, they are exhibiting syntactic interoperability. Specified data formats, communication protocols and the like are fundamental. In general, standards such as XML or SQL support syntactic interoperability. Syntactic interoperability is required for any higher level interoperability, such as semantic interoperability.
Semantic interoperability	Beyond the ability of two or more computer systems to exchange information, semantic interoperability is the ability to automatically interpret the information exchanged meaningfully and accurately to produce useful results as defined by the end users of both systems. To achieve semantic interoperability, both sides must share a common information exchange reference model. The semantic content of the information exchange requests are defined unambiguously: what is sent is the same as what is understood.
Ontology	For the purpose of public health surveillance, ontology reflects an explicit way of categorizing reality, arranging hierarchies of those categories, defining terms and relationship among those categories, all of which lead to the ability to share knowledge across domains.
Requirements analysis	A document encompassing those tasks that go into determining the needs or conditions to meet for a new or altered product, taking account of the possibly conflicting requirements of the various stakeholders, such as beneficiaries or users (*see* Fig. 5–1).
Requirements specification (for a system)	A complete description of the behavior of the system to be developed. It includes a set of use cases that describe all the interactions the users will have with the software.

(continued)

Table 5–1 (*continued*)

Informatics term or tool	Description for relevance of the term to data management for surveillance
Use case	In software engineering and systems engineering, a description of a system's behavior as it responds to a request that originates from outside of that system (i.e., how exactly does a case of Acute Flaccid Paralysis get detected, by whom, and how does it become a statistic in a Polio Surveillance System?). In other words, a use case describes "who" can do "what" with the system in question. The use case technique is used to capture a system's behavioral requirements by detailing scenario-driven threads through the functional requirements.
Reference model	A model, example, or concrete implementation of something that effectively serves a basic goal or serves a basic function and can then be looked at as a shared point of reference for various purposes. For example, Microsoft's Excel could serve as a reference model or shared reference point for a software spreadsheet function, or Google search as a reference model for an internet search function.
Stewardship	A responsibility to take care of something that one does not own.
Enterprise architecture	Enterprise Architecture is an abstract depiction of the organizing logic for all of an enterprise's business processes reflecting the enterprise's operating model and how all the business processes interact. Enterprise Architecture typically then describes enterprise IT infrastructure, applications, and systems and their relationships to enterprise business processes and goals.
Standard Operating Procedures	A standard operating procedure is a set of instructions having the force of a directive, covering those features of operations that lend themselves to a definite or standardized procedure without loss of effectiveness. Standard Operating Policies and Procedures can be effective catalysts to drive performance improvement and improve organizational results. Every good quality system is based on its standard operating procedures.

*Adapted from UNAIDS 2007; Jernigan 2003; Lumpkin 2003, among other sources, with definitions adapted from Wikipedia.

evolution of data management for surveillance is described in detail in the next section. One special standards-related term that is essential for understanding the future of public health surveillance and data management is the concept of "interoperability." This refers to the property of different processes or systems that are enabled to interact meaningfully and efficiently because each adheres to a common rulebook. For example, vehicular traffic is interoperable across state lines in the United States because all states agree to enforce the same rules about driving on a particular side of the road, interpreting traffic lights and road signs the same way, and so on. The beauty is that drivers do not need to negotiate with each other how to use the shared roadways, or even speak the same language—they simply need to adhere to the same roadway rules. The effort to promote interoperability in governance among societies is reflected in institutions such as the United Nations. Corresponding efforts to promote inter-operability among nations in improved surveillance and response to diseases and health threats are reflected in the International Health Regulations, which were revised in 2005 (*see* Chapter 17). Definitions for several important but more abstract concepts related to interoperability of health and surveillance information systems are included in Table 5–1. In the future we predict a focus on interoperability that results from the constantly growing pressure to share health information more quickly and comprehensively and to link it with envi-ronmental data, travel history data, and many other sectors and domains of information.

A more familiar element of the informatics lexicon for the average surveil-lance practitioner might be the concept of a "data dictionary" that expresses the semantic content and the data format for each data element of a surveillance database. A comprehensive data dictionary is often documented in the form of columns and rows, where rows represents data elements and the corresponding columns of each row express the *values* and *rules* pertaining to that particular data element. The values can be *variable name*, character type (alphanumeric, numeric, alphabet, or object/image), and so on, whereas the rules may include relevant limitations (range values), applicable skip patterns, controlled vocabu-laries, and other relevant validation rules. Data type is a characteristic of a data element that determines what kind of data it may hold. For example, the name of one data type could be "date." For this example, the date value can be required to be expressed as YYYY-MM-DD (where YYYY represents *year* in four dig-its, MM represents *month* in two digits, and DD represents *day* in two digits). For each data type in the data dictionary, various additional components can be listed, such as value ranges, validation rules, and skip patterns, to provide addi-tional clarity to the data type. Explicit data dictionaries that represent solutions that effectively meet public health surveillance requirements should be docu-mented and shared more actively as part of knowledge management for public health surveillance. This is an example of a "standards-based approach" that is offered below as part of the general strategy for drawing on public health and informatics disciplines to strengthen data and information management capaci-ties for public health surveillance.

Additional concepts of increasing importance at the boundaries between public health and informatics are ideas from general management and systems thinking. In particular, explicit *standard operating procedures* (SOPs) is a clas-sic term from early management theory and science that is increasingly resurgent as a concept, in part as a necessary guide for quality operations of surveillance data management but also as a typical first step of abstraction leading to the busi-ness process abstraction and modeling that is the basis for all systems analysis (Table 5–2).

Table 5-2 Selected Standards, Standards-Development Processes (SDPs), and Standards Developing Organizations (SDOs) Relevant to Management of Public Health Surveillance Data

Standards or SDP	Description	References	Home URL
WHO Recommended Surveillance Standards, Second edition—1999	Jointly produced by technical clusters of WHO and UNAIDS, this document provides recommended case definition standards for the surveillance of notifiable diseases and serves as a guide to good practice and harmonize surveillance activities.	World Health Organization, ed. *WHO Recommended Surveillance Standards.* Second edition. http://www.who.int/csr/resources/publications/surveillance/WHO_CDS_CSR_ISR_99_2_EN/en/. Accessed September 7, 2009.	http://www.who.int/csr/resources/publications/surveillance/WHO_CDS_CSR_ISR_99_2_EN/en/
A Guide to Establishing Event-based Surveillance—2008	Developed by the WHO Western Pacific Regional Office, this guide describes event-based surveillance systems and rapid capture of information about events that are a potential risk to public health.	World Health Organization, ed. *A guide to establishing event-based surveillance.* http://www.wpro.who.int/internet/resources.ashx/CSR/Publications/eventbasedsurv.pdf. Accessed September 7, 2009.	http://www.wpro.who.int/internet/resources.ashx/CSR/Publications/eventbasedsurv.pdf
Guidelines on Protecting the Confidentiality and Security of HIV Information—2007	This document by UNAIDS provides guidelines on protecting the confidentiality and security of HIV information, and to produce a plan to field test them within countries. The content serves for non-HIV-related diseases as well.	UNAIDS, ed. Guidelines on Protecting the Confidentiality and Security of HIV Information http://data.unaids.org/pub/manual/2007/confidentiality_security_interim_guidelines_15may2007_en.pdf. Accessed September 7, 2009.	http://data.unaids.org/pub/manual/2007/confidentiality_security_interim_guidelines_15may2007_en.pdf

(continued)

Table 5–2 (continued)

Standards or SDP	Description	References	Home URL
National Public Health Performance Standards Program (NPHPSP)	Developed by National Association for Country and City Health Officials (NACCHO), Association of State and Territorial Health Officials (ASTHO), and CDC, NPHPSP provides performance assessment instruments for state public health systems, local public health systems, and local governing entities.	CDC. *National Public Health Performance Standards Program (NPHPSP)*. http://www.cdc.gov/od/ocphp/nphpsp/cdcocphpnews.htm#end Accessed September 7, 2009.	http://www.cdc.gov/od/ocphp/nphpsp/cdcocphpnews.htm#end
The Council to Improve Foodborne Outbreak Response (CIFOR) Guidelines for Foodborne Disease Outbreak Response (for the United States)—2009	The guidelines, developed by the Council of State and Territorial Epidemiologists (CSTE), provide model practices used in foodborne disease outbreaks.	Council to Improve Foodborne Outbreak Response (CIFOR). *Guidelines for Foodborne Disease Outbreak Response.* Atlanta: Council of State and Territorial Epidemiologists, 2009. http://www.cste.org/dnn/. Accessed September 7, 2009.	http://www.cste.org/dnn/
Public Health Informatics Network (PHIN) and PHIN Implementation Guides	CDC's PHIN is a national initiative to improve the capacity of public health to use and exchange information electronically by promoting the use of standards and defining functional and technical requirements. PHIN strives to improve public health by enhancing research and practice through best practices related to efficient, effective, and interoperable public health information systems.	CDC. *Guides (PHIN Implementation)* http://www.cdc.gov/phin/resources/guides.html. Accessed September 7, 2009.	http://www.cdc.gov/PHIN/;http://www.cdc.gov/phin/resources/phin-facts.html

Public Health Data Standards Consortium (PHDSC)–*Health Information Technology Standard*	The PHDSC, together with public health agency representatives, has compiled health information technology standards to provide guidelines for data standards, information content standards, information exchange standards, identifiers standards, privacy and security standards, and functional standards for health data.	Public Health Data Standards Consortium. *Health Information Technology Standard. http://phdsc. org/standards/health-information-tech-standards. asp.* Accessed September 7, 2009.	http://www.phdsc.org/
International Statistical Classification of Diseases and Related Health Problems (ICD)–Terminology Standard	Currently in 10th revision, The International Classification of Diseases and Related Health Problems (ICD) was developed by WHO is a widely used vocabulary standard in the collection, processing, classification, and presentation of morbidity and mortality data.	WHO, ed. *International Statistical Classification of Diseases and Related Health Problems 10th Revision.* http://apps.who. int/classifications/apps/ icd/icd10online/. Accessed September 7, 2009.	http://apps.who.int/ classifications/apps/icd/ icd10online/
Logical Observation Identifiers Names and Codes (LOINC)–Terminology Standard	Developed by the Regenstrief Institute and the voluntary LOINC committee, LOINC is a widely used vocabulary standard that provides a list of codes to describe specific universal identifiers for laboratory and other clinical observations to facilitate the exchange and pooling of results for clinical care, outcomes management, and research.	Regenstrief Institute, Inc. *Logical Observation Identifiers Names and Codes (LOINC). http://loinc.org/.* Accessed September 7, 2009.	http://loinc.org/
Systematized Nomenclature of Medicine—Clinical Terms (SNOMED-CT)–Terminology Standard	Originally developed by the College of American Pathologists (CAP), SNOMED-CT is a comprehensive clinical terminology (vocabulary) to provide computational semantic interoperability to exchange data. It is maintained, and distributed by the International Health Terminology Standards Development Organization (IHTSDO), a non-for-profit association in Denmark.	International Health Terminology Standards Development Organisation. *SNOMED CT.* http://www. ihtsdo.org/. Accessed September 7, 2009.	http://www.ihtsdo.org/

(*continued*)

Table 5–2 *(continued)*

Standards or SDP	Description	References	Home URL
RxNorm–Terminology Standard	Produced by the National Library of Medicine (NLM), RxNorm provides a standardized nomenclature for clinical drugs and drug delivery devices. It is used in pharmacy management and drug interaction software.	National Library of Medicine. *RxNorm* http://www.nlm.nih.gov/research/umls/rxnorm/overview.html. Accessed September 7, 2009.	http://www.nlm.nih.gov/research/umls/rxnorm/overview.html
SQL (Structured Query Language)	SQL is a database computer language design for managing data in relational database management systems (RDBMS). Its scope includes data query and update, schema creation and modification, and data access control.	SQL is an American National Standards Institute (ANSI) standard, and and official U.S. standard can be located at the ANSI website www.ansi.org Accessed September 21, 2009.	*Information can be accessed at multiple sites, including* www.sql.org/, www.mysql.com, *and others. Definition and main concepts can be seen at* http://en.wikipedia.org/wiki/SQL
Health Level 7 (HL-7)–Messaging Standard	Health Level Seven is one of several ANSI-accredited SDO in the area of healthcare that provides standards for electronic interchange of clinical, financial, and administrative information among computerized health information systems.	Health Level Seven, Inc. *HL-7. http://www.hl7.org/about/index.cfm.* Accessed September 7, 2009.	http://www.hl7.org/

ANALYSIS OF SURVEILLANCE DATA FLOW, WORK FLOW, AND INFORMATION FLOW: AN EXAMPLE OF INFORMATICS APPLIED TO PUBLIC HEALTH SURVEILLANCE

Excellent data management requires comprehensive understanding of the entire surveillance process. Depending on the level of complexity, surveillance systems involve various data collection rules, logical orders of data flow, work flow, and information flow within the context of the data capture environment. In addition, substantial variability in data collection methods exists between data capture activities in clinical facilities and laboratories compared with community-based and other non-health facility settings. Although these concepts are different, they can be represented in a single illustration (*see* illustration of a prototype national surveillance system, accounting for national and subnational data flow [from the start of data capture to its intended final destination], feedback on analyzed data [information flow], and the role of health workers [work flow]); (Fig. 5–2).

Data flow, work flow, and information flow are three distinct conceptual pathways within any surveillance system. By process of abstraction, flow diagrams should provide a simplified yet rich view of the critical transactions that occur from the point of original capture of data all the way through the final dissemination of findings for public health action. During the course of routine data management, surveillance flow pathway diagrams can serve as a quick reference manual to identify the critical domains that require monitoring and intervention to assure data quality and data integrity. Periodic updating of these diagrams is especially useful in guiding complex and long-term data management activities.

Data capture involves all ways in which signals might first enter the surveillance system that ultimately contribute to messages or other critical outputs from the system. For structured surveillance systems, data capture modalities are usually few, predefined, and explicit. For unstructured surveillance systems represented by what has been widely termed as *event-based surveillance* (*17*; *see* Chapter 17), the data capture modalities are sometimes more numerous and are adaptive and responsive rather than explicit and predefined. Informal and unstructured reports from local clinicians, health authorities, traditional healers, public security officers, other civil authorities, and individual citizens are critical to timely detection of health threats. Nevertheless, even for event-based surveillance, a few main types of methods for data capture, such as automated scanning of mass media and of internet data sources, result in the great majority of signals that ultimately are verified to be of substantial public health interest (*18,19*). Validated processes of data capture are needed to assure that the health phenomena that public health officials intended to be captured and reflected as the fundamental data in the system are indeed being represented accurately when first captured into the system.

Data flow encompasses the transition of captured data between various agents (e.g., between health-care providers and surveillance officers); translation of data formats (e.g., translating hardcopy reports into digital formats, or between different platforms for data representation, such as between a storage on a computer

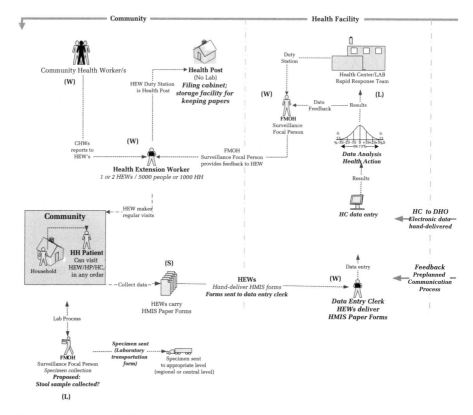

Figure 5–2 Generalized Flow of Data, Work, and Information of a National Public Health Surveillance System.

drive to uploaded to an internet-based database); transmission between levels of the health system; feedback loops reflecting data quality checks, corrections, and updates; and analytic transformations of data (e.g., calculation of rates or creation of maps from aggregate reports of disease). Well-documented, valid data flow pathways are needed to assure that the integrity of data captured in the system are maintained at all times and that an audit trail is established for all changes to or transformations of the raw data.

Work flow refers to the systematic human activities in the collecting and processing of surveillance data. Data captured at the point of its origin by a health worker reflects specific activities or actions associated with his or her daily work. Similarly, the health officer at the district, states, or regional health facility level has predefined work practices related to data analysis and information dissemination for public health action. At the highest level of a national health system, the central health authorities have predefined roles in managing health information. Documentation of these work flow activities as they relate to a surveillance system is important to successful data management.

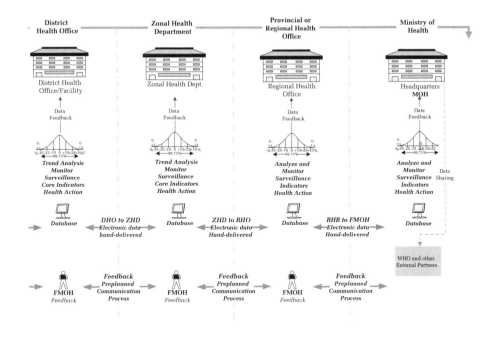

Codes:
Work Flow Process **(W)**
Surveillance Data Flow Process **(S)**
Laboratory Data Flow Process **(L)**
Text in bold italics represents new/proposed approach

Information flow refers to the critical logical processes, transactions, inputs, and decision points along the movement of information from the first capture of data, through all chains of transmission and transformation, through analysis and dissemination as information and knowledge. This process is analogous to the "chain of custody" for fungible evidence in legal proceedings where the careful custodianship for evidence collected at a crime scene must be guarded carefully and documented to allow a jury to know that spurious evidence was not introduced nor good evidence destroyed. The additional challenge for surveillance is that the data, usually in electronic format at some early point in the surveillance process, are transformed continuously as they move toward public health information and knowledge.

Flow pathway diagrams allow chemical, aeronautical, and other engineers to identify the critical hazards to quality outcomes and to continually pursue improved processes and quality. We have found that collaboratively assembling a surveillance information flow diagram as represented in Figure 5–2 can be transformative in bringing all stakeholders, contributors, and consumers of surveillance data to better appreciate their own and their partners' roles. Moreover, such a diagram can provide a complete "radar screen" for the surveillance data manager to use in pursuing ever higher quality of surveillance information.

THE ROLE OF STANDARDS IN DATA MANAGEMENT FOR PUBLIC HEALTH SURVEILLANCE

Agreement to adopt consensus standards represents one of the most powerful forces for efficient sharing among individuals and societies. For example, consider the ability to step off a plane almost anywhere in the world, switch on a cell phone, and have a conversation with someone 8,000 miles away, and then—with a small plastic card—quickly withdraw from a cash machine a handful of the local currency, the name of which you might not even know. To date, health and surveillance data have clearly failed to keep pace with the information revolution observed in the domains of telecommunications and banking.

A large number and diverse types of standards are relevant to surveillance data management. These range from the specific "business" standards for surveillance scientific practice through informatics standards for: terminology or semantics of health conditions under surveillance; syntactical and database structure; and messaging for transportation of information for disease reporting. Examples of a business standard for surveillance include WHO's Standards for Surveillance of Reportable Diseases and the national reporting requirements published by any national government. An example of a terminology or semantic standard is the use of the International Classification of Diseases and Health Related Problems (ICD-9 and ICD-10) to represent health conditions and used for official mortality statistics. The use of ICD-9 codes, which have been translated into the official national languages of all countries in the world, functions like the red traffic light, which likewise has been adopted as a standard throughout the world to provide common semantic messaging regardless of the tremendous variation in spoken and written language and in cultural understanding and interpretation of events (*20*). Other especially important examples of terminology standards applicable to public health surveillance data are the Logical Observation Identifiers Names and Codes (LOINC) and the Systematized Nomenclature of Medicine–Clinical Terms (SNOMED–CT) (Table 5–2).

Public health surveillance data must be stored, and data storage should be governed by an appropriate database or data storage standard. The selection of the type of database depends on the type of surveillance activity. Some of the commonly used relational databases include Structured Query Language (SQL) (used in MySQL and Microsoft SQL), Microsoft Access, and Oracle. Once data are coded and stored, messaging standards such as Extensible Markup Language (XML) or Health Level Seven (HL7) allow data to be transmitted to another system that is configured to receive and parse (i.e., to deconstruct the message into its components) HL7 data and store in a database. To date, data interchange standards for billing and reimbursement in the clinical environment have had relatively limited use in public health information systems. The Uniform Bill 92 (UB92) was used for paper-based transactions until that standard was enhanced by new billing and reimbursement standards for medical procedures issued by the American National Standards Institute (ANSI). Many other standards exist, and most countries have a national standards institute corresponding to ANSI to guide the administration and use of health data standards within a country. The standards listed in Table 5–2 are among the most common entryways to the universe and practice of the application of standards to one's work that will be encountered by the typical public health surveillance data manager.

ROLES, RESPONSIBILITIES, AND PERSONNEL FOR PUBLIC HEALTH SURVEILLANCE DATA MANAGEMENT

Modern public health surveillance systems require diverse types of expertise. Depending on the scope of the data collection and data management activity, a project manager, a database manager, data entry personnel, software developers, and other categories of personnel might be needed to develop and manage an information system. At a minimum, each surveillance information management system needs to have a designated, responsible surveillance data manager. The role of a data manager includes managing the surveillance database and ensuring its integrity, security, and completeness. In addition, the data manager provides detailed guidance for the daily operation of the information management system, manages access to the database, and provides reports as required within the scope of the surveillance activity. When a surveillance system is larger—especially when multiple surveillance needs are managed by a common surveillance information system unit—areas of special expertise within the larger domain of data management and informatics commonly will be addressed by specialists. Examples of specialized roles involve database administrators, data modelers, geospatial data or geographic information systems (GIS) experts, and webmasters (Table 5–3). When only one person is hired to serve as a public health surveillance data manager for a surveillance system, this person takes on all of these roles and responsibilities. In that case, it is essential to negotiate a clear statement of the highest priority responsibilities and expectations for that officer.

"Surveillance Data Modeling and Database Design" As an Example of Informatics Application to a Surveillance Task

In the process of designing a database, one constructs a data model that describes how data are represented and accessed within the database. Most database applications provide a database management layer that offers the ability to write small programs (sometimes called "scripts") to create data input, data editing, data storage, data retrieval, and data export. Although databases generally are not designed for advanced statistical analysis, most database applications provide ability for simple statistical analysis and allow datasets to be exported for analysis using separate statistical software application packages. Often, scripts can be written to support simple statistical analysis such as summary statistics.

Table 5–3 Roles and Responsibilities of Public Health Data Management and Informatics to be Distributed Among Data Management Staff

Data manager	Has responsibility for daily operation and management of data/information system/s; creates new databases and log-ins as appropriate, administers data security, and establishes and monitors database backup and recovery processes; plans capacity requirements for disk storage and other server hardware; and coordinates with appropriate internal or external entities for hardware and software upgrades and maintenance.
Database administrator	Has responsibility for ensuring the confidentiality, integrity, and availability of physical databases and datasets; accepts and processes requests for data or database access from internal and external users. Develop and document internal data standards according to the need; keeps abreast of data and metadata standards to ensure adherence where applicable.
Database designer	Translates the data requirements into a physical implementation using the available standard database management technologies.
Data modeler	Creates and maintains visual models and textual documents for data requirements. Analyzes business requirements to determine data types and relationships to properly define and represent the underlying data structures.
Document manager	Administers and assists program areas with the implementation of Document Management and other commercial content management software. Analyzes workflow processes and develops custom processes for organizing, sharing, routing, and storing content.
Geospatial and temporal data	Manages the content of the geo-spatial databases. Supports surveillance requirements to acquire new spatial datasets for visualization of data. (these requirements apply primarily to spatial data created for GIS applications but might also be applied to any dataset that contains a geographic component or locator information).
Metadata manager	Creates and maintains metadata or "data about data". Essential for efforts to make governmental data (such as public health surveillance data) widely, uniformly, and rapidly accessible, through efforts such as Data.Gov.
Webmaster	Coordinates within entities to provide technical services and support for the Web server environment; manages the overall Web server architecture; administers Web server support utilities, applications, and scripts.

Modified after National Center for Environmental Health, CDC. http://intranet.cdc.gov/nceh-atsdr/is/datamanagement.html. Accessed June 22, 2009.

Database applications must support various types and levels of interfaces—the images shown on a computer screen or cell phone screen that guide a person to put information in or withdraw information from the computer and the various databases to which it provides access. In addition to user interfaces to access the data, hardware interfaces, software interfaces, and, where applicable, relevant communication interfaces also need to be constructed and quality-controlled. User interfaces are provided through a set of log-in screens and associated data entry, search, and retrieval capabilities. Hardware interfaces have to be documented to provide the logical structure and physical address of the device where the data are stored. For devices such as smart phones, personal digital assistants, or other mobile computing devices, user interfaces must be developed to upload the original data from these devices to the database. Communications interfaces include documentation of appropriate network interface information (such as local area network address) to the hardware devices used in the surveillance information system. Each aspect of database design and management can be addressed explicitly through database modeling and design, or—ideally—they have been designed systematically and defined explicitly for the overall enterprise or public health activity through the enterprise architecture (*see* Table 5–1 for definition).

"Rolled Up" (Centralized or Consolidated) Versus Decentralized Informatics Support

There is a tension between the surveillance epidemiologist who typically prefers his or her "own" data manager, who can be immediately and exclusively responsive to the needs of her or his specific public health surveillance system, and the informatics-savvy manager who perceives the advantages of "rolling up" data managers across many units into a consolidated informatics service unit that can gain economies of scale and thus provide a higher level of information systems service to each of the individual surveillance systems. Different ways of addressing the ever-increasing demands for quality and timeliness of surveillance information and different ways of solving the interoperability question need to be documented carefully so that we make as much progress as possible in serving the needs of public health rather than the needs of entrenched factions. For example, this tension can be minimized by considering the institutions that contribute data to the system as users rather than simply data sources by allowing epidemiologists and analysts in subnational institutions access to the data they have entered at their level to conduct their own analyses and produce their own reports to answer local questions. It is also helpful for the central system to provide reports to subnational managers that compare their districts (or other area) with other similar areas or with national standards. These reports can be invaluable tools for local managers to quantify and address perceived needs and to advocate for resources. Public health surveillance epidemiologists who acquire depth of understanding of informatics and informaticians who immerse themselves in understanding and solving problems in surveillance and public health will be key facilitators in the synergy of disciplines, which is needed for the best outcomes in public health.

Surveillance Teamwork—Informatics, Epidemiology, and Laboratory Expertise

Overall management of surveillance data requires an information management team that represents the data management team but also includes other domains of expertise, including at least surveillance epidemiologists and laboratory scientists (for any surveillance system that involves laboratory data). Three dimensions of public health surveillance—coverage, quality, and timeliness—form an excellent framework around which to organize teamwork among practitioners of these different disciplines. Additional disciplines (such as behavioral science, communications, and geography) might be drawn in according to the nature of the health problem and the surveillance activities implemented in response to a specific problem. Weekly, multidisciplinary meetings among at least epidemiologists, laboratory scientists, and data managers are an excellent basis on which to build the needed teamwork.

The Role of Institutions

Public health surveillance systems should be thought of as partnerships between individual health workers and the institutions they represent. It is not uncommon for local institutions to feel that surveillance is yet another chore imposed from the central level, and they are only too familiar with central level institutions calling them "partners" without really treating them as partners. Surveillance managers must overcome this cynicism by building and maintaining trust within the system, including among all those who have responsibility for any aspect of the handling of public health surveillance data. This can be done through transparency (while respecting privacy and bureaucratic sensitivities), and shared ownership of as much of the data and analysis is feasible. It is well worth the expense to train local surveillance teams and provide yearly national or international meetings where teams can share ideas and present their results. Each of the different disciplines that contribute to public health surveillance, including the informatics and data management disciplines, should have an opportunity to highlight their expertise and contributions to the systems and be appreciated by their partners in other disciplines.

Public health surveillance data have limited value unless they are transformed into high-quality information and are disseminated in a timely manner to serve as the basis for public health action (21,22). The most essential roles of a surveillance data manager are to (1) maintain the integrity of the original surveillance data; (2) improve the quality of the surveillance database; and (3) increase the availability of surveillance information, so that it yields the most valid, useful, timely information to guide the improvement of the public's health. A useful way to frame and conceptualize the job of the data manager is as a surveillance data quality officer.

Eleven elements of a quality assurance process for public health surveillance data management can be applied to the systematic and ongoing collection, collation, analysis, and dissemination of public health surveillance data (Table 5–4). These elements are adapted from several frameworks and from the authors' experience and represent a work in progress rather than a final, definitive set of dimensions. Notably, these are relatively independent of, complement, and extend the criteria outlined in "Guidance for Evaluation of Surveillance Data" (see Chapter 7 and reference 23). Once again, a general movement toward what might be called an "information standards-based approach" is at the heart of this effort, where

Table 5–4 Dimensions of Quality Improvement and Promotion as Applied to Public Health Surveillance Data Management

1. Accuracy	Extent to which electronic surveillance data reflect data captured into the system and are validated
2. Accountability	Extent to which a "chain of custody" can reconstruct the process for each surveillance finding or statistic from its original sources, including any modifications and transformations
3. Completeness	Extent to which the completeness of surveillance reports and data are characterized and managed over time
4. Security	Assurance of security of electronic data and associated objects (reports in hardcopy, specimens, etc.) against a range of unintentional, environmental, data tampering, and malicious effects that could corrupt or inadvertently allow release of data
5. Confidentiality and privacy	Maintenance of the privacy of individuals and the confidentiality of data are maintained within every requirement of law, regulation, and policy
6. Accessibility	Maximal user access to data that can help to inform and promote the public health, while preserving all confidentiality, privacy, and security requirements for the surveillance data
7. Reliability	The day-to-day consistency of operations, including meeting maintenance requirements for hardware, necessary updates of software, and maintenance of the human capacity needed to conduct surveillance data management at a high level
8. Adherence to standards	Consistent efforts to learn about and adhere to an expanding sphere of relevant standards for data management; best practices for surveillance in general; best practices for informatics; quality management in general
9. Interoperability	Ability to exchange data across different computing environments through adoption of data exchange standards and standardized vocabularies
10. Documentation	Maintenance of written standard operating procedures (SOP) for all key components of surveillance data operations, and assurance that those SOPs are a central tool for management and that all employees have full cognizance of SOPs governing the functions on which they work
11. Stewardship of the surveillance data system	Provision of responsible and accountable management for of all aspects of the surveillance information system

surveillance data collection and management is performed using widely accepted information standards (*see* Table 5–2).

Among these dimensions of data quality, data integrity warrants particular attention; data integrity is a value that pervades a high-functioning data management enterprise. The first element of data integrity—validation of the observation recorded and translation into digital format—is highly vulnerable and always warrants the particular attention of the informatician and data manager. Subsequent corrections of or changes to those data should be documented and justified. Similarly, transformations of those data through aggregation, calculation of rates by meshing with population statistics, portrayal on maps or other visualization platforms, and other modifications should be carried out through explicit and transparent processes that the data manager can guarantee have guarded the integrity of the information. From another perspective, data represented in summary national surveillance reports should be traceable to the original cases detected and reported in each jurisdiction.

Issues regarding quality and integrity of data are often identified when more intensive analysis is done, and when unexpected or counterintuitive findings are produced. In this setting, the epidemiologist and data manager must track down the source of the error or unexpected finding. These are often the most important exercises of all in the investigation of surveillance data, potentially leading, for example, either to the detection of a heretofore-unrecognized flaw in data processing within the surveillance data management system or, on the other hand, to a new disease or an unrecognized manifestation of a public health problem.

Just as the epidemiologist must be trained, prepared, and vigilant in observing the epidemiologic signals coming from the population, the data manager and informatician must be vigilant in monitoring surveillance data quality, data integrity, and information system performance. In the exponentially increasing complexity and volume of information potentially accessible to practitioners of public health surveillance, these two disciplines and likely other disciplines will need to innovate in how they manage vast streams of digital information to guide public health action.

REFERENCES

1. Williams F. The role of electronic medical record in care delivery in developing countries. *Int J Info Mgmt* 2008;28(6):503–507.
2. World Health Organization ed. *Electronic Health Records: Manual for Developing Countries.* Geneva, Switzerland: World Health Organization; 2006.
3. Brennan PF, Yasnoff WA. Medical informatics and preparedness. *J Am Med Inform Assoc* 2002;9(2):202–203.
4. Demchak B, Chan TC, Griswold WG, Lenert LA. Situational awareness during mass-casualty events: command and control. *AMIA Annu Symp Proc* 2006:905.
5. Kunapareddy N, Mirhaji P, Zhang J, Michea Y, Srinivasan A. Information visualization for quality control in health data exchange platforms. *AMIA Annu Symp Proc* 2005:1013.
6. Mandl KD, Overhage JM, Wagner MM, *et al.* Implementing syndromic surveillance: a practical guide informed by the early experience. *J Am Med Inform Assoc* 2004;11(2):141–150.
7. Al-Shorbaji NM. WHO EMRO's approach for supporting e-health in the Eastern Mediterranean Region. *East Mediterr Health J* 2006;12(Suppl 2):S238–S252.
8. Nguyen QT, Naguib RN, Abd Ghani MK, Bali RK, Lee IM. An analysis of the healthcare informatics and systems in Southeast Asia: a current perspective from seven countries. *Int J Electron Healthc* 2008;4(2):184–207.

9. Araujo J, Pepper C, Richards J, Choi M, Xing J, Li W. The profession of public health informatics: still emerging? *Int J Med Inform* 2009;78(6):375–385.

10. Hersh WR. Medical informatics: improving health care through information. *JAMA* 2002;288(16):1955–1958.

11. Hills RA, Turner AM. Informatics and communication in a state public health department: a case study. *AMIA Annu Symp Proc* 2008:970.

12. O'Carroll PW, Yasnoff WA, Ward EM, Ripp LH, Martin EL. *Public Health Informatics and Information Systems*. New York: Springer; 2003.

13. Healthcare Information and Management Systems Society. Stakeholder Analysis. 2008; http://www.himss.org/content/files/deviceSecurity/StakeholderAnalysisMedicalDeviceSecurity.pdf. Accessed March 11, 2010.

14. Kumar Y, Chaudhury N, Vasudev N. Stakeholder Analysis: The Women and Children's Health Project in India. *Health Systems 20/20*. 1997.

15. Fairchild AL, Bayer R, Colgrove JK, Wolfe D. *Searching Eyes: Privacy, the State, and Disease Surveillance in America*. Berkeley; New York: University of California Press; Milbank Memorial Fund; 2007.

16. Bayer R, Fairchild A. The limits of privacy: surveillance and the control of disease. *Health Care Anal* 2002;10(1):19–35.

17. Paquet C, Coulombier D, Kaiser R, Ciotti M. Epidemic intelligence: a new framework for strengthening disease surveillance in Europe. *Euro Surveill* 2006;11(12):212–214.

18. Brownstein JS, Freifeld CC, Madoff LC. Digital disease detection–harnessing the Web for public health surveillance. *N Engl J Med* 2009;360(21):2153–2155, 2157.

19. Grein TW, Kamara KB, Rodier G, *et al.* Rumors of disease in the global village: outbreak verification. *Emerg Infect Dis* 2000;6(2):97–102.

20. World Health Organization. International Classification of Diseases 2008. http://www.who.int/classifications/icd/en/. Accessed March 11, 2010.

21. Ma H, Rolka H, Mandl K, Buckeridge D, Fleischauer A, Pavlin J. Implementation of laboratory order data in BioSense Early Event Detection and Situation Awareness System. *MMWR* 2005;54(Suppl):27–30.

22. U.S. Government. Homeland security presidential directive/HSPD 21, Public Health and Medical Preparedness. 2007.

23. German RR, Lee LM, Horan JM, Milstein RL, Pertowski CA, Waller MN. Updated guidelines for evaluating public health surveillance systems: recommendations from the Guidelines Working Group. *MMWR Recomm Rep* 2001;50(RR-13):1–35; quiz CE31–37.

6

Analyzing and Interpreting Public Health Surveillance Data

PATRICK S. SULLIVAN, MATTHEW T. McKENNA,
LANCE A. WALLER, G. DAVID WILLIAMSON,
AND LISA M. LEE

It is a very sad thing that nowadays there is so little useless information.
—Oscar Wilde

Surveillance is information for action. Analyzing and interpreting public health surveillance data are the links between the design and operation of a surveillance system and the use of data from the system to implement public health action and disease control programs (*1*).

Surveillance data have many uses (*2,3*), and the approaches to analysis and interpreation of surveillance data are tied to both the design of the surveillance system and to the intended uses of the data. For example, surveillance data are used to detect epidemics, suggest hypotheses, characterize trends in disease or injury, evaluate prevention programs, and project future public health needs. In this chapter, we address practical and methodologically sound approaches to analyzing surveillance data from different types of surveillance systems and discuss the presentation of surveillance data by person, place, and time. We emphasize a wide variety of analytical methods that can be used with surveillance data of different types, including case surveillance data and data from supplemental and syndromic surveillance systems. We also discuss the systematic interpretation of surveillance data and presentation of the results of surveillance analyses through graphical presentation.

TYPES OF SURVEILLANCE SYSTEMS AND RELATIONSHIP TO ANALYSIS

To approach methods for analysis of surveillance data, it is important to note the ways in which public health surveillance has expanded, in terms of scope and methods, in recent years. Historically, public health surveillance has been concerned primarily with *case surveillance systems*, in which individual case reports are assembled on a census (or as close to a census as possible, given resource contraints) of all cases of a disease or health event. Over the past several decades, public health surveillance has expanded its scope and methods in several ways. First, surveillance increasingly measures not only individual cases of disease but also behavioral or environmental precedents and outcomes of disease. *Supplemental surveillance systems* collect more in-depth data on risk behaviors and clinical outcomes of those with disease from a smaller number of persons—in some cases, a probability sample of those at risk for disease or under care for a disease or condition. In response to bioterrorisim and preparedness concerns, *syndromic surveillance systems* (see Chapter 14), which ascertain not diagnosed cases of disease but clusters of symptoms and clinical findings that might be suggestive of disease, have proliferated. Syndromic surveillance systems often use existing data sources, such as data from medical records systems, as a source of data flow.

The anaysis of data is guided largely by the purpose and design of the surveillance system. Data from case surveillance traditionally are analyzed in a descriptive way, emphasizing person, place, and time, but with minimal statistical analysis or inference. Surveillance systems that use probability samples are analyzed most appropriately using methods that take into account the sampling design, and use sampling weights to increase the scope of inference. In response to the needs of preparedness programs, analysis of data from some syndromic surveillance systems places a premium on abberation detection in "real time," featuring continuous analysis of incoming data streams.

Analytic practices for data from surveillance systems have changed as new tools and increased computational capacity of computers have become available. For example, technology for Geographic Information Service (GIS) methods, originally developed for military applications, have been integrated into many commercially available electronic devices, and software for the analysis of spatial information has been developed for commercial markets (4). Surveillance systems thus increasingly incorporate locating data, and analysis of spatial data has become feasible in many state and local health department settings.

We conceptualize the variety of analytic approaches that can be applied to data from surveillance systems relative to the design of systems—including case surveillance systems, supplemental surveillance systems such as behavioral and clinical outcomes surveillance systems, and syndromic surveillance systems. Table 6–1 presents a review of these designs, examples, and related analytic methods.

Table 6–1 also relates the types of surveillance systems to the types of analyses—descriptive analysis, inferential analysis, aberration detection, and demographic analyses—that might be performed using the data from those systems. *Descriptive analyses* focus on the observed patterns in the data and might also seek to compare the relative occurrence of disease in different subgroups. *Interential analyses* seek to make statistical conslusions about the patterns of disease, predicates of disease, or outcomes of disease. *Aberration detection analytic methods* seek to make judgements in "real time" about whether there is significant clustering of disease in space or time; the goal of such analyses is to

Table 6–1 Types of Surveillance Systems and Associated Analysis Types and Methods

Data collection design	Analysis type	Analysis methods	Examples
Case surveillance	Case counts/rates (D)	Rate calculation, rate ratios, standardized rates	Number and rates of violent deaths in the US (5); age-standardized projected rates of arthritis (6)
	Trend over time (I)	Regression analysis to describe estimated annual percent change in case reports	Trends in HIV diagnoses in men who have sex with men (7); trends in pancreatic cancer (8)
	Geographic clustering (A)		Clustering of road injuries in Rome (9)
Syndromic surveillance	Geographic clustering/ aberration (A)		Pesticide exposure (10)
	Temporal aberration (A)		Symptoms in companion animals after an industrial chemical release (11)
Supplemental surveillance systems			
Behavioral surveillance	Prevalence of behaviors (D)	Related to design (e.g., weighted analyses from probability surveys)	HIV testing from among men who have sex with men (12)
	Trends in prevalence of behaviors over time (I)	Age-adjusted rates, linear regression analysis for monotonic trends	Prevalence of smoking in the United States (13)
Clinical outcomes surveillance	Rates of clinical outcomes (D)	Incidence rates from probability sample	Prevalence of anemia among renal dialysis patients (14)
	Factors associated with clinical outcomes (I)		Factors associated with thrombosis in patients with HIV infection (15)

D: Descriptive; I: Inferential; A: Aberration detection.

determine when public health follow-up is needed to confirm whether an outbreak is occurring and, if so, to shed light on the causes of clusters of a condition and recommend public health interventions where needed. *Demographic data* are used to provide critical population-level contexts for other types of analyses.

A PRACTICAL APPROACH

Regardless of the type of surveillance system or the type of analysis to be performed, there are certain overriding principles that should guide analyses. In general, analyzing and interpreting surveillance data should be of primary importance, resisting the urge to allow the time-consuming problems of collecting, managing, and storing surveillance data to supersede the analysis itself. Thus, analyses should be implemented as part of a routine surveillance program so results can be monitored over time. General steps to analyzing surveillance data include:

1. **Know the inherent idiosyncracies of the surveillance data set**. It is tempting to begin immediately to examine trends over time. However, intimate knowledge of the strengths and weaknesses of the data collection methods, understanding of the reporting process, and knowledge of changes in surveillance system and practices can provide a critical context in which to interpret the trends that emerge.

   For the analyst conducting a one-time analysis of surveillance data, it is important to ask those knowledgable of the system what evaluations are done routinely and to review the results of those analyses (*16*). What are the key indicators of performance for this system, how are they measured, and have they been stable over time? For public health scientists who will be working over time with data from a surveillance system, being engaged in evaluation activities, or initiating them if they do not already exist, is an important long-term activity.

2. **Proceed from the simplest to the most complex**. Using the concepts of exploratory data analysis, examine each condition and characteristic separately. Are there apparent issues in data quality or completeness? How many cases were reported each year? How many cases were reported in each age group each year? Perform subgroup analyses to determine whether trends vary by factors such as race/ethnicity or sex.

3. **Recognize limitations of the data that preclude more sophisticated analyses**. Erratically collected or incomplete data cannot be corrected fully by complex analytic techniques. Differential reporting by regions or health facilities render the resulting surveillance data set liable to misinterpretation. Again, routine evaluation will help identify such issues.

4. **Report findings to stakeholders and to those who run the surveillance system**. Dissemination is a key aspect of surveillance practice and is discussed elsewhere in this book (*17*). Part of the process of surveillance is using the results of evaluations and findings of analyses to provoke improvements to the functioning of the system; the practice of feeding back to surveillance staff about how data collection can be improved is both a responsibility of the analyst and a way to promote higher quality data for future analyses.

The remainder of this chapter focuses on these broad topics—descriptive, inferential, and aberration detection analytic methods and uses of demographic data in surveillance analysis. We do not attempt to provide exhaustive methods for each analytic approach; rather, we seek to describe how and when certain methods can be used and provide references to more detailed methodologic sources.

DESCRIPTIVE ANALYSIS OF SURVEILLANCE DATA

Descriptive analyses are especially important in the routine monitoring and reporting of surveillance data. Officials responsible for making program and policy decisions, and in turn for explaining their decisions to elected authorities, the public, or other stakeholders, often have limited background in statistical or epidemiologic analytic methods. Therefore, routine analyses of surveillance data should report estimates of basic epidemiologic parameters that can be explained intuitively to lay audiences. Descriptive analyses meet many of these criteria and answer questions such as: "How much disease is occurring in the population?" or "What proportion of the population has an important risk factor for disease?"; "What are the key demographic characteristics of cases or persons at risk for a condition?"; "Is one subgroup of the population more affected than another?"; "How do the number of cases this year compare to case counts in the previous years?"

This section focuses on calculating and interpreting common epidemiologic parameters used to analyze surveillance data, and the statistical methods that provide the framework to guide interpretation. Standard analyses of surveillance data focus on questions of who, where, and when (i.e., person, place, and time). When unexpected results occur, more in-depth studies and analyses can be done to identify the underlying causes of those unexpected results. In this way, descriptive analyses might lead to hypotheses or inferential analyses, which can provide invaluable etiologic clues, as well as a deeper understanding of disease processes (18).

Measurements and Parameters

Public health surveillance data focus on outcomes that are either (1) discrete phenomena in humans, animals, or their environments or (2) continuous characteristics of these same entities. Examples of the discrete phenomena include vital events (i.e., births and deaths), disease and injury diagnoses, knowledge about health information, and contaminant levels that exceed predetermined levels. Continuous characteristics include physiological attributes such as height, weight, blood pressure, antibody levels against pathogens such as West Nile virus, and particulate matter (e.g., smog) in the atmosphere. To examine trends in these outcomes, the results usually are aggregated across the dimensions of person, place, and time.

Because epidemiology and public health focus on populations and their environments, rather than individuals, individually measured values must be aggregated and transformed into epidemiologic *parameter estimates*, such as rates and averages, to be useful in guiding appropriate action (19). The procedures for constructing the most common parameters and the relevant statistical methods used to assess important differences across epidemiologic dimensions are explained below. Simple equations for the statistical testing, and calculating 95% confidence

intervals (CIs) can be used in the majority of analyses (Table 6–2). Other calculation methods should be used when the numbers of observations available for the
analysis are small; consultation with a statistician is recommended in the case of
small numbers of observations.

Frequency (Counts)

Surveillance of disease diagnoses, deaths, and other discrete events frequently are
assessed by reporting counts of events overall and within subgroups. For events that
are relatively uncommon (e.g., affect less than 5% of the population in 1 year), the
Poisson probability distribution can be used to evaluate the probabilities associated
with the differences between groups. For pairwise comparisons of such counts
that have large numbers (>50 events), there is a simple formula available based on
approximations to the normal distribution that commonly is used (Table 6–2); with
sufficient numbers of events, a CI can also be computed around the count.

Rates

When the counts of events vary, it might be because of differences in the underlying probability, or risk, of an event occurring or because of differences in the
size of the population groups being evaluated. For example, larger numbers of
persons will die of lung cancer in California than Kentucky because the population of California is much larger, whereas the risk of lung cancer mortality is
lower. Aggregating the number of events over a defined period (usually 1 year) by
the population size at the midpoint of the period provides a ratio parameter called
a rate—for example, the number of cases in a given year per 1,000 persons.[a] To
illustrate differences in rates between two groups, the relative rate (or ratio of the
rates), for two the groups commonly is used. In cases where the rate of the event is
relatively small (e.g., the probability is 0.05 where the number of opportunities is
at least 20), the Poisson probability distribution can be used to describe the probability in differences between the two rates because the relative contributions of
the disease counts to the variance are much greater than the contributions of the
relatively large population counts to the variance (Table 6–2).

Age is a powerful, nonmodifiable, biological determinant for the risk of many
health events. Therefore, rates are often age-standardized to avoid confounding
caused by differences in the distribution of this variable between comparison
groups or populations. The details of age-standardization are discussed in detail in
this chapter's section on uses of demographic methods in surveillance analysis.

Statistical comparison of rates, or probabilities, of common events, or characteristics requires the use of other statistical distributions such as the binomial and
hypergeometric. Frequently, when comparing the prevalence or incidence of common events odds ratios are used, because the odds ratio has more stable statistical
properties than relative risks or rates (20). In the interpretation of these analyses,

---

[a] Though the word "rate" is often used to refer to proportions that do not include an element of time, in this
description it is assumed that a defined period is used to assess the time over which events are ascertained for the
numerator of the ratio, and the denominator represents person time of observation.

Table 6–2 Types and Examples of Public Health Data and Parameters With Frequently Used Formulas for Computing Statistical Significance Tests, and Calculating Confidence Intervals for Large Samples (i.e., $n > 50$)

Type of data or parameter	Examples	Formulas for p-values of a pairwise comparison*	95% Confidence interval (CI) formulas
Events affecting < 5 % of the group of interest			
Frequency counts	Case counts Death counts Cancer cases Tuberculosis cases AIDS/HIV cases Number of pedestrian injuries	Two count values of x_1 and x_2 from groups being compared $$Z = \frac{x_1 - x_2}{\sqrt{x_1 + x_2}}$$	For any count x: $95\% \text{ CI} = x \pm 1.96\sqrt{x}$
Rates	Computed from cohorts, or populations: Death rates Incidence rates	Two rates of R_1 and R_2 computed from two groups with event counts of x_1 and x_2: $$Z = \frac{R_1 - R_2}{\sqrt{\dfrac{R_1^2}{x_1} + \dfrac{R_2^2}{x_2}}}$$	For any rate, R, with event counts of x: $95\% \text{ CI} = R \pm 1.96 \times \dfrac{R}{\sqrt{x}}$
Relative rate or risk	Ratio of two rates	Differences in rate ratios are rarely compared. A simple, approximate method is to visually evaluate the overlap in 95% confidence intervals	For a rate ratio (RR) of two rates with event count values of x_1 and x_2: $95\% \text{ CI} =$ $$\exp\left\{ \ln(RR) \pm 1.96 \times \sqrt{\frac{1}{x_1} + \frac{1}{x_2}} \right\}$$

Events affecting >5% of the group of interest

Frequency counts	Number of smokers Number of children appropriately immunized Number of children with lead poisoning	Comparison of two count values x_1 and x_2 with total populations of n_1 and n_2 $$Z = \frac{x_1 - x_2}{\sqrt{x_1\left(1 - \dfrac{x_1}{n_1}\right) + x_2\left(1 - \dfrac{x_2}{n_2}\right)}}$$	For any count x from a total population size n $$95\% \text{ CI} = x \pm 1.96\sqrt{x\left(1 - \frac{x}{n}\right)}$$
Proportions†	Smoking prevalence Mammography utilization Immunization coverage Screened children with lead poisoning	Comparison of two proportions p_1 and p_2 with total populations of n_1, n_2 $$Z = \frac{p_1 - p_2}{\sqrt{\dfrac{p_1(1-p_1)}{n_1} + \dfrac{p_2(1-p_2)}{n_2}}}$$	For a proportion, p, with a total population size of n. $$95\% \text{ CI} = p \pm 1.96\sqrt{\frac{p(1-p)}{n}}$$
Odds ratio	Ratio of two odds‡	Differences in odds ratios are rarely compared. A simple, approximate method is to visually assess the overlap in 95% confidence intervals.	For an ratio of two odds (OR) with event counts of x_1 and x_2, respectively, and population counts of n_1 and $n2$: $$95\% \text{ CI} =$$ $$\exp\left\{\ln(OR) \pm 1.96\sqrt{\frac{1}{x_1} + \frac{1}{n_1 - x_1} + \frac{1}{x_2} + \frac{1}{n_2 - x_2}}\right\}$$

(continued)

Table 6-2 (continued)

Type of data or parameter	Examples	Formulas for p-values of a pairwise comparison*	95% Confidence interval (CI) formulas
Means or medians	Body mass index Blood pressure Ambient air particulates Serum Cholesterol	The estimate of the mean (μ) of measured values x_j in a population size n is: $$\frac{\sum_{j=1}^{n} x_j}{n}$$ The test of the significance of the difference between 2 means, μ_1 and μ_2 is: $$Z = \frac{\mu_1 - \mu_2}{\sqrt{\frac{\sum_{j=1}^{n_1}(x_{j1}-\mu_1)^2}{(n_1-1)} + \frac{\sum_{j=1}^{n_2}(x_{j2}-\mu_2)^2}{(n_2-1)}}}$$	The confidence interval of the mean, μ, for measurements x made on a population size n is: $$95\% \text{ CI} = \mu \pm 1.96\sqrt{\frac{\sum_{j=1}^{n}(x_j-\mu)^2}{(n-1)}}$$ For non-normally distributed data, median tests (e.g., Wilcoxon rank–sum tests) may be used to test for differences between groups.

*Z is the standardized normal deviate that denotes the tail probability for the normal distribution. For a two-sided test probability of 0.05, Z = 1.96. Therefore, values of Z greater than 1.96 suggest differences that are significant at the α=0.05 level.

†An alternative test of significant differences is the Chi-square test for a 2×2 table. Formulas for this test are available in standard statistical texts (20).

‡Odds are the ratio of the probability (p) of an event occurring divided by the event not occurring (i.e., $\frac{p}{1-p}$). This ratio is equivalent to the ratio of the *counts* enumerating the numbers of events (x) divided by the number of members of the population (n) without events (i.e., for a population of size n with x events: $\frac{p}{1-p} = \frac{x}{n-x}$).

care must be taken not to equate the magnitude of the odds ratio to the relative risk or rate. Odds ratios are only an approximation for risk when the number of events of interest is relatively small in comparison to the size of the population from which the event emerges (21). Thus, it is important that reports of associations determined by odds ratios be reported as differences in the odds of an event, rather than differences in the risk of an event. Computational methods have been proposed to obtain valid estimates of the relative risk from odds ratios, but these methods depend on statistical modeling assumptions and require complex statistical evaluations that might be beyond the training of some surveillance data analysts (22,23).

Proportions

For frequently occurring events such as arthritis in the elderly or visits to a medical provider in a year, the ratio of the events divided by the defined population is a proportion, and the probabilities in differences between proportions are determined by the binomial distribution (Table 6–2).

Measures of Central Tendency

Describing the populations monitored through public health surveillance often involves reporting a measure of central tendency, such as the average or mean value of an ordinal variable. Pairs of averages derived from large numbers of measured observations can usually be compared using the Z-test based on the normal probability distribution (Table 6–2). When the data do not follow a normal distribution, other approaches are used to describe the central tendency (median) and test for differences between groups (median tests such as the Wilcoxon rank–sum test).

Although the average value for a population often provides a concise quantitative summary of the attribute of that population, it is also important to inspect the distribution of the measured value of interest across the population. For example, Figure 6–1 presents the age distributions of the populations of Texas and Pennsylvania based on data from the 2000 U.S. Census. In 2000, the average age of Texans was 33.4 years and the average age of Pennsylvanians was 38 years. The distributions presented in the figure demonstrate that the proportion of older residents was greater in Pennsylvania, as suggested by the single, average value. However, without reviewing the distributions of these variables, an analyst would miss the more severe dip in the number of persons ages 20 to 30 years in Pennsylvania when compared with Texas. These distributional properties of continuous or ordinal data that frequently are compared using means can be important, and conclusions about differences or similarities in these types of variables across populations should include analyses of distributions as well as means.

Categories

Surveillance data based on continuous measures such as age, weight, and height are often used to group populations based on intervals of the continuous measures. The number of groups is usually based on the sample size available for dividing the

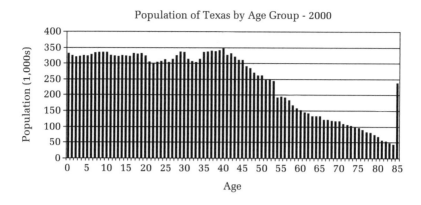

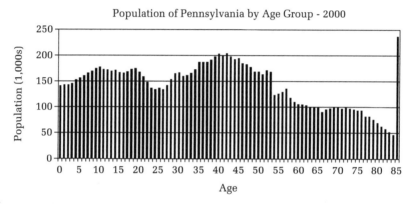

Figure 6–1 Distributions of the populations of Texans and Pennsylvanians, by year of age, in 2000 (*24*).

population sample into categories such that each group has sufficient numbers to provide reasonable statistical precision—ideally at least 25 observations per group. Other standard variables used in surveillance to categorize populations include sex, race, and ethnicity. These values obviously do not have ordinal properties, and the analyst frequently is required to combine data from multiple years, or across geographic area, to obtain adequate statistical precision to assess differences between populations in these groups. Chi-square statistics are used to analyze differences between the distributions of these values between groups (Table 6–2).

Descriptive Analyses of Data From Surveillance Systems Based on Survey Sample Designs

For surveillance systems using complex sampling strategies, alternative approaches are needed to analyze the data, taking into account the sampling schemes. An example of such surveillance systems is the Behavioral Risk Factor Surveillance System (BRFSS). This surveillance system measures the self-reported frequency of health determinants such as smoking and physical activity. Analyses of pairwise and multiple category differences between proportions is the cornerstone for analyzing this kind of survey data. The main methods for generating adjusted estimates from complex samples include simulation procedures (e.g., jackknife and bootstrap), generalized estimating equations, and Taylor series approximations. There are several statistical software packages (STATA, SAS modules, and SUDAAN) available for executing these methods. The interested reader should consult texts devoted to these methods (25) and manuals for the available software packages. Similarly, computing means and their standard errors of parameters obtained through sampling surveys require specialized statistical methods and analytic packages (e.g., PROC SURVEYMEANS in SAS).

INFERENTIAL ANALYSIS OF SURVEILLANCE DATA

Inferential analyses test a hypothesis using statistical methods. Although the primary mode of presenting surveillance data and using data for disease prevention and control has been descriptive analysis, surveillance data also have a number of features that lend themselves to inferential analyses. Surveillance data often have high quality and high representativeness of the underlying population. In some cases, surveillance systems collect data at multiple time-points in the disease process, allowing for longitudinal analyses.

There are several reasons an epidemiologist might want to conduct inferential analyses with surveillance data. First, it might be desirable to make a statistical conclusion about data, because a statistical conclusion can be more persuasive to motivate policy changes. For example, if reported cases of a disease have increased from year to year, it might be desirable to illustrate not just the reported numbers of cases over time but also to conclude that the increases are not explained by random fluctuations in the data. Such analyses might allow the epidemiologist to detect an epidemic (i.e., a greater than expected number of cases). Second, inferential analysis methods allow controlling for important variables that might confound outcomes. Third, inferential approaches allow multivariable analyses of longitudinal data.

Trend Analyses

A question that arises in the analysis of surveillance data is the relationship between the risk of events and whether this risk increases or decreases systematically over time. Practically, the most common question asked of surveillance programs by policymakers is: "Are things getting better, worse, or staying the same?" When things are getting better, public health and other officials sometimes will try to relate improvements to their own governmental or programmatic actions. If things are getting worse, they often will develop or strengthen programmatic responses.

A commonly used inferential analytic approach is trend analysis over time. Here, the null hypothesis is typically that no change in the number of case reports or events has occurred over time. The alternate hypothesis is that a change in case reports has occurred over time. Analytic approaches are different in situations where the trend is consistent over time (monotonic trends), and situations where the trend changes at one or more inflection points over the time period (non-monotonic trends).

Monotonic Trends

After decades of stable cigarette smoking behaviors, New York City implemented a series of tobacco control measures from 2002 through 2006 that included raising the average price of the product through taxes, prohibiting smoking in essentially all indoor workplaces, and implementing a multimillion-dollar media campaign aimed at discouraging smoking. The authors attributed the decline between 2002 and 2006 to the series of public health interventions (26).

To make statistical conclusions about the trend in smoking, surveillance staff analyzed the decline using two methods. First, they simply described the relative difference in the proportion of smokers in the populations in 2002 and 2006; the result was a 19% decline. The statistical assessment of the significance of this change is a simple pairwise comparison of proportions.

However, such an approach does not account for potential deviations from a monotonic trend in the intervening years between the start and end years. To assess both the overall extent of the fall in cigarette smoking during the period, as well as the consistency of this trend, the analysts also conducted another trend analysis that used all the data across the period (Fig. 6–2). Known as the average annual percent change (AAPC; ref. 27), this analysis involves a regression analysis of the natural log transformation of the outcome of interest and the independent variable is the year the outcome is assessed. The AAPC is estimated from the regression coefficient for the year variable; the significance of the linear trend over the period examined is assessed by the probability that the regression coefficient for year is equivalent to 0. In the New York City example, the AAPC was –5% or consistent with a 5% decline for each year that was statistically significant over the period. These results indicate that the decline was consistent and significant. There is growing consensus that this method of describing monotonic trends, and testing for statistical significance in rates over time, is the preferred analytic approach in this situation.

Non-Monotonic Trends

Analyses of time trend data derived from surveillance information often reveal temporal trends that are non-monotonic. An example that has received much attention was the fluctuation in prostate cancer incidence rates observed in the United States from 1975 through 2005 (Fig. 6–3). These observed increases in rates after 1990 have been attributed to greater diagnoses of asymptomatic disease resulting from advances in relatively noninvasive surgical and diagnostic procedures for urinary obstruction that can result from prostatic hypertrophy, as well as greater use of the prostate specific antigen (PSA) blood test to screen for early prostate cancer (28). An important issue was whether the widespread implementation of these early detection technologies was effective in reducing deaths from prostate cancer—a topic that is debated vigorously (29,30).

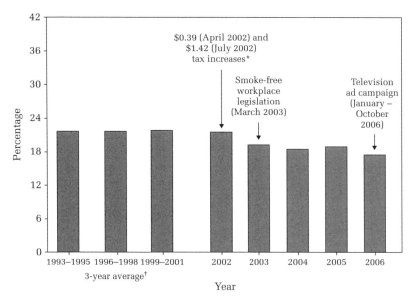

Figure 6–2 Estimated adult smoking prevalence, by year—New York City, 1993–2006 (*26*).
Sources: New York State Behavioral Risk Factor Surveillance System (1993–2001); New York City Community Health Survey (2002–2006); New York State Department of Health; New York City Department of Health aand Mental Hygiene.
*Specific (rather than percentage) tax, not indexed to inflation, resulted in decreasing real price of tobacco during 2003 to 2006.
†Because of small sample sizes specific to New York City for individual years from 1993 to 2001 (range: 794–1665 respondents annually), BRFSS data for these years were grouped into 3-year data sets (1993–1995, 1996–1998, and 1999–2001).

To analyze such non-linear and non-monotonic data, regression analyses can be used that transform the outcome data using exponential or geometric functions and polynomial regression equations that include higher order (e.g., cubic or quadratic) terms for the independent variable denoting time (*30*). However, these techniques are often difficult to interpret and frequently quite challenging to communicate to policymakers. A conceptually simpler approach to such non-linear data is a technique known as joinpoint analysis developed at the U.S. National Cancer Institute (*31*). This method models the trends using statistical criteria to determine the number of times and when the trends change. The result is a series of linear segments that describes the overall data. An AAPC can be calculated for each segment.

The lines connecting annual data points show the results from a joinpoint analysis of prostate cancer incidence by race/ethnicity groups (Fig. 6–3). The joinpoint analysis indicates that there were four segments overall (*8*): in some periods (e.g., 1989–1992), incidence rates increased, whereas in others (e.g., 1992–1995), incidence rates declined. The ability of such an analysis to provide discrete information that can be related to contemporaneous events such as the introduction of new technologies (e.g., PSA in 1989) or program interventions can provide useful surveillance information to evaluate events and programs pertinent to the health of populations.

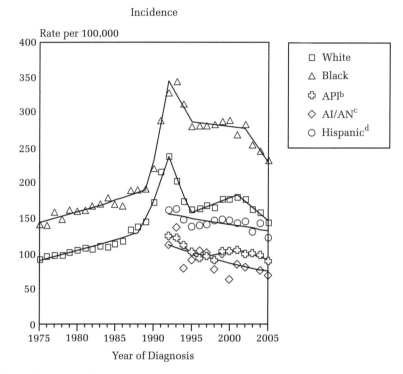

Figure 6–3 Annual prostate cancer incidence rates by race in areas covered by the Surveillance, Epidemiology, and End Results cancer registry system, 1975–2005 (8).

Survival Analyses

Survival analyses are useful in surveillance systems that collect data at multiple points in the disease process. For example, HIV and some cancer surveillance systems collect diagnosis date as well as date of death. The null hypothesis is typically that no difference exists between survival between two groups in the population, and the alternate hypothesis is that a survival difference does exist. Analytic methods are typically time-to-event analyses, such as Kaplan-Meier univariate analyses and Cox proportional hazards regression for multivariate analyses (30). The results are expressed as proportions surviving at a certain follow-up interval with a *p*-value for difference in survival between strata or as a hazard ratio with confidence intervals.

There are some special considerations for the application of these standard methods of survival analyses to surveillance data. One has to do with the starting point of the survival analysis. If date of diagnosis or report to the surveillance system is used as the starting point, there is some concern as to whether there are important differences in the stage of disease at diagnosis or report among the subgroups in the analysis. For example, if one group is diagnosed with HIV later in their course of infection than another, the then starting point of "diagnosis date" systematically will show shorter survival among those diagnosed later. This can

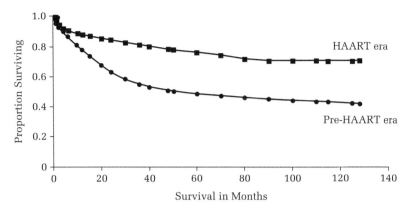

Figure 6–4 Adjusted survival curves of AIDS patients in Chicago before (1993–1995) and after (1996–2001) the introduction of highly active antiretroviral therapy (*32*).

be addressed by using for such analyses an alternative starting point that relates to stage of disease. In this example, survival can be calculated from the first CD4 count at or below 200 cells/μL. Alternatively, analyses stratified by CD4 count at diagnoses might be conducted (*34*).

Survival analysis of data from the HIV/AIDS Surveillance System in Chicago illustrates several important aspects of survival analyses from surveillance data (Fig. 6–4). The figure illustrates survival from a clinically meaningful starting point—AIDS diagnosis—and shows the proportion of cases surviving stratified by whether the AIDS diagnosis occurred before or after the availability of highly effective antiretroviral therapy. To make statistical conclusions about whether the differences illustrated in the graph were significant, the authors used stratified Cox proportional hazards analysis, controlling for race/ethnicity and age. They concluded that survival was significantly better for those diagnosed after improved therapies were available, and that black, non-Hispanic persons had a higher risk of death in both periods (*33*).

Analyses of Associations in Cross-Sectional Data

Logistic regression analyses are appropriate when surveillance data take a cross-sectional form for analysis. The null hypothesis is that some disease outcome (e.g., a clinical event, the strain of infectious agent, receipt of indicated health care service, or engaging in a disease-related risk behavior) is not related to demographic factors, other clinical factors, or some historical exposure. The results are expressed as adjusted odds ratios for the relationship between the explanatory factors and the outcome.

For example, data from a supplemental clinical outcomes surveillance system for persons in care for HIV infection were used to describe the receipt of influenza vaccine, a recommended preventive health service for those living with HIV. The analysis found that most HIV-infected persons in care did not receive an influenza vaccine as recommended; the odds of receiving a vaccine were higher for those with more frequent care visits, and for older patients (*35*).

Analysis of Data From Complex Survey Sample Designs

An advantage of surveillance systems that use survey sample designs is that the data can be used to make inference to broad populations by taking advantage of sampling weights in the analytic process. Specific procedures within statistical software packages allow logistic regression analyses of weighted survey data, with automated calculation of appropriate variances and CIs.

For example, scientists at the U.S. Centers for Disease Control and Prevention (CDC) recently reported an analysis of data on receipt of influenza vaccine among smokers (35). The data were from the BRFSS, an ongoing, state-based, landline telephone survey that uses probability sampling methods to collect information on health risk behaviors, preventive health practices, and access to and use of health services related to chronic conditions among U.S. adults. By using logistic regression accounting for the survey sample design, the authors concluded that the odds of receiving an influenza vaccine were lower for current smokers, compared with nonsmokers (adjusted odds ratio 0.75, 95% CI: 0.71–0.80).

Spatial and Temporal Aberration Detection

Maps of disease incidence and prevalence have long captured the imagination of medical researchers and the general public (36). The story of John Snow's maps of cholera outbreaks in mid-19th century London is often used to motivate increased use of spatial analysis in public health, although the story is more complex than the usual "Snow mapped the cases, noted a cluster around the Broad Street pump, had the handle removed, and stopped the outbreak" version of the story (37,38).

The advent of GIS provide a convenient mechanism for storing, linking, and displaying georeferenced data, and many health agencies have integrated GIS data into disease surveillance efforts. In this section, we briefly review spatial methods for the analysis of disease surveillance data.

Spatial questions quickly arise once surveillance data are mapped. We review three general categories of such questions:

1. Are there unusual aggregations (or deficits) of cases in particular areas? In other words, are there "clusters" of disease?
2. Are there patterns in local rates observed in specific small administrative areas (e.g., counties or census tracts)?
3. Are there links between the spatial pattern of a particular exposure (e.g., levels of air pollution, or more general notions of "exposure" such as socioeconomic or demographic summaries from local or neighboring populations) and that of a particular health outcome (e.g., emergency room visits for asthma)?

Although each category involves questions regarding the spatial pattern of disease, each addresses particular aspects of the spatial pattern and methods to address one category will only address part of the questions in other areas. For example, although questions in category 1 (are there clusters?) are related to those in category 2 (where are local rates the highest?), sufficiently answering questions in category 2 requires good estimates of *all* local rates, not simply the highest ones. Similarly, adequate answers to questions from categories 1 and 2 will fall short of assessing associations with local exposure values which are of primary importance in category 3.

Data Requirements

A close look at each category of questions reveals that each will require different types of data to address the question at hand. Data addressing category 1 typically includes geocoded locations (residence, occupation, or other relevant locations) for each case as well as geocoded locations for all persons at risk or a sample of "controls" (non-cases). The control locations are particularly important because a cluster of cases is not particularly interesting if it occurs in an area with a large number of individuals at risk. Rather, an interesting cluster is one where there are considerably more (or fewer) cases in an area than the number of local controls would suggest under some null model of disease distribution, for example, if national age-specific rates hold for the population under study.

Often, confidentiality requirements preclude release of individual-level data and analysts resort the use of counts from small administrative areas. In such cases, census counts are often used to define the population at risk and the number of cases expected under the null model of disease. Regional counts and census data also form the basis for most methods addressing questions in regarding patterns by small area (category 2).

In addition to data regarding disease counts and regarding the population at risk, questions associated with category 3 require exposure data for this population under study. For sociodemographic exposures, these might include census data, but for environmental data, these often include an additional set of data, collected by different individuals and/or agencies than the original data.

Analytic/Statistical Methods

The methods used to analyze the different types of data differ between categories of spatial questions of interest. In addition, there are subtleties within each category driving the development and applications of analytic methods.

The determination of whether significant clusters of disease events are occurring in space caught renewed epidemiologic interest in the late 1980s and early 1990s following a highly publicized cluster of childhood leukemia deaths in Woburn, Massachusetts (*39,40*), and reviews of available analytic techniques (*41,42*) note several concepts important for applying analytic methods properly. First, the reviews note the distinction between approaches that test for *clustering*, a general tendency for cases to occur near other cases, and tests *to detect clusters* that seek to define which cases define the collection least consistent with the null model, that is, the most unusual cluster. Waller and Gotway (*43*) note that tests of clustering often provide a single significance value for the entire data set while tests to detect clusters often provide significance values for each suspected cluster.

Methods to Detect Clustering

An example of a test of clustering is Tango's index (*44*), detailed in Waller (*45*). Tango's index contains elements similar to Pearson's chi-square test of goodness of fit but also incorporates a measure of geographic closeness between pairs of regions. A higher index indicates more evidence for clustering (*46*).

In contrast to indices of clustering, the software package SaTScan offers a popular test to detect the most likely cluster(s) within a data set. SaTScan, uses spatial (or spatio-temporal) scan statistics wherein one defines a (large) set of potential clusters and evaluates them to find the most unusual one in the set. In the case of the SaTScan software, we consider the set of circular (or elliptical) collections of cases and controls (for point-level data) or small regions whose centroids fall within a given distance of each region's centroid (for regional data) as potential clusters. We allow the radius to vary from the smallest interpoint (or inter-centroid) distance up until some user-defined limit is reached (typically, one-half of the study area). For each potential cluster, we evaluate its "unusualness" by calculating the likelihood ratio test statistic defined by considering a model where the disease risk within the potential cluster is higher (or lower) than that outside versus that where the disease risk is the same inside and outside of the potential cluster. The potential cluster least consistent with the constant risk model has the highest likelihood ratio test statistic and is the "most likely cluster."

To evaluate the statistical significance of the most likely cluster, Kuldorff considers the following permutation procedure (*47*). Fixing the locations of all cases and controls (for point-level data) or regions (for regional data), we permute the cases among the population at risk, find the most likely cluster for the permuted data, and store its associated likelihood ratio test statistic. We randomly permute the cases a large number of times, create a histogram of the stored likelihood ratio test statistics and compare the likelihood ratio statistic observed in the data to this distribution. The proportion of test statistic values from the permutations which exceed the value from the observed data represents the *p*-value or probability of observing a more extreme likelihood ratio test statistic in the most likely cluster. Note that the *p*-value is not defined for each potential cluster but across random permutations of cases, thereby avoiding a multiple comparisons problem. Also note that the scan statistic is a bit unusual in that the most likely cluster is compared with most likely clusters at any location arising under the permutation model, not only against clusters at the same location. Applications of the spatial scan statistic appear in the medical, veterinary, and surveillance literature, with a current bibliography maintained on the SaTScan website (www. satscan.org).

Methods to Detect Clusters/Disease Mapping

Tests of clustering and tests to detect cluster address question 1 above by helping to identify general tendencies and aberrant collections of cases. To address question 2, one needs methods to provide a set of accurate estimates of local incidence rates, prevalence, or proportions from small areas within a larger map. This goal straddles two competing issues: the need for geographic precision through small areas and the need for statistical precision through large local sample sizes. This issue is addressed through the use of *small-area estimation*, a collection of techniques designed to provide model-based estimates for subsets of the data via a weighted average of the data within each small area (the local data) and the same estimate for the entire data set. Such models typically use a random effects structure and are often implemented in a Bayesian framework (*43*). The resulting estimators consist of a compromise between the local data (good geographic precision but poor statistical precision resulting from the small sample size) and the entire data set (poor geographic precision but better statistical precision).

Such estimates are often referred to as *spatial smoothing* approaches as the weighted average tends to bring extremely high and/or low local rates back toward the overall average. This adjustment is accompanied by a reduction in the variance of the local estimates and reflects an improvement in variation by accepting a small amount of bias in the estimates. Such statistical approaches are common in Bayesian modeling and are gaining support in epidemiology (*48,49*). When applied to regional disease rates, the approach often is referred to as *disease mapping*. Lawson and Williams (*50*), Lawson, Browne, and Vidal Rodeiro (*51*), and Waller and Gotway (*43*) provide detailed introductions to the approach illustrate advantages over competing approaches.

The Bayesian framework also is appealing in addressing question 3 above—namely, investigating the association between observed spatial patterns and locally observed covariate values. Traditional linear, logistic, and Poisson regression approaches all suffer from an assumed independence between observations from different regions and do not allow for residual spatial correlation between observations in neighboring regions. The disease mapping methods above might be framed as regression models (typically logistic or Poisson regressions) with spatially correlated random effects where the observed rate in each region depends on the rates observed in neighboring regions. A Bayesian approach allows estimation of model parameters, including the impact of locally measured exposures, adjustments for potential confounders and effect modifiers, as well as parameters defining the amount and extent of residual spatial correlation. Although the all-in-one nature of a Bayesian approach is appealing, the model description and computational implementation are somewhat more advanced than that typically covered in introductory courses in epidemiology and biostatistics and often require implementation by a statistician. Waller and Gotway (*43*) and Lawson (*52*) offer introductions to such methods and illustrate the approaches on a variety of data sets.

Reporting and Interpretation of Results

Methods to detect clusters or clustering (answers to question 1) typically are reported in a hypothesis testing framework wherein the analyst obtains an observed value of test statistic based on the data and assesses the probability (under the null hypothesis) of observing a more extreme value than that observed (the *p*-value). As noted above, tests to detect clustering (such as Tango's test) typically report a single *p*-value summarizing clustering across the entire data set, whereas tests to detect clusters typically report a separate *p*-value for each suspected cluster.

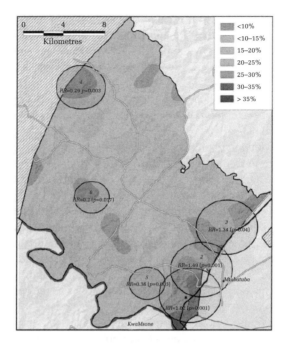

Figure 6–5 An example of the use of spatial depiction of health events, in this case the clustering of HIV prevalence in an area of South Africa. Kuldorrf's spatial scan statistic was used to identify independent clusters of high or low HIV prevalence (*53*).

Spatially smoothed rates (answers to question 2) are typically reported through the use of chloropleth maps where local estimates define the color or shading of each small area. Areas of clustering might overlay the choropleth map. For example, Kuldorff's spatial scan statistic was used to identify clusters of HIV in a surveillance system in South Africa; clusters are indicated by circles on the map (Fig. 6–5; ref. *53*). Sometimes such maps are accompanied by maps of estimates of local variation (variance or standard deviation) to identify unusual local departures from the overall rate. In a Bayesian framework, one can map local posterior probabilities of exceeding a given value (e.g., a given level of relative risk or odds ratio).

Question 3 requires estimates of associations between the outcome and the exposure of interest and a map of local estimated rates. Associations typically are reported as regression parameters or odds ratios associated with given changes in the exposure and local rates are presented as in the answers to question 2. Again, a Bayesian framework requires care in model definition and implementation but provides a complete set of inference for both model parameters and model predictions.

Temporal Aberration Detection

Because the definition of surveillance includes ongoing collection of data, perhaps the most fundamental question suggested by the analysis of surveillance data is: When does the value of reported events signal a change from past patterns? Note that this question, framed in the language of aberration detection, is a functionally different one than questions posed earlier in the discussion of trend analysis. Here, the practical question is: At what point do we have sufficient data to suggest that what we are seeing represents an increase in disease and that public health action is required?

The analysis required to address this question suggests additional questions: How are "past patterns" defined? If an outbreak occurred in the past, should this affect the historical (baseline) frequency of disease for the purposes of identifying changes? Other than the disease or injury process itself, what other factors could cause a change? In the conception of this analysis, the term *baseline* denotes historical data used to define past patterns and current report denotes the most recent data on which the assessment of an aberration is based. Details of three techniques for assessing deviations from baseline follow.

Graph of Current and Past Experience
In the United States, state health departments report the numbers of cases of about 50 notifiable diseases each week to CDC's nationally notifiable disease surveillance system (NNDSS). The list of reportable health events is determined collaboratively by the Council of State and Territorial Epidemiologists and CDC (*54,55*). Each week, provisional reports are published in the *Morbidity and Mortality Weekly Report* (*MMWR*) and are made available to epidemiologists, clinicians, and other public health professionals in a timely manner. Although the tables of the *MMWR* continue to provide important information, the volume of data and the need for ease of interpretation encouraged the development of a graphic display to highlight unusually high or low numbers of reported cases.

An analytic and graphical method was adopted for this system to achieve the following objectives: *(a)* to portray in a single comprehensible figure the weekly reports of data for multiple diseases and to compare those data with past results, and *(b)* to highlight for further analysis the results most likely to reflect either long-term trends or epidemics. These objectives were formulated to reflect most recent behavior in as short a period as possible for weekly publication but a period long enough to assure stable results. To facilitate comprehension, the same method is used for all diseases portrayed.

The analytic method currently used for constructing the weekly notifiable disease figure in the *MMWR* (Fig. 6–6) compares the number of reported cases in the current 4-week period for a given health event with historical data on the same condition from the preceding 5 years (*56,57*). Numbers of cases in the current month are listed to facilitate interpretation of instability caused by small numbers.

The choice of 4 weeks as the "current period" is based on evidence that weekly fluctuations in data from disease reports usually reflect irregular reporting practices rather than actual incidence of disease. The use of 5 years of history achieves the objective of using the same model for all conditions portrayed, as some health events were made notifiable more recently. Also, modeling of data from influenza mortality surveillance has shown that more accurate forecasts

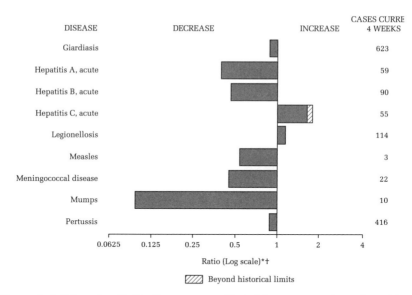

Figure 6–6 Selected notifiable disease reports, United States, comparison of provisional 4-week totals (June 27, 2009), with historical data (*58*).

are based on more recent data (*47*). To increase the historical sample size and to account for any seasonal effect, the baseline is taken to be the average of the reported number of cases for the preceding 4-week period, the corresponding 4-week period, and the following 4-week period for the previous 5 years. This yields 15 correlated observations, referred to as the historical observations, or baseline (Fig. 6–7).

The deviation from unity of the ratio of the current 4-week total to the historical average indicates a departure from past patterns. This ratio is plotted on a logarithmic scale so that an n-fold increase projects to the right the same distance as an n-fold decrease projects to the left, and no change from past patterns (a ratio of 1:1) produces a bar of zero length (*59*). To distinguish the conditions that might require further epidemiologic investigation, the hatching on the bars begins at a point based on the mean and standard deviation of the historical observations. Historical limits of the ratio of current reports to the historical mean are calculated as 1 plus or minus 2 times the standard deviation divided by the mean, where the mean and the standard deviation are calculated from the 15 historical 4-week periods. An evaluation of this method shows that it has good statistical robustness and high sensitivity and predictive value positive for epidemiologically confirmed outbreaks (*60,61*).

Scan Statistic
The scan statistic (*62*) offers a relatively simple approach to determining whether the number of cases reported for a certain period is excessive. The scan statistic is an estimate of the probability that at least a certain number of reported cases (i.e., events) will occur in a time interval of predetermined length. It is used to test

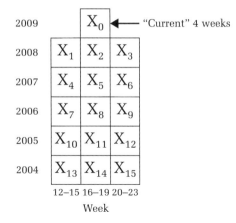

Figure 6–7 Example: Data used to report notifiable diseases (May, 2009).

the null hypothesis of uniformity of reporting against an alternative of temporal clustering. The statistical question addressed by the scan statistic is: "What is the probability that the maximum number of cases in a time interval is equal to or exceeds the number of cases observed?"

If the results of the scan statistic are to be useful, the lengths of the entire time frame and the scanning time interval must be determined *a priori*. The method is intended to detect relatively infrequent elevations in a series of relatively small numbers of events. Recently, open source software has been made available through the Realtime Outbreak Detection project (https://www.rods.pitt.edu/site/), which can perform scan statistic calculations. Approximations to the exact distribution can be helpful in providing associated significance levels in a timely manner (*63,64*).

Time-Series Methods
Another alternative approach to determine whether the number of observed events represents a true incease uses time-series methods. In 1979, CDC proposed a new method to estimate expected deaths using a group of methods called time series; the method of time series is appropriate for data available sequentially over time (*65*). Time-series methods refer to a number of modeling approaches, in which data from previous years can be used to account for seasonal or other cyclical changes in the occurrence of diseases or conditions. Accounting for these changes might allow analysts to recognize important, concurrent trends in the occurrence of the condition. Time-series methods are referred to by numerous descriptive names and include the modeling of moving averages and autoregressive integrated moving average (ARIMA) models. In moving averages procedures, each observation in a data series is replaced by an average of that value and a specified number of preceding and following values; this procedure has the effect of "smoothing" random variations in the data. Autoregressive methods are more sophisticated and estimate coefficients for the relationships between individual data points and data points from specific, earlier time-points.

Most common methods of time-series analysis, such as ARIMA models (66), are available in commercial statistical software packages and are appropriate for relatively long series of data that exhibit certain regular properties over the entire series. Differencing, or forming a new series by subtracting adjacent observations, is generally used to create a series with a stationary mean—that is, without trend. An additional property, stationarity of the variance, is generally required, so that the process does not become more or less variable over time. An autoregressive model includes terms that predict data at one point in time as a function of previous data and estimated temporal autocorrelations. A moving-average term creates a series from averages of adjacent observations and is used to model cycles in the data.

The advantage for surveillance of time-series models over other modeling methods, such as regression is that the estimation process accounts for period-to-period correlations and seasonality, as well as long-term secular trends. The process of model fitting consists of identification, estimation, and diagnostic validation. One then evaluates competing models on the basis of the fit of the models to the observed data and of the accuracy of the forecasts (67). These methods also have some important limitations. For example, to construct optimal models, many years of data are sometimes required (68) and other properties of the data are required for some models.

The uses of time-series methods are illustrated by several examples of their uses in the context of surveillance systems. Expected, cause-specific numbers of deaths have been estimated by the median number of deaths during a non-epidemic year (69), and regression modeling of incidence data (70). Several time-series methods were used to evaluate the incidence of nosocomial infections in a hospital (71). Various time-series models were used to desribe historical data and to estimate the impact of a training program to reduce nosocomial infections (estimated to have decreased infections by 3.6% monthly) and of a medical strike (estimated to have increased infections by 4.3% monthly).

A report of the use of electronic medical records data from a chain of veterinary hospitals describes the use of time-series methods for analysis of syndromic surveillance data (11). Researchers examined time-series data for a specific disease syndrome—gastrointestinal disease in dogs—during a period that spanned a known chemical release from a production plant in Georgia. Data were collected in an ongoing, systematic data collection system (electronic medical records). The results indicated that the number of diagnosed cases of the gastrointestinal syndrome in the days after the chemical release was higher than the number of reported cases in the weeks preceeding the release and higher than the number predicted based on historical patterns in the data (Fig. 6–8). ARIMA methods were used to demonstrate that the increase in gastrointestinal syndrome diagnoses occurred after the chemical release.

DEMOGRAPHIC DATA AND METHODS FOR ANALYSIS

Surveillance data typically consist of event counts or "numerator" data. As described earlier, epidemiologists often want to know how these events compare

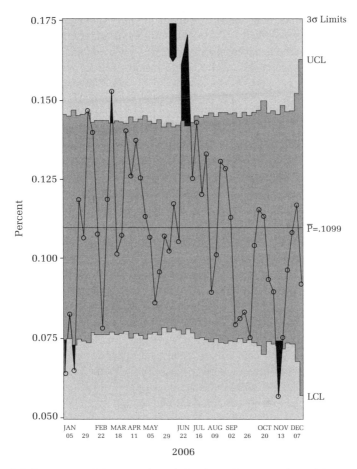

Figure 6–8 Percentage of dogs seen in a chain of veterinary practices with a respiratory syndrome 6 months before and after an accidental release of propyl mercaptan, Fairburn Georgia, 2006 (*11*). A suspected release of the chemical propyl mercaptan occurred on June 29, 2006, as indicated by the arrow. UCL: upper confidence limit; LCL: lower confidence limit.

across populations, subgroups or time. This requires denominator data, which come from demographic data collections of census or intercensal estimates. Other demographic data and methods can be used to complement the analyses of surveillance data. In general, demographic data describe basic characteristics and dynamics of populations, including size and growth; age, race, sex, and geographic distribution; natality and mortality; immigration; and other characteristics of special interest. Typical demographic methods that might be helpful in analyzing public health surveillance data include direct and indirect standardization; life table probability estimates; population estimates and projections; methods to attribute proximate determinants of events; and methods to separate age, period and cohort effects on changes in rates of disease or risk factors observed over time.

Using demographic data and demographic methods in conjunction with public health surveillance data helps address numerous important questions that otherwise would remain unanswered. Demographic data, which generally cover an entire population, can be especially useful in low-resource settings where public health surveillance systems do not provide complete population-based coverage or where systems have not been evaluated for timeliness, completeness, and accuracy.

Another way demographic methods can be useful, especially in low-resource settings, is in providing context for findings from detailed sentinel surveillance systems. Sentinel surveillance systems, which rely on a limited number of geographic or clinical settings for detailed case data, are often used when population-based case reporting systems are not feasible. Comprehensive case identification is traded for level of detail, sometimes including expensive laboratory testing information. In this situation, population-based demographic and health surveys, a long-standing staple of representative health information in the developing world, can provide useful comparisons of disease estimates from population-based surveys with wider coverage and representativeness. These surveys might provide less detailed information about a particular disease or condition than a sentinel surveillance system but can be useful in comparing overall background level and general comparisons.

An important consideration when examining population health, as public health surveillance attempts to do, is the effect of population changes on disease dynamics. Populations are not static, especially under the pressure of morbidity and mortality of disease effects, and these changes, in turn, affect disease transmission. Demographic methods can shed light on the effect of changes in a population, such as changes in age, on disease rates and transmission. Additionally, demographic methods have been critical in helping epidemiologists separate the age, period, and cohort effects of disease dynamics. These effects direct public health interventions for prevention and control.

The converse is also true: Disease has an effect on population dynamics. Demographic data and methods have been used in conjunction with public health surveillance data to examine the effect of diseases and disease-specific mortality on population dynamics—fertility, mortality, growth, and orphans, to name a few.

Data Requirements

Demographic analyses require data both from the public health surveillance system itself as well as data from outside sources. Sometimes the analyses combine data from numerous sources; other times analyses are separate and results are compared. A key factor in these types of analyses is partnership with the data owners. Many demographic data sets are available as public-use data files or published information accessible to epidemiologists and other researchers. Data files not publicly available require contact with data owners and usually require an agreement outlining uses, protections, and disposition of the data before the files are released for use. Most organizations that collect demographic data are motivated to ensure their wide use and have a user-friendly process for accessing data.

In general, demographic data are supplied as counts of events, or numerators, and populations at risk, or denominators. Often public health officials are interested in certain population characteristics that are not collected in the surveillance system (e.g., socioeconomic characteristics of a community or number of persons in specific age groups in a population) or in background rates of events not captured in a disease reporting system (e.g., age-specific fertility rates). Demographic data systems or surveys (72) can provide these types of population attributes to help epidemiologists interpret surveillance data (Table 6–3).

Several demographic analytic methods have been used in conjunction with public health surveillance data. Some methods, like direct and indirect standardization, are used so commonly in public health that they are no longer considered unusual or even attributed to demography. Others, like life table probabilities and disaggregation of proximate determinants, remain closely tied to their demographic roots.

Standardization

Like other methods of controlling for confounding, standardization enables comparison of rates while removing the effect of another variable. Elimination of the effect of the third extraneous variable allows for more accurate examination of the effect of the variable of interest. Age-standardized rates are the most commonly calculated because age has an impact on most things that public health surveillance scientists study. Comparing crude disease or death rates in two groups with different age structures would not be an accurate way to characterize the differences, because age will have an influence on the rate in each population. Standardizing or controlling for age removes the effect of age and allows for a more equal comparison. There are two types of standardized (or adjusted) rates: direct and indirect. Specific examples of these calculations are available in most demography, epidemiology, or statistics textbooks (73,74).

Direct Standardization

Direct standardization uses the rates measured in populations under observation and applies them to a standard population distribution. For example, an age-standardized rate might be calculated using death rates observed in a population and the age distribution of the U.S. standard population (75). From this multiplication, an age-standardized rate is calculated and can be compared with other rates standardized to the same standard population. The interpretation of the absolute value of the standardized rates is unimportant; it is the relative ranking of the rates that is of interest—that is, the rates with the effect of age or other confounding variable of interest removed. For example, direct standardization was used to compare cigarette smoking rates among two cohorts of United States Air Force recruits with rates from the national BRFSS, controlling for demographic differences between the groups (76). When standardized for age and gender, smoking rates were higher among Air Force recruits compared with the general public as represented in the national surveillance system.

Table 6–3 Typical Demographic Measures Available From Census, Vital Registration, and Demographic Surveys

Category	Measure	Description
Population		The residents or residents and visitors in a specific area at a specific time
	Population size	The number of people in a specific area at a specific time
	Population distribution	The spread of a population over a specific area at a specific time
	Population density	The number of people per each unit of land
	Percent distribution by demographic characteristic (age, race, sex, family composition, educational attainment, economic characteristics)	The percentage of persons by specific characteristic in population over specific area at specific time
	Sex ratio	A measure of the male to female composition of a population
	Urbanicity	Concentration of persons living in large locality comprising a city and suburban surroundings
	Lorenz curve	A graphical measurement of the inequality in distribution of two variables
	Gini concentration ratio	A measurement of the degree of inequality between two variables used to measure population concentration
	Population change	A measure of the difference (increase, decrease, or zero) in the number of inhabitants in a specific area over time
	Absolute change	The magnitude of change calculated as a difference between ending population count and starting population count
	Percent change	The magnitude of change calculated by dividing the absolute change by the starting population count and multiplying by 100

(continued)

Table 6–3 *(continued)*

Category	Measure	Description
	Rate of change	The average annual percentage change in a population expressed as arithmetic, geometric, or exponential approximation
	Time required for population to double	The number of years it takes for a population to double in size, measured as a function of increases (fertility and in-migration) and decreases (mortality and out-migration)
	Population momentum	The tendency of a population to increase for up to 70 years after fertility replacement level is reached
Vital events		Events recorded in registration systems related to mortality, fertility, marriage, and divorce
Natality		A general term that represents the contribution of births to population change
	Crude birth rate	The number of births in 1 year for each 1000 people in the mid-year population
	General fertility rate	The number of births in 1 year for each 1000 women of childbearing age during the same period of time
	Age-specific birth rate	The number of births to women in a specific age group in 1 year for each 1000 women in that age group
	Birth-order-specific birth rate	The number of births of a specific sequence of child to the mother in 1 year for each 1000 women of childbearing age during the same period of time
	Marital fertility rate	The number of births to legally married women in 1 year for each 1000 women of childbearing age during the same period
	Total fertility rate	A measure of the average number of children a cohort women would have based on age-specific fertility rates and assuming zero mortality among women of childbearing age

(continued)

Table 6–3 (*continued*)

Category	Measure	Description
	Gross reproduction rate	A measure of the average number of daughters a cohort of women would have based on age-specific fertility rates and assuming zero mortality among women of childbearing age
	Net reproduction rate	A measure of the number of daughters a cohort of newborn females will have based on age-specific fertility rates and assuming a fixed schedule of age-specific mortality rates
	Cumulative fertility rate	The total number of children born to a cohort of women up to a particular age
	Completed fertility rate	The number of children born to a cohort of women through the end of childbearing age for each 1000 women
	Parity distribution	The distribution or division of women in a cohort by the number of live births to a woman
	Birth probabilities by age and parity	The chance that a women of a specific parity and age at the beginning of the year will have a child during the course of the year
	Children ever born	The number of live births to a woman
	General paternal fertility rate	The number of births for each 1000 males between the ages of 15 and 54
	Replacement index	A measure approximating the net reproduction rate calculated by division of the ratio of children under age 5 to females in reproductive ages in the actual population by the corresponding ratio in the life table stationary population
Mortality		The number of deaths in a specified group
	Crude death rate	The number of deaths in 1 year for each 1000 people in the mid-year population

(*continued*)

Table 6–3 (*continued*)

Category	Measure	Description
	Age-specific death rate	The number of deaths of persons a specific age in 1 year for each 1000 people of that age in the mid-year population
	Cause-specific death ratio	The percentage of total deaths resulting from a specific cause or group of causes
	Cause-specific death rate	The number of deaths from a specific cause or group of causes during 1 year for each 100,000 people in the mid-year population
	Endogenous death rate	The death rate for deaths arising from genetic makeup and prenatal and birth circumstances
	Exogenous death rate	The death rate for deaths arising from environmental and external causes
	Standardized mortality ratio	A measure of the number of deaths that occur in a specific population relative to the number of deaths expected based on the age-specific death rate of a reference population
	Infant mortality rate	The number infant deaths prior to age 1 during 1 year for each 1000 live births during the same period of time
	Adjusted infant mortality rate	A form of the conventional infant mortality rate that accounts for fluctuations in birth rate from the prior year
	Child mortality rate	The number of deaths of children under age 5 for each 1000 live births averaged over the previous 5 years
	Maternal mortality rate	A cause-specific morality rate representing the deaths resulting from complications related to pregnancy, childbirth, and the puerperium
	Age-standardized death rates (direct and indirect)	A hypothetical death rate that would have occurred if the observed age specific rates were associated with a population whose age distribution equaled that of the standard population

(*continued*)

Table 6–3 (*continued*)

Category	Measure	Description
	Comparative mortality index	A measure indicating change in mortality of a population based on a ratio of the population-weighted sum of age-specific death rates at the end of a specific period relative to the beginning of the same period
	Fetal mortality	Death prior to the complete expulsion or extraction from its mother through stillbirths, miscarriages, and abortions
	Fetal death rate	The number of reported late fetal deaths during 1 year for each 1000 live births and late fetal deaths during the same period of time
	Fetal death ratio	The number of reported late fetal deaths during 1 year for each 1000 live births during the same period of time
	Perinatal mortality rate	The number of reported deaths under 1 week and late fetal deaths during 1 year for each 1000 live births and late fetal deaths during the same period of time
	Perinatal mortality ratio	The number of reported deaths under one week and late fetal deaths during 1 year for each 1000 live births during the same period of time
Life table measures		A demographic statistical model that measures mortality of a cohort or estimates a stationary population
	Life expectancy at birth (at age x)	The average remaining number of years of life at birth (or age x) assuming survival to the beginning of the age interval
	Median age at death	The age at which half of the cohort is surviving
	Life table death rate	An age-adjusted death rate that results from weighting of age-specific death rates by life table stationary population
	Life table survival rates	A rate expressing the probability of survival of an age group from one date and age to another

Source: Preston SH, Heuveline P, Guillot M. *Demography: Measuring and modeling population processes.* Blackwell Publishers. Malden, MA: 2001.

Indirect Standardization

There are situations when only crude rates and no age-specific rates are available in the populations of interest, yet one would like to compare the number of observed events to the number of expected events. Indirect standardization uses the age-specific rates from a standard population and applies them to the population distribution of the observed population to calculate the total number of events one would expect if the observed population behaved the way the standard population behaved. The total number of observed events is then compared with the total number of expected events; this ratio is called the standardized mortality/incidence/prevalence ratio, depending on the measure being compared. Again, the interpretation is the relative rate with the effect of age (or other confounder of interest) removed. Epidemiologists examined the complicated associations between healthy worker effect, exposures associated with steel and iron production, and injury risk with the risk for death among Korean iron and steel workers using a combination of methods, including indirect standardization (*77*). The healthy worker effect, which arises from the healthiest in the population selecting into the worker cohort, yielded an all-cause standardized mortality ratio (SMR) of 0.59 indicating that steel workers experienced lower mortality than the general population. However, when comparing steel producers to other types of workers (removing those who were too sick to self-select into the workforce), the SMR was elevated (1.14), indicating that the steel workers' risk for mortality was actually higher than other workers.

Life Table Probabilities

Life tables are one of the oldest tools of demographic analysis. Most broadly, a life table is a statistical method used to model changes in a population caused by decrements, or departures. Life tables can model the probability of a single decrement like mortality or morbidity, or their complements: survival, life expectation at birth or any age, or disease-free years lived. They can also be used to model multiple decrements while incorporating other demographic or socioeconomic characteristics.

There are two interpretations of life table models—cohort and period. A cohort interpretation is based on observing the experience of a particular cohort—for example, observing mortality of a cohort of persons born in a particular year. In public health, a more useful interpretation is a period life table, where the model estimates what would happen if persons were subject for their entire lives to the force (or probability) of the event that exists in the current period. Construction of single decrement life tables is straightforward. Instructions, formulas, and examples are available in introductory demographic methods texts (*72,73*), and calculation is made especially easy with simple spreadsheet programs available in basic computing software packages.

Multiple decrement life tables are more complex to calculate and yield more sophisticated analyses that are quite useful in public health. These models describe the probability of an event (usually death) with a series of related tables showing the conditional probability of dying of one cause of interest in one table and all other causes in another. An analysis of death registration data and multiple decrement life table methods showed potential gains and losses in life expectancy for a variety of causes among working adults in Italy, providing data to inform effective allocation of public health resources (78). The benefits of reducing mortality from cardiovascular disease and malignant neoplasms by implementing effective screening programs, for example, are easily seen in this analysis of public health data. Similarly, the devastating impact of HIV/AIDS on life expectancy is demonstrated using these methods (78).

Cause-eliminated life tables model the probability of death with a given cause removed, which have been used in combination with surveillance data to estimate the effect of HIV on under-5 mortality in urban and rural Africa (79). Increment–decrement life tables allow one to model entry and exit into the population and are useful in public health when describing recurrent morbidity or risk behaviors. Using data from several large population-based surveys and a four-state increment–decrement life table model, analysts estimated the lifetime years a U.S. citizen would spend in their community, in a hospital, and in a nursing home (80). This type of information is extremely useful for public health planning and resource allocation decisions.

Population Estimation and Projections

Accurate counts of populations at risk are of great interest to demographers and epidemiologists as they ensure more accurate rates and comparisons between subgroups. A complete enumeration of a population is done infrequently, usually every 10 years, partly because of cost and logistics of counting and characterizing every person in a population. Between decennial censuses, demographers use census information collected earlier along with information on births, deaths, and migration to estimate the population at a past or current time. Estimation is generally referred to a measure that uses two census counts as its anchors, and projection is used to describe a number derived for a future date based on a set of assumptions about how a population will behave. Population estimates and projections are often used in surveillance as the denominator for rates and sometimes as standard populations in direct standardization. Epidemiologists have paired surveillance data with various estimation and projection methods to estimate HIV prevalence and AIDS deaths in Tanzania (81), the population size of orphans left motherless in the United States by AIDS (82), and the population of U.S. adults with a lifetime experience of depression through 2050 (83).

Attribution of Age, Period, and Cohort Effects

Demography is concerned with the behavior of rates across age, time, and cohorts. Measuring events across these dimensions provides answers to questions that differ in important ways. Examining data across only one of these dimensions can lead to misinterpretations of data that might ultimately lead to an ineffective public health response. To address this concern, age-period-cohort (APC) analyses have been developed to provide quantitative models of the separate effects of these three factors (*84*). In 1939, Wade Hampton Frost provided an elegant parsimonious APC analysis of tuberculosis mortality showing the erroneous conclusion one might make if one stopped with a simple analysis of age-specific mortality rates over time (*85*). The conclusion that the risk of death from tuberculosis was highest at older age groups in more recent years was shown to be false once one looked at the rates of deaths in successive cohorts. The true story was, as Frost stated, "…the group of people who were children 0 to 9 years of age in 1880 and who are now aged 50 to 60 years…have, in two earlier periods, passed through *greater* risks."

Disaggregation of Proximate Determinants of Disease

Initially developed to study socio-economic impact on changes in fertility levels, the proximate determinants framework was outlined by demographers in the 1950s (*86*). Its widespread application is attributed, however, to demographer John Bongaarts (*87,88*), who simplified the method, casting its broad appeal to fertility and, ultimately, other outcomes. In the broadest sense, the method models the smallest number of most proximate, distinct, and quantitatively important explanatory variables for an outcome. It is known, for example, that many things affect fertility, including nutritional status, socio-economic status, and cultural and environmental variables. These are considered distal factors. Using a simple model of four indices, Bongaarts determined that 96% of variation in fertility across populations was explained by four proximate factors: exposure to intercourse, contraception, induced abortion, and postpartum infecundability. Using similar approaches for other health events, public health scientists and epidemiologists have developed proximate determinant models for childhood psychosocial stress (*89*), diarrheal-related infant mortality (*90*), and HIV transmission (*91*).

Demographers and public health surveillance scientists continue to share an interest in the characteristics and dynamics of populations. Shared methods will continue to allow innovative approaches to address challenging questions about population health.

VISUAL DISPLAY OF SURVEILLANCE INFORMATION

Visual tools also play a critical role in analysis of public health surveillance data. Data graphics visually display measured quantities using points, lines, a coordinate system, numbers, symbols, words, shading, and color (*92*). As has already been highlighted in the preceding sections, inspections of graphic displays of surveillance data can be an important step in data analysis, giving rise to hypotheses and providing direction to analysis steps. Data graphics are also essential to summarizing and communicating information clearly and effectively. The design and quality of such graphics largely determine how effectively scientists can communicate their information.

Table 6–4 Types of Data Graphics and When to Use Them

Type of chart or graph	When to use
Arithmetic-scale line graph	Trends in numbers or rates over time
Semilogarithmic-scale line graph	1. Emphasize rate of change over time
	2. Display values ranging >2 orders of magnitude
Histogram	1. Frequency distribution of continuous variable
	2. Number of cases during an epidemic (i.e., epidemic curve) or over time
Cumulative frequency	Show accumulation of number or percent of observations over time
Simple bar chart	Compare size or freqeuncy of different categories of a single variable
Grouped bar chart	Compare size or frequency of different categories of 2–4 series of data
Stacked bar chart	Compare totals and illustrate component parts of the total among different groups
Pie chart	Show components of the whole
Spot map	Show location of cases or events
Chloropleth map	Display events or rates geographically
Interactive data displays	Provide intuitive display of data for stakeholders with different levels of interpretive skills; provide broad access to the public

Many visual tools are available to assist in analysis and presentation of results. The data to be presented and the purpose for the presentation are the key factors in deciding which visual tools should be used (Table 6–4). Further discussion and guidance in producing effective, high-quality data graphics are available from numerous sources (*92–97*).

Tables

A table arranges data in rows and columns and is used to demonstrate data patterns and relationships among variables and to serve as a source of information for other types of data graphics (*94*). Table entries can be counts, means, rates, or other analytic measures.

A table should be simple; two or three small tables are simpler to understand than one large one. A table should be self-explanatory so that, if taken out of context, readers can still understand the data. The guidelines below should be used to increase effectiveness of a table and to ensure that it is self-explanatory (*95*):

- Describe what, when, and where in a clear, concise table title.
- Label each row and column clearly and concisely.
- Provide units of measure for the data.
- Provide row and column totals.
- Define abbreviations and symbols in a footnote.
- Note data exclusions in a footnote.
- If the data are not original, then reference the source.

Single-Variable Tables

One of the most basic tables is a frequency distribution by category for a single variable. For example, the first column of the table contains the categories of the factor of interest, and the second column lists the number of persons or events that appear in each category and gives the total count. Subsequent columns contain percentages or rates of total events in each category (Table 6–5).

Multivariable Tables

Most phenomena monitored by public health surveillance systems are complex and require analysis of relationships between several factors. When data are available on more than one variable, multivariable cross-classified tables can elucidate associations. These tables are also called contingency tables when all the primary table entries (e.g., frequencies, persons, or events) are classified by each of the variables in the table (Table 6–6).

Graphs

A graph is a visual display of quantitative information involving a system of coordinates. Two-dimensional graphs are generally depicted along an *x*-axis (horizontal orientation) and *y*-axis (vertical orientation) coordinate system. Graphs are primary analytic tools used to assist the reader to visualize patterns, trends, aberrations, similarities, and differences in data.

Simplicity is the key to designing graphs. Simple, uncluttered graphs are more likely than complicated presentations to convey information effectively. Although current graphics and presentation software allow many options for presentation of data using three-dimensional graphs should be avoided to improve clarity. Several specific principles should be observed when constructing graphs (95):

- Ensure that the graph is self-explanatory by clear, concise labeling of title (including what, when, and where), source, axes, scales, and legends.
- Clearly differentiate variables by legends or keys.
- Minimize the number of coordinate lines.
- Portray frequency on the vertical scale, starting at zero, and the method of classification on the horizontal scale.
- Ensure that scales for each axis are appropriate for the data.
- Clearly indicate scale division, any scale breaks, and units of measure.
- Define abbreviations and symbols in a footnote.
- Note data exclusions in a footnote.
- If the data are not original, reference the source.

Arithmetic-Scale Line Graphs

An arithmetic-scale line graph is one in which equal distances along the *x*- and *y*-axes represent equal quantities along that axis. This type of graph typically is used to demonstrate an overall trend over time rather than focus on particular observation values. It is most helpful for examining long series of data or for comparing

Table 6–5 Example of a Single-Variable Table Depicting the Estimated Number, Percentage and Rate of Pool Chemical-Associated Injuries Treated in Emergency Departments, by Selected Characteristics—United States, 2007 (*98*)

Characteristic	No.	Weighted estimate	(95% CI)	%1	Annual rate	(95% CI)
Total	115	4,635	(2,929–6,341)	100	1.5	(1.0–2.1)
Injury diagnosis						
Poisoning	47	1,944	(1,216–2,472)	40	0.6	(0.4–0.8)
Dermatitis conjunctivitis	31	1,245	(691–1,799)	27	0.4	(0.2–0.6)
Chemical burns	16	820	(187–1,454)	18	—	—
Other	21	725	(282–1,189)	16	—	—
Affected body part						
All parts of the body (more than 50% of body)	59	2,255	(1,704–2,807)	49	0.7	(0.6–0.9)
Eye	41	1,938	(1,123–2,752)	42	0.6	(0.4–0.9)
Other (e.g., upper trunk [not shoulder], hand, or foot)	15	442	(74–809)	10	—	—
Patient disposition						
Treated and released, or examined and released without treatment	111	4,391	(3,230–5,551)	95	1.5	(1.1–1.8)
Treated and admitted for hospitalization (within same facility)	2	160	(0–369)	3	—	
Left without being seen, or left against medical advice	1	69	(0–208)	1	—	—
Treated and transferred to another hospital	1	15	(0–46)	0	—	—
Incident location						
Residence	51	2,010	(1,125–2,896)	43	—	—
Place of recreation or sports	11	486	(98–874)	10	—	—
School	1	15	(0–46)	0	—	—
Other identified location	6	311	(30–592)	7	—	—
Unknown	46	1,912	(935–2,689)	39	—	—

(continued)

Characteristic	No.	Weighted estimate	(95% CI)	%1	Annual rate	(95% CI)
Patient age (yrs)						
≤5	22	442	(86–798)	10	—	—
6–11	18	808	(279–1,337)	17	—	—
12–17	18	445	(167–723)	10	—	—
19–45	39	1,975	(1,180–2,789)	43	17	(1.0–2.4)
46–64	18	966	(477–1,455)	21	—	—
≥65	0	0		0	—	—
Patient sex						
Male	65	2,537	(1,695–3,379)	55	17	(1.1–2.4)
Female	50	2,098	(1,383–2,813)	45	14	(0.9–1.8)
Patient race/ethnicity						
White	57	2,429	(1,364–3,494)	52	—	—
Hispanic	9	152	(0–308)	3	—	—
Black	8	136	(0–324)	3	—	—
American Indian/ Alaska Native	2	140	(0–423)	3	—	—
Unknown	39	1,778	(780–2,776)	38	—	—

several data sets (Fig. 6–9). The scale of the *x*-axis is usually presented in the same increments as the data are collected or reported (e.g., weekly, monthly, or annually). Several factors should be considered when selecting a scale for the *y*-axis.

- Choose a length for the *y*-axis that is suitably proportional to that of the *x*-axis. A common recomendation is a 5:3 ratio for the ratio of *x*-axis to *y*-axis.
- Start the *y*-axis at 0.
- Identify the maximum *y*-axis value and round the value up slightly.
- Select an interval size that provides enough detail for the purpose of the graph.

Scale breaks can be used for either or both axes if the range of the data is excessive. However, care should be taken to avoid misrepresentation and misinterpretation of the data when scale breaks are used.

Semilogarithmic-Scale Line Graphs

A semilogarithmic-scale line graph or semilog graph is characterized by one axis being measured on an arithmetic scale (usually the *x*-axis) and the other being measured on a logarithmic scale (Fig. 6–10). A logarithm is the exponent expressing the power to which a base number is raised (e.g., log 100 = log 10^2 = 2 for base 10). The axis portraying the logarithmic scale on semilog graph is divided into several cycles, with each cycle representing an order of magnitude and values 10 times greater than the preceding cycle (e.g., a three-cycle semilog graph could represent 1 to 10 in the first cycle, 10 to 100 in the second cycle, and 100 to 1,000 in the third cycle).

A semilogarithmic-scale line graph is particularly valuable when examining the rate of change in surveillance data, because a straight line represents a constant rate of change. For absolute changes, an arithmetic-scale line graph would

Table 6–6 Example of a Multivariable Table Depicting the Estimated Average Annual Number of Persons With Self-Reported Current Asthma, by Age, Sex, Race, Ethnicity, Region, and Poverty Level—National Health Interview Survey, United States, 2001–2003 (*99*)

				Age (yrs)		
Characteristic	Total	<18	≥18	0–4	5–14	15–34
Sex						
Male	**8,418,000**	3,583,000	4,835,000	682,000	2,321,000	2,393,000
Female	**11,630,000**	2,616,000	9,013,000	480,000	1,557,000	3,439,000
Race*						
White	**15,283,000**	**4,142,000**	**11,141,000**	**636,000**	**2,674,000**	**4,375,000**
Male	**6,273,000**	2,366,000	3,907,000	383,000	1,572,000	1,792,000
Female	**9,010,000**	1,777,000	7,233,000	253,000	1,102,000	2,584,000
Black	**3,121,000**	**1,339,000**	**1,782,000**	**351,000**	**780,000**	**929,000**
Male	**1,303,000**	757,000	545,000	186,000	474,000	350,000
Female	**1,819,000**	582,000	1,237,000	165,000	306,000	580,000
Other races NTA	**1,643,000**	**717,000**	**926,000**	**174,000**	**425,000**	**528,000**
Male	**842,000**	460,000	382,000	112,000	275,000	252,000
Female	**801,000**	258,000	544,000	62,000	150,000	275,000
Ethnicity						
Hispanic or Latino	**1,978,000**	**885,000**	**1,093,000**	**203,000**	**538,000**	**603,000**
Male	**874,000**	493,000	381,000	113,000	300,000	251,000
Female	**1,104,000**	392,000	712,000	90,000	237,000	351,000
Puerto Rican	**532,000**	**226,000**	**305,000**	**38,000**	**145,000**	**169,000**
Male	**226,000**	122,000	104,000	20,000	84,000	59,000
Female	**306,000**	104,000	202,000	18,000	61,000	109,000
Mexican	**903,000**	**417,000**	**485,000**	**104,000**	**257,000**	**277,000**
Male	**407,000**	239,000	168,000	59,000	141,000	121,000
Female	**495,000**	178,000	317,000	45,000	116,000	156,000
Not Hispanic or Latino	**18,070,000**	**5,314,000**	**12,756,000**	**959,000**	**3,341,000**	**5,229,000**
Male	**7,544,000**	3,090,000	4,454,000	569,000	2,021,000	2,142,000
Female	**10,526,000**	2,224,000	8,302,000	390,000	1,320,000	3,087,000
Region						
Northeast	**4,282,000**	1,347,000	2,935,000	241,000	852,000	1,141,000
Midwest	**5,058,000**	1,494,000	3,564,000	311,000	896,000	1,586,000
South	**6,890,000**	2,210,000	4,680,000	440,000	1,380,000	1,979,000
West	**3,818,000**	1,148,000	2,670,000	170,000	751,000	1,126,000
Ratio of family income to poverty threshold						
0–.99	**2,697,000**	1,014,000	1,683,000	288,000	562,000	851,000
1.00–2.49	**4,603,000**	1,513,000	3,090,000	346,000	915,000	1,362,000
2.50–4.49	**4,249,000**	1,287,000	2,962,000	175,000	866,000	1,355,000
≥4.50	**4,157,000**	1,023,000	3,134,000	124,000	666,000	1,080,000
Total	**20,047,000**	**6,199,000**	**13,849,000**	**1,162,000**	**3,878,000**	**5,832,000**

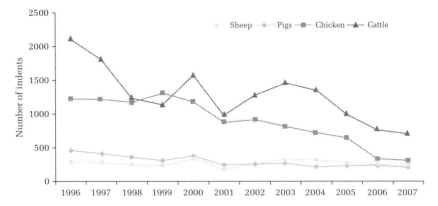

Figure 6–9 Example of an arithmetic scale graph depicting the number of *Salmonellosis* events in livestock and chickens by year, by affected species—Great Britain, 1996–2007 (*100*).

be more appropriate. The semilog scale is also useful when large differences in magnitude or outliers occur because this type of graph allows the plotting of wide ranges of values. With semilog graphs, the slope of the line indicates the rate of increase or decrease; thus a horizontal line indicates no change in rate. Also, parallel lines for two conditions demonstrate identical rates of change (*95*).

Histograms

A histogram is a graph in which a frequency distribution is represented by adjoining vertical bars. The area represented by each bar is proportional to the frequency for that interval (i.e., the height multiplied by the width of each bar yields the number of events for that interval). Thus, scale breaks should never be used in histograms because these misrepresent the data.

Histograms can be constructed with equal- and unequal-class intervals. Equal-class intervals occur when the height of each bar is proportional to the frequency of the events in that interval. Using histograms with unequal class intervals is not recommended because they are difficult to construct and interpret correctly.

The epidemic curve is a special type of histogram in which time is the variable plotted on the *x*-axis. The epidemic curve represents the occurrence of cases of a health problem by date of onset during an epidemic, (e.g., an outbreak of H1N1 influenza infections in the United States; Fig. 6–11; ref. *101*). Usually the class intervals on the *x*-axis should be less than one-fourth of the incubation period of the disease, and the intervals should begin before the first reported case during the epidemic to portray any identified background cases of the condition being graphed.

Cumulative Frequency and Survival Curves

A cumulative frequency curve is used for both continuous and categorical data. It plots the cumulative frequency on the *y*-axis and the value of the variable on the *x*-axis. Cumulative frequencies can be expressed either as the number of cases or

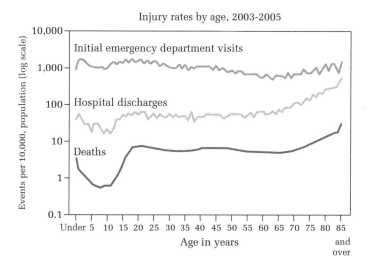

Figure 6–10 Injury Rates By Age, 2003–2005. Example of a semi-logarithmic-scale graph depicting injury rates by age—United States, 2003–2005 (*102*). *Source:* Centers for Disease Control and Prevention, National Center for Health Statistics, *Injury in the United States: 2007 Chartbook.*

as a percentage of total cases. For categorical data, the cumulative frequency is plotted at the right-most end of each class interval (rather than at the mid-point) to depict more realistically the number or percentage of cases above and below the *x*-axis value (Fig. 6–12). When percentages are graphed, the cumulative frequency curve allows easy identification of medians, quartiles, and other percentiles of interest.

A survival curve (Fig. 6–4) is useful in a follow-up study for graphing the percentage of subjects remaining until an event occurs in the study. The *x*-axis represents time, and the *y*-axis is percentage surviving. A difference in orientation exists between cumulative frequency and survival curves (Figs. 6–4 and 6–12).

Charts

Charts are useful graphics for illustrating statistical information. Many types of charts can be used (*94–96*). They are most suited and helpful for comparing magnitudes of events in categories of a variable. In the paragraphs below, we describe several of the most frequently used types of charts.

Bar Charts

A bar chart is one of the simplest and most effective ways to present comparative data. A bar chart uses bars of the same width to represent different categories of a factor. Comparison of the categories is based on linear values because the length of a bar is proportional to the frequency of the event in that category. Therefore, scale breaks could cause the data to be misinterpreted and should not be used in bar charts. Bars from different categories are separated by spaces (unlike the

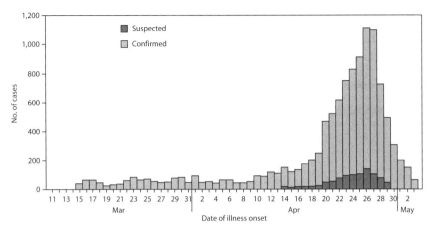

Figure 6–11 An example of a histogram chart depicting the number of confirmed and suspected cases of novel influenza A (H1N1) virus infection, by date of illness onset—Mexico, March 11–May 3, 2009 (*103*).

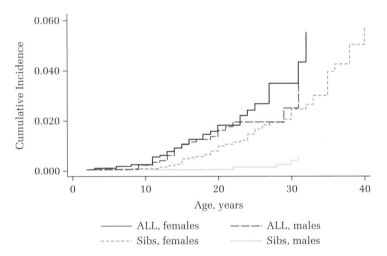

Figure 6–12 An example of a cumulative frequency plot depicting the cumulative incidence of hypothyroidism among 5-year acute lymphoblastic leukemia (ALL) survivors versus siblings, stratified by sex—United States and Canada, 1970–2008 (*104*).

bars in a histogram). Although most bar charts are presented in the vertical orientation, they can be depicted horizontally as well. They are usually arranged in ascending or descending length or in some other systematic order. Many computer graphics programs offer a three-dimensional option for bar charts, but these are often difficult to read accurately and are not recommended.

Several commons variations of the bar chart are used. The grouped or multiple-unit bar chart compares units within categories (Fig. 6–13). Generally, the number of units within a category is limited to 3 for effective presentation and understanding.

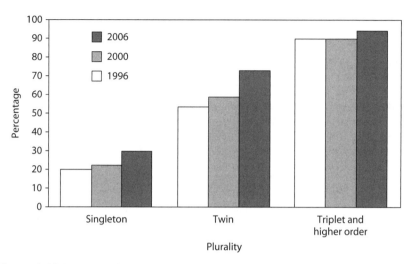

Figure 6–13 Example of a grouped bar chart depicting percentage of live births by Caesarian section, by plurality and year, United States, 1996–2006 (*105*).

A stacked bar chart is also used to compare different groups within each category of a variable. However, it differs from the grouped bar chart in that the different groups are differentiated not with separate bars, but with different segments within a single bar for each category. The distinct segments are illustrated by different types of shading, hatching, or coloring, which are defined in a legend (Fig. 6–14).

Pie Charts

A pie chart represents the different percentages of categories of a variable by proportionally sized pieces of pie (Fig. 6–15). The pieces are usually denoted with different colors or shading, and the percentages are written inside or outside the pieces to allow the reader to make accurate comparisons.

Maps

Maps are the graphic representation of data using location and geographic coordinates (*106*). A map generally provides a clear, quick method for grasping data and is particularly effective for readers who are familiar with the physical area being portrayed. A few popular types of maps that depict incidence or distribution of health conditions are described below.

Spot Maps

A spot map is produced by placing a dot or other symbol on the map where the health condition occurred or exists (Fig. 6–16). Spot maps can be very useful for generating hypotheses and focusing investigations. Different symbols can be used for multiple events at a single location. Although a spot map is beneficial

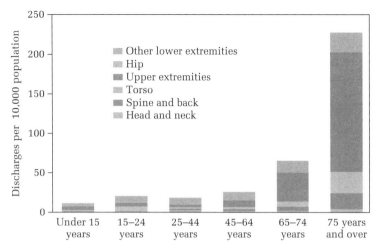

Figure 6–14 An example of a stacked bar chart depicting hospital discharge rates for fracture, by age and anatomical site of fracture, United States, 2004–2005 (*102*).

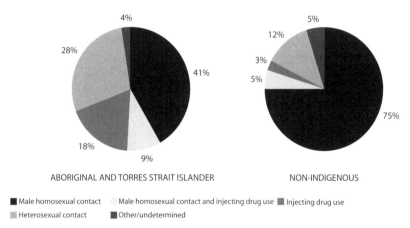

Figure 6–15 Examples of pie charts depicting the proportional distribution of risk factors for HIV acquisition in indigenous and non-indigenous persons with HIV infection in Australia, 2003–2007 (*107*).

for displaying the geographic distribution of an event, generating hypotheses, and focusing investigations geographically, it does not provide a measure of risk because population size is not taken into account. In Figure 6–16, this limitation is clear, as the pattern of spots—each representing 50 AIDS diagnoses—appear in a pattern that overlies major U.S. cities, where more people live, and therefore more people are at risk for HIV infection.

Chloropleth Maps

A chloropleth map, also called a shaded or area map, is a frequently used statistical map involving different types of shading, hatching, or coloring to portray

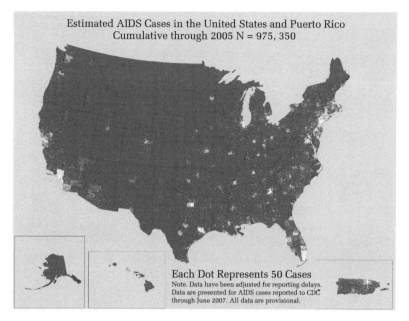

Figure 6–16 Estimated AIDS Cases in the United States and Puerto Rico, Cumulative through 200. An example of a spot map depicting estimated AIDS cases, United States and Puerto Rico, through 2005.

range-graded values (Fig. 6–17). Chloropleth maps are useful for depicting rates of a health condition in specific areas.

Care must be taken in interpreting chloropleth maps because each area is shaded uniformly regardless of any demographic differences within an area. For example, although most of a county might be relatively sparsely populated by low-income persons and a small portion of that county might be densely inhabited by persons with higher incomes, the rate at which a particular health condition occurs might falsely appear to be evenly distributed by location and by socio-economic status throughout the county. Chloropleth maps can also give the false impression of abrupt change in number or rate of a condition across area boundaries when, in fact, a gradual change might have occurred from one area to the next.

Interactive Displays of Data

Increased access to the Internet and improved computing resources have also given rise to new, interactive modalities for displaying surveillance data. These systems feature interactive maps where users can zoom in and out to see surveillance data depicted as chloropleth maps or allow custom queries of surveillance databases. Current examples include an interactive atlas of HIV/AIDS surveillance (www.maphiv.org) and "WISQARS," an interactive system for queries of injury surveillance data maintained by CDC. (http://www.cdc.gov/injury/wisqars/index.html).

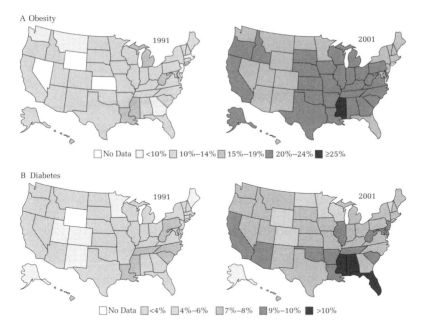

A Obesity

1991 2001

☐ No Data ☐ <10% ☐ 10%–14% ☐ 15%–19% ■ 20%–24% ■ ≥25%

B Diabetes

1991 2001

☐ No Data ☐ <4% ☐ 4%–6% ☐ 7%–8% ■ 9%–10% ■ >10%

Figure 6–17 Examples of chloropleth maps depicting prevalence of obesity and diagnosed diabetes among U.S. adults, 1991 and 2001 (*108*).

INTERPRETIVE USES FOR SURVEILLANCE DATA

Interpretation of Surveillance Findings

Throughout this chapter, we have empahsized the importance of understanding the surveillance systems that give rise to data. An important aspect of interpretation of surveillance information is to bring to bear the understanding of the system and its attributes as well as a deep understanding of the disease or condition in question and the ability to consider a comprehensive set of alternate hypotheses to explain observed surveillance findings and use these in the critical interpretation of findings.

Considering Alternate Hypotheses

A recent study reported increasing HIV case reports among men who have sex with men (MSM) in eight countries (Fig. 6–18; ref. 7). Joinpoint analysis was used to illustrate declining rates of new HIV notifications in the countries from 1996 through 2000; statistically signifcant increases in rates of HIV notifications to surveillance were observed in all countries from 2000 through 2005. The authors considered several alternate hypotheses that might explain the findings of increased case reports after 2000. Was this a true increase in the occurrence of disease, or had surveillance practices changed or case definitions been expanded? Did reporting of male–male sex risk increase over the period? Were

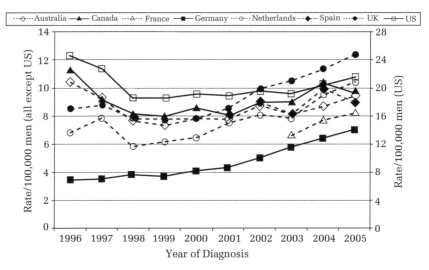

Figure 6–18 Rates of HIV notifications among men who have sex with men aged 15–65 in eight countries, 1996–2005 (7).

there changes in HIV testing among MSM during this period? Other data were considered that might support the interpretation of true rises in HIV among MSM—for example, were there other indicators of increased sexual risk, such as diagnoses of sexually transmitted diseases, that showed consistent trends? The authors concluded that, based on the correlative data, changes in HIV testing or case reporting procedures did not wholly account for the increases in new case reports.

Identifying Epidemics

An important use of surveillance data is in determining whether increases in numbers of cases of a health condition at the local or national level represent outbreak (i.e., epidemic) situations that require immediate investigation and intervention. Thus, a surveillance system can function as an early warning for public health officials. Some of the methodological issues involved in defining an epidemic have been discussed already.

A few examples of outbreaks and the responses they triggered include the documented increases in numbers of cases of hepatitis B among military recruits that provided the stimulus to intervene with drug-prevention programs (109). CDC's Birth Defects Monitoring System identified increases in renal agenesis (110) during the 1970s and 1980s, which prompted an investigation. Monitoring of regional trends in rubella and congenital rubella identified outbreaks among an Amish community in 1989 through 1990 (111). A national registry of anti-abortion-associated violence clearly documented an "epidemic" of attacks in the mid-1980s, which have varied depending on the level of prosecution permitted (112). Documentation of the number of fatal car trunk entrapments involving children over the past decade resulted in evaluation of design changes to auto trunk locks, allowing lock release from within the trunk (*113*).

The utility of surveillance data in detecting epidemics is highest in situations in which cases of the health condition occur over a wide geographic area or gradually over time. In such situations, the person–place–time links among cases probably would not be recognized by individual practitioners (*114*). Typical examples occur with infectious diseases when laboratory monitoring of unusual serotypes or antibiotic-resistance patterns identify outbreaks of specific microorganisms that otherwise might have gone unnoticed. Widespread epidemics of Salmonella have been detected through surveillance (*115,116*).

Identifying New Syndromes

The most dramatic use of surveillance data occurs when a "new" syndrome emerges from an ongoing monitoring system. Legionnaires' disease was detected and subsequently characterized as the result of an outbreak of non-influenza pneumonia within a specific place and population (*117*). AIDS was recognized both because of rapid increases in requests for CDC's pentamidine supply and because it occurred in a specific time (early 1981), in two specific places (California, New York), and among specific subpopulations (men having sex with men and injection drug users) (*118*). Finally, the national scope of the epidemic of eosinophilia myalgia syndrome was noticed because its unique features were like those of toxic oil syndrome (*119*).

Monitoring Trends

Even if specific outbreaks or new syndromes cannot be identified by tracking surveillance data, changes in the the baseline level of the health condition being monitored over time might demonstrate important changes in well-understood conditions. This purpose is relevant especially to assessing events associated with reproductive health (e.g., ectopic pregnancy or neonatal mortality), chronic disease, or infections with a long latency. The upward trend in obesity rates in New Jersey from 1996 through 2006 reflects this monitoring function (Fig. 6–17; ref. *101*).

Evaluating Public Policy

Surveillance data are used to assess the health impact of specific interventions (either biomedical or structural) and public policy. The rapid fall in numbers of cases of poliomyelitis and measles after national vaccination campaigns were instituted is a classic example of the usefulness of surveillance data (*120,121*). More recently, the Florida Youth Tobacco Survey was used to test the effectiveness of the Florida Pilot Program on Tobacco Control, a youth-oriented, countermarketing media campaign developed to reduce the allure of smoking (*122*). Following implementation of the program, evidence of a significant decline in tobacco use among middle and high school students has spurred adoption of similar programs in other states. Creative interpretation of surveillance data has also been applied to other non-infectious conditions; however, the impact in such situations is somewhat more difficult to assess. For example, in Washington, D.C., the adoption of a gun-licensing law coincided with an abrupt decline in firearm-related homicides and suicides (*123*). No similar reductions occurred in the number of homicides or suicides committed by other means, nor did states adjacent to the District experience any reductions in their rates of firearm-related homicides or suicides. Also, surveillance of legal abortions and of deaths associated with illegal abortion has helped trace the public health impact of this controversial health problem (*122–126*). After legal abortions became widely available, deaths from illegal abortions decreased markedly; however, restriction of federal funds for abortions had a negligible effect on health parameters (*127*).

Alhough it is tempting to use trends in disease and injury to monitor the impact of community interventions, such evaluation is prone to ecologic fallacy and becomes increasingly suspect when several factors contribute to the occurrence of the disease or health condition being monitored. In addition, if only a portion of the population accepts an intervention, analysis and interpretation of surveillance data are made even more difficult. Frequently, surveillance of process measures or other health problems act as proxies for the intended outcome. For example, decreases in unsafe sexual behaviors or other sexually transmitted diseases after HIV campaigns have been used as surrogates for trends in HIV incidence. Moreover, finding comparability in data from several populations that have attempted similar public health programs strengthens evidence that the interpretation is correct. For example, to evaluate the effectiveness of allowing people to exchange used hypodermic needles for new ones as a means of preventing AIDS, epidemiologists could examine simultaneously trends in numbers of needles distributed, surveys of needle use, and incidence of higher-prevalence infections such as hepatitis C.

Projecting Future Needs

Mathematical models based on surveillance data can be used to project future trends. This tool helps health officials determine the eventual need for preventive and curative services. Recently, such modeling assisted in estimating state-specific increases in arthritis and arthritis-attributable activity limitations through 2030 (*6*). The analysis used estimates of arthritis prevalence derived from analysis of weighted data from the BRFSS; the results indicated that because of growth in the numbers of older Americans projected through 2030, certain states such as Arizona and Florida will need increased public health capcity for prevention of arthritis-related activity limitations. In addition, models based on surveillance data can predict the decline of morbidity and mortality when there are changes in risk factors among the population at risk. Examples of this application include projecting the decline in cardiovascular disease on the basis of decreased smoking of cigarettes (*128*), the decline in cirrhosis-related mortality in the presence of lower levels of alcohol use (*129*) and decreased rates of mortality from cervical cancer associated with an increase in the prevalence of hysterectomy (*130*). In addition, extensions of projection methods are used to describe what to expect in the presence or absence of an intervention or to identify changes in the momentum of dynamic public health concerns. For example, obesity is an increasing trend in the United States, so a slowing of the increase might be an indicator of programmatic success. Conversely, the prevalence of smoking is dereasing in the United States, and a slowing of the decrease in prevalence would represent a programmatic concern.

CONCLUSIONS

The process of analysis and interpretation of surveillance data is a rich endeavor, encompassing a wide variety of system designs, analytic methods, modes of presentation, and interprative uses. In general, descriptive methods are the foundation of routine reporting of surveillance data, and more specialized hypotheses are explored using inferential methods. The most critical elements of an analytic activity in a surveillance system are a thorough understanding of the underlying data, a routine process for disseminating reports of surveillance data (usually descriptive in nature), and careful interpretation of observed trends or other findings to avoid unfounded causal inference.

REFERENCES

1. Thacker SB, Berkelman RL. Public health surveillance in the United States. *Epidemiol Rev* 1988;10:164–190.
2. Buehler JL, Rothman KJ, Greenland S. Surveillance. *Modern Epidemiology* Philadelphia, PA: Lippencott–Raven; 1998:435–457.
3. Berkelman R, Sullivan PS, J. B. Public Health Surveillance. In: Detels *et al.*, ed. *Oxford Textbook of Public Health,* 5th ed. London: Oxford University Press; 2009.
4. Cromley EK. GIS and disease. *Annu Rev Public Health* 2003;24(1):7–24.
5. Centers for Disease Control and Prevention. Surveillance for Violent Deaths— National Violent Death Reporting System, 16 States, 2006. *MMWR Surv Summ.* 2009;58(SS01):1–44.
6. Centers for Disease Control and Prevention. Projected state-specific increases in self-reported doctor-diagnosed arthritis and arthritis-attributable activity limitations– United States, 2005–2030. *MMWR* 2007;56(17):423–425.
7. Sullivan PS, Hamouda O, Delpech V, *et al.* The reemergence of the HIV epidemic among men who have sex with men in North America, Western Europe, and Australia, 1996–2005. *Ann Epidemiol* 2009;19(6):423–431.
8. Ries LAG, Eisner MP, Kosary CL, *et al.* eds. SEER Cancer Statistics Review, 1973–1999. http://seer.cancer.gov/csr/1973_1999/, 2002. Accessed December 1, 2008.
9. Chini F, Farchi S, Ciaramella I, *et al.* Road traffic injuries in one local health unit in the Lazio region: results of a surveillance system integrating police and health data. *Int J Health Geograph* 2009;8(1):21.

10. Sudakin DL, Power LE. Regional variation in the severity of pesticide exposure outcomes: applications of geographic information systems and spatial scan statistics. *Clin Toxicol* 2009;47(3):248–252.

11. Maciejewski R, Glickman N, Moore G, *et al.* Companion animals as sentinels for community exposure to industrial chemicals: the Fairburn, GA, propyl mercaptan case study. *Public Health Rep* 2008;123(3):333–342.

12. Centers for Disease Control and Prevention. Human immunodeficiency virus (HIV) risk, prevention, and testing behaviors—United States, National HIV Behavioral Surveillance System: men who have sex with men, November 2003–April 2005. *MMWR Surveill Summ* 2006;55(6):1–16.

13. State-specific prevalence among adults of current cigarette smoking and smokeless tobacco use and per capita tax-paid sales of cigarettes—United States, 1997. *MMWR* 1998;47(43):922–926.

14. U.S. Renal Data System, USRDS 2007 Annual Data Report: Atlas of Chronic Kidney Disease and End-Stage Renal Disease in the United States, National Institutes of Health, National Institute of Diabetes and Digestive and Kidney Diseases, Bethesda, MD, 2007.

15. Sullivan PS, Dworkin MS, Jones JL, Hooper WC. Epidemiology of thrombosis in HIV-infected individuals. The Adult/Adolescent Spectrum of HIV Disease Project. *AIDS* 2000;14(3):321–324.

16. Centers for Disease Control and Prevention. Updated guidelines for evaluating public health surveillance systems: recommendations from the guidelines working group. *MMWR* 2001;50(NoRR–13):1–51.

17. Remington PL, Nelson DE. Communicating public health surveillance information for action. In: Lee LM, Teutsch SM, Thacker SB, St Louis ME. eds. *Principles and Practice of Public Health Surveillance.* 3rd ed. NewYork, NY: Oxford University Press; 2010.

18. Brookmeyer R, Stroup DF, eds. *Monitoring the Health of Populations.* New York: Oxford University Press; 2004.

19. Clayton D, Hills M. *Statistical Models in Epidemiology.* New York: Oxford University Press; 1993.

20. Breslow NE, Day N. *Statistical Methods in Cancer Research: Analysis Of Case-control Studies.* Vol 1. Lyon, France: International Agency for Research on Cancer; 1980.

21. Miettinen O. Estimability and estimation in case-referent studies. *Am J Epidemiol* 1976;103:226–235.

22. Zhang J, Yu KF. What's the relative risk?: A method of correcting the odds ratio in cohort studies of common outcomes. *JAMA* 1998; 280:1690–1691.

23. McNutt L-A, Wu C, Xue X, Hafner JP. Estimating the relative risk in cohort studies and clinical trials of common outcomes. *Am J Epidemiol* 2003;157(10):940–943.

24. United States Census Bureau. US Census, 2000. www.census.gov. Accessed September 30, 2005.

25. Lehtonen R, Pahkinen E. *Practical Methods for Design and Analysis of Complex Surveys.* New York: John Wiley & Sons; 2004.

26. Centers for Disease Control and Prevention. Decline in smoking prevalence–New York City, 2002–2006. *MMWR* 2007;56(24):604–608.

27. Etzioni R, Kessler L, di Tommaso D. Using public health data to evaluate screening programs: application to prostate cancer. In: Brookmeyer R, Stroup DF, eds. *Monitoring the Health of Populations.* New York: Oxford University Press; 2004: 147–166.

28. Andriole GL, Crawford ED, Grubb RL, 3rd, *et al.* Mortality results from a random-ized prostate–cancer screening trial. *N Engl J Med* 2009;360(13):1310–1319.
29. Schroder FH, Hugosson J, Roobol MJ, *et al.* Screening and prostate-cancer mortality in a randomized European study. *N Engl J Med* 2009;360(13):1320–1328.
30. Kleinbaum D, Kupper L, Muller K, Nizam A. *Applied Regression Analysis and Other Multivariable Methods.* Pacific Grove, CA: Brooks/Cole Publishing; 1998.
31. Surveillance Epidemiology and End Results Program. Joinpoint regression pro-gram. *Statistical Research and Applications,* 2008. http://srab.cancer.gov/joinpoint/. Accessed September 23, 2008.
32. Woldemichael G, Christiansen D, Thomas S, Benbow N. Demographic characteris-tics and survival with AIDS: health disparities in Chicago, 1993–2001. *Am J Public Health* 2009;99(S1):S118–S123.
33. Sullivan PS, Hanson DL, Chu SY, Jones JL, Ciesielski CA. Surveillance for thrombocytopenia in persons infected with HIV: results from the multistate Adult and Adolescent Spectrum of Disease Project. *J Acquir Immune Defic Syndr Hum Retrovirol* 1997;14(4):374–379.
34. Gallagher KM, Juhasz M, Harris NS, Teshale EH. Predictors of influenza vac-cination in HIV–infected patients in the United States, 1990–2002. *J Infect Dis* 2007;196(3):339–346.
35. Pearson WS, Dube SR, Ford ES, Mokdad AH. Influenza and pneumococcal vacci-nation rates among smokers: Data from the 2006 behavioral risk factor surveillance system. *Prev med* 2008.
36. Koch T. *Cartographies of Disease.* Redlands, CA: ESRI Press; 2005.
37. Johnson S. *The Ghost Map: The Story of London's Most Terrifying Epidemic–and How It Changed Science, Cities, and the Modern World.* New York: Riverhead Books; 2007.
38. Brody H, Rip MR, Vinten–Johansen P, Paneth N, Rachman S. Map–making and myth–making in Broad Street: the London cholera epidemic, 1854. *Lancet* 2000;356(9223):64–68.
39. Lagakos SW, Wessen BJ, Zelen M. An analysis of contaminated well water and health–effects in Woburn, Massachusetts. *J Am Stat Assoc* 1986;81:583–596.
40. Harr J. *A Civil Action.* New York: Random House; 1996.
41. National Conference on Clustering of Health Events. Atlanta, Georgia, February 16–17, 1989. *Am J Epidemiol* 1990;132(1 Suppl):S1–S202.
42. Besag J, Newell J. The detection of clusters in rare diseases. *J Royal Stat Soc, Series A* 1991;154:327–333.
43. Waller LA, Gotway CA. *Applied Spatial Statistics for Public Health Data.* Hoboken, NJ: Wiley Interscience; 2004.
44. Tango T. An index for cancer clustering. *Environ Health Perspect* 1990;87:157–162.
45. Waller LA. Methods for detecting disease clustering in time or space. In: Brookmeyer R, Stroup DF, eds. *Monitoring the Health of Populations: Statistical Principles and Methods and in Public Health Surveillance.* New York: Oxford University Press; 2003:167–201.
46. Tango T. A class of tests for detecting "general" and "focused" clustering of rare dis-eases. *Stat Med* 1995;14(21–22):2323–2334.
47. Kuldorff M. A spatial scan statistic. *Commun Stat Theory Methods* 1997;26:1481–1496.
48. Steenland K, Bray I, Greenland S, Boffetta P. Empirical Bayes adjustments for mul-tiple results in hypothesis–generating or surveillance studies. *Cancer Epidemiol Biomarkers Prev* 2000;9(9):895–903.

49. Greenland S. Smoothing observational data: a philosophy and implementation for the health sciences. *Int Stat Rev* 2006;74:31–46.

50. Lawson AB, Williams FLR. *An Introductory Guide to Disease Mapping*. Chinchester: Wiley; 2001.

51. Lawson AB, Browne WJ, Vidal Rodeiro CL. *Disease Mapping with WinBUGS and MNwiN*. Chinchester, PA: Wiley; 2003.

52. Lawson AB. *Statistical Methods in Spatial Epidemiology*, 2nd ed. Chinchester: Wiley; 2006.

53. Tanser F, Barnighausen T, Cooke GS, Newell M-L. Localized spatial clustering of HIV infections in a widely disseminated rural South African epidemic. *Int J Epidemiol* 2009;148.

54. Thacker SB, Choi K, Brachman PS. The surveillance of infectious diseases. *JAMA* 1983;249(9):1181–1185.

55. McNabb SJ, Jajosky RA, Hall–Baker PA, *et al.* Summary of notifiable diseases—United States, 2006. *MMWR* 2008;55(53):1–92.

56. Stroup DF, Williamson GD, Herndon JL, Karon JM. Detection of aberrations in the occurrence of notifiable diseases surveillance data. *Stat Med* 1989;8(3):323–329; discussion 331–322.

57. Centers for Disease Control and Prevention. Proposed changes in format for presentation of notifiable disease report data. *MMWR* 1989;38(47):805–809.

58. Centers for Disease Control and Prevention. Notifiable diseases/deaths in selected cities weekly information. *MMWR* 2009;58(17):474–485.

59. Morgenstern H, Greenland S. Graphing ratio measures of effect. *J Clin Epidemiol* 1990;43(6):539–542.

60. Stroup DF, Wharton M, Kafadar K, Dean AG. Evaluation of a method for detecting aberrations in public health surveillance data. *Am J Epidemiol* 1993;137(3):373–380.

61. Wharton M, Price W, Hoesly F, *et al.* Evaluation of a method for detecting outbreaks of diseases in six states. *Am J Prev Med* 1993;9(1):45–49.

62. Wallenstein S. A test for detection of clustering over time. *Am J Epidemiol* 1980;111(3):367–372.

63. Naus JI. Approximations for distributions of scan statistics. *J Am Stat Assoc* 1982;77:560–566.

64. Glaz J. Approximations and bounds for the distribution of the scan statistic. *J Am Stat Assoc* 1989;84:560–566.

65. Choi K, Thacker SB. An evaluation of influenza mortality surveillance, 1962–1979. I. Time series forecasts of expected pneumonia and influenza deaths. *Am J Epidemiol* 1981;113(3):215–226.

66. Devine O, Parrish RG, Stroup DF, Teutsch SM. Monitoring the health of a population. In *Statistics in Public Health*. Oxford: Oxford University Press; 1998.

67. Kafadar K, Andrews Jr. JS. Investigvating health effects and hazards in the community. In: Stroup DF, Teutsch SM, eds. *Statistics in Public Health*. Oxford: Oxford University Press; 1998:93–122.

68. Hutwagner L, Browne T, Seeman GM, Fleischauer AT. Comparing aberration detection methods with simulated data. *Emerg Infect Dis* 2005;11(2):314–316.

69. Collins SD. Excess mortality from causes other than influenza and pneumonia during the influenza epidemics. *Public Health Rep* 1932;(47):2159–2180.

70. Serfling RE. Methods for current statistical analysis of excess pneumonia–influenza deaths. *Public Health Rep* 1963;78:494–505.

71. Fernandez–Perez C, Tejada J, Carrasco M. Multivariate time series analysis in nosocomial infection surveillance: a case study. *Int J Epidemiol* 1998;27(2):282–288.

72. Siegel JS, Swanson DA. *Methods and Materials of Demography,* 2d ed. San Diego, CA: Elsevier Academic Press; 2004.

73. Preston SH, Heuveline P, Guillot M. *Demography: Measuring and Modeling Population Processes.* Malden, MA: Blackwell Publishers; 2001.

74. Szklo M, Nieto FJ. *Epidemiology: Beyond the Basics.* Sudbury, MA; 2004.

75. Anderson RN, Rosenberg HM. Age standardization of death rates: implementation of the year 2000 standard. *Nat Vital Stat Rep* 1998;47(3):1–16.

76. Haddock CK, Pyle SA, DeBon M, *et al.* Cigarette use among two cohorts of U.S. Air Force recruits, compared with secular trends. *Mil Med* 2007;172(3):288–294.

77. Park RM, Ahn YS, Stayner LT, Kang SK, Jang JK. Mortality of iron and steel workers in Korea. *Am J Ind Med* 2005;48(3):194–204.

78. Conti S, Farchi G, Masocco M, Toccaceli V, Vichi M. The impact of the major causes of death on life expectancy in Italy. *Int J Epidemiol* 1999;28(5):905–910.

79. Nicoll A, Timaeus I, Kigadye RM, Walraven G, Killewo J. The impact of HIV–1 infection on mortality in children under 5 years of age in sub-Saharan Africa: a demographic and epidemiologic analysis. *AIDS* 1994;8(7):995–1005.

80. Liang J, Liu X, Tu E, Whitelaw N. Probabilities and lifetime durations of short-stay hospital and nursing home use in the United States, 1985. *Med Care* 1996;34(10):1018–1036.

81. Somi GR, Matee MI, Swai RO, *et al.* Estimating and projecting HIV prevalence and AIDS deaths in Tanzania using antenatal surveillance data. *BMC Public Health* 2006;6:120.

82. Lee LM, Fleming PL. Estimated number of children left motherless by AIDS in the United States, 1978–1998. *J Acquir Immune Defic Syndr* 2003;34(2):231–236.

83. Heo M, Murphy CF, Fontaine KR, Bruce ML, Alexopoulos GS. Population projection of US adults with lifetime experience of depressive disorder by age and sex from year 2005 to 2050. *Int J Geriatr Psychiatry* 2008;23(12):1266–1270.

84. Kupper LL, Janis JM, Karmous A, Greenberg BG. Statistical age-period-cohort analysis: a review and critique. *J Chronic Dis* 1985;38(10):811–830.

85. Frost WH. The age selection of mortality from tuberculosis in successive decades. 1939. *Am J Epidemiol* 1995;141(1):4–9; discussion 3.

86. Davis K, Blake J. Social stucture and fertility: an analytic framework. *Econ Devel Cultural Change* 1956;4(4):211–235.

87. Bongaarts J. A framework for analyzing the proximate determinants of fertility. *Population Devel Rev* 1978;4(1):105–132.

88. Bongaarts J. The fertility-inhibiting effects of the intermidiate fertility variable. *Stud Family Plan* 1982;4:179–189.

89. Nyamukapa CA, Gregson S, Lopman B, *et al.* HIV-associated orphanhood and children's psychosocial distress: theoretical framework tested with data from Zimbabwe. *Am J Public Health* 2008;98(1):133–141.

90. De Souza AC, Petersont KE, Cufino E, do Amaral MI, Gardner J. Underlying and proximate determinants of diarrhoea–specific infant mortality rates among municipalities in the state of Ceara, north–east Brazil: an ecological study. *J Biosoc Sci* 2001;33(2):227–244.

91. Lopman B, Nyamukapa C, Mushati P, et al. HIV incidence in 3 years of follow-up of a Zimbabwe cohort—1998–2000 to 2001–03: contributions of proximate and underlying determinants to transmission. *Int J Epidemiol* 2008;37(1):88–105.

92. Tufte ER. *The Visual Display of Quantitative Information.* Cheshire, CT: Graphics Press; 1987.

93. Tufte ER. *Envisioning Information.* Chershire, CT: Graphics Press; 1990.

94. *Principles of Epidemiology*, 2nd-(developmental) ed. Washington, DC: American Public Health Association; 1992.

95. Peavy J, Dyal WW, Eddins DL. *Descriptive Statistics: Tables, Graphs, and Charts.* Department of Health and Services, Centers for Disease Control; 1986.

96. Schmid CF. *Statistical Graphics Design Principles and Practices.* New York: John Wiley and Sons; 1983.

97. Chambers JM, Cleveland WS, Kleiner B, Tukey PA. *Graphical Methods for Data analysis.* Boston: Duxbury Press; 1983.

98. Centers for Disease Control and Prevention. Pool chemical–associated health events in public and residential settings—United States, 1983–2007. *MMWR.* 2009;58(18):489–493.

99. Centers for Disease Control and Prevention. National surveillance for asthma, 1980–2004. *MMWR* 2007; 56(No SS–8).

100. Department for Environment, Food and Rural Affairs. Zoonoses report, 2007. http://www.defra.gov.uk/animalh/diseases/zoonoses/zoonoses_reports/zoonoses2007.pdf.

101. Jafa K, McElroy P, Fitzpatrick L, *et al.* HIV transmission in a state prison system, 1998–2005. *PLoS One* 2009;4(5):e5416.

102. US Department of Health and Human Services. Injury in the United States: 2007. http://www.cdc.gov/nchs/data/misc/injury2007.pdf.

103. Centers for Disease Control and Prevention. Update: novel influenza A (H1N1) virus infections—worldwide, May 6, 2009. *MMWR.* 2009;58(17):453–458.

104. Chow E, Friedman D, Stovall M, *et al.* Risk of thyroid dysfunction and subsequent thyroid cancer among survivors of acute lymphoblastic leukemia: A report from the Childhood Cancer Survivor Study. *Pediatric Blood Cancer* 2009;9999(9999):n/a.

105. Centers for Disease Control and Prevention. Percentage of live births by cesarean delivery, by plurality—United States, 1996, 2000, and 2006. *MMWR.* 2009;58(19):542.

106. Haggett P, Cliff AD, Frey A. *Locational Analysis in Human Geography.* Bristol, England: J.W. Arrowsmith; 1977.

107. National Centre in HIV Epidemiology and Clinical Research. Bloodborne viral and sexually transmitted infections in Aboriginal and Torres Strait Islander People: Surveillance Report 2008. National Centre in HIV Epidemiology and Clinical Research, The University of New South Wales, Sydney, NSW.

108. New Jersey Department of Health and Senior Services. Obesity Trends in New Jersey Counties: 1992–2006. June 2008. http://www.state.nj.us/health/chs/documents/obesity_brief.pdf.

109. Cowan DN, Prier RE. Changes in hepatitis morbidity in the United States Army, Europe. *Mil Med* 1984;149(5):260–265.

110. Edmonds LD, James LM. Temporal trends in the prevalence of congenital malformations at birth based on the birth defects monitoring program, United States, 1979–1987. *MMWR CDC Surveill Summ* 1990;39(4):19–23.

111. Outbreaks of rubella among the Amish–United States, 1991. *MMWR Morb Mortal Wkly Rep* 1991;40(16):264–265.

112. Grimes DA, Forrest JD, Kirkman AL, Radford B. An epidemic of antiabortion violence in the United States *Am J Obstet Gynecol* 1991;165(5 Pt 1):1263–1268.

113. Centers for Disease Control and Prevention. Fatal car trunk entrapment involving children—United States, 1987–1998. *MMWR* 1998;47(47):1019–1022.

114. Berkelman RL, Buehler JL, Holland WW, Detels R, Knox G. Surveillance. In: *Oxford Textbook of Public Health,* Vol 2. Oxford: Oxford University Press; 1991: 161–176.

115. Centers for Disease Control and Prevention. Multistate outbreaks of Salmonella infections associated with live poultry–United States, 2007. *MMWR* 2009;58(2):25–29.

116. Centers for Disease Control and Prevention. Outbreak of Salmonella serotype Saintpaul infections associated with eating alfalfa sprouts—United States, 2009. *MMWR* 2009;58(18):500–503.

117. Fraser DW, Tsai TR, Orenstein W, *et al*. Legionnaires' disease: description of an epidemic of pneumonia. *N Engl J Med* 1977;297(22):1189–1197.

118. Centers for Disease Control and P. Pneumocystis pneumonia—Los Angeles. *MMWR* 1981;30(21):1–3.

119. Swygert LA, Maes EF, Sewell LE, Miller L, Falk H, Kilbourne EM. Eosinophilia-myalgia syndrome. Results of national surveillance. *JAMA* 1990;264(13):1698–1703.

120. Centers for Disease Control and Prevention. Progress toward eradicating poliomyelitis from the Americas. *MMWR* 1989;38(31):532–535.

121. Centers for Disease Control and Prevention. Measles prevention: recommendations of the Immunization Practices Advisory Committee (IPAC). *MMWR* 1989(38(No. S–9)):1–18.

122. Centers for Disease Control and Prevention. Tobacco use among middle and high school students—Florida, 1998 and 1999. *MMWR* 1999;48(12):248–253.

123. Loftin C, McDowall D, Wiersema B, Cottey TJ. Effects of restrictive licensing of handguns on homicide and suicide in the District of Columbia. *N Engl J Med* 1991;325(23):1615–1620.

124. Cates W, Jr, Rochat RW, Grimes DA, Tyler CW Jr. Legalized abortion: effect on national trends of maternal and abortion-related mortality (1940 through 1976). *Am J Obstet Gynecol* 1978;132(2):211–214.

125. Cates W, Jr. Legal abortion: the public health record. *Science* 1982;215(4540):1586–1590.

126. Robinson WS. Ecological correlations and the behavior of individuals. *Am Sociol Rev* 1950;15:351–357.

127. Cates W, Jr. The Hyde Amendment in action. How did the restriction of federal funds for abortion affect low-income women? *JAMA* 1981;246(10):1109–1112.

128. Kullback S, Cornfield J. An information theoretic contingency table analysis of the Dorn study of smoking and mortality. *Comput Biomed Res* 1976;9(5):409–437.

129. Skog OJ. The risk function for liver cirrhosis from lifetime alcohol consumption. *J Stud Alcohol* 1984;45(3):199–208.

130. Hysterectomy prevalence and death rates for cervical cancer—United States, 1965–1988. *MMWR* 1992;41(2):17–20.

7

Communicating Public Health Surveillance Information for Action

PATRICK L. REMINGTON AND DAVID E. NELSON

The data speak for themselves.

—Unknown

INTRODUCTION

Surveillance has been defined as "the ongoing systematic collection, analysis, and interpretation of health data that are essential to the planning, implementation, and evaluation of public health practice" (*1*). Surveillance activities must be closely integrated with the timely dissemination of these data for public health action. Thus, a public health surveillance "system" not only includes a capacity for data collection and analysis but also for *communication* with those who need to know. Because the data rarely speak for themselves, public health professionals must serve to "translate" the findings to the general public or to policymakers (*2*).

Effective communication of surveillance information requires learning from the field of health communication by understanding the importance of knowing audiences and developing new skills in communication planning, social marketing, media communications, and risk communication. Reaching audiences with public health surveillance information can be challenging, as this information is often complex and technical. Too often, public health agencies simply analyze the data and report the results in agency reports or occasionally in local or state publications that are long and contain technical jargon. In addition, information is seldom linked to program priorities, and reports are seldom used to promote public health practice or as a vehicle for setting priorities for action (*3*).

In addition, public health professionals charged with the collection and analysis of data might not have the expertise, experience, and incentives necessary to communicate findings effectively, leaving policymakers to develop health policies without input from existing surveillance systems. Even when information is communicated, many people—an estimated 60 million Americans—have difficulty understanding even the most basic health information (*4*).

The importance of public health communication has been increasingly recognized with the publication of several textbooks and the recent competency

146

established by the Association of Schools of Public Health and the Council on Linkages that describes how students and practitioners (5) should have the ability to collect, manage, and organize data and to communicate this information to different audiences in person, through information technologies, and through media channels.

As a result of fundamental changes in public health priorities, programs at all levels require innovative approaches to convey surveillance findings to new and diverse constituencies. This chapter does not attempt to provide an exhaustive review of the many health communication strategies—such a review is provided elsewhere (*see* Resources at the end of this chapter). Rather, we focus on information collected during public health surveillance and (*1*) describe the history of approaches to health communication; (*2*) present models and approaches for communicating surveillance information; and (*3*) discuss several important challenges and opportunities for effective communication.

BACKGROUND AND PURPOSE

History of Surveillance Communication

Traditionally in the United States, surveillance findings have been disseminated through written reports produced by public health agencies at the local, state, and national level. The flagship publication for surveillance information is the Centers for Disease Control and Prevention (CDC) *Morbidity and Mortality Weekly Report* (*MMWR*). The *MMWR's* history is almost synonymous with the evolution of public health in the United States, dating back to 1878, when Congress passed the first National Quarantine Act requiring U.S. consuls to report sanitary conditions abroad and on vessels bound for U.S. ports (*6*). By 1952 the *MMWR* acquired its present name and began to be published by the then Communicable Disease Center in 1961. Since that time, the *MMWR* has filled that critical time gap between the immediate public health need for information and the long wait for publication in the scientific journals.

Over the past 50 years, the scope of public health surveillance has changed as the definition of public health has broadened, increasingly recognizing the role of multiple determinants of population health. As recently as the 1970s, public health surveillance in the United States focused almost exclusively on the detection and monitoring of cases of specific communicable diseases, and surveillance data were disseminated primarily in a basic tabular format to state and local health departments. However, surveillance efforts have expanded rapidly and now include problems as diverse as health-related behavior (e.g., cigarette smoking and seatbelt use); environmental insults (e.g., hazardous materials incidents); and preventive practices (e.g., Papanicolaou [Pap] tests and mammographic screening) (*7*). Most recently, public health surveillance includes the multiple determinants of population health, including health-care quality and access and measures of socioeconomic status, such as income and education (*see* Chapter 13).

Purpose of Communication: Dissemination versus Communication

The longstanding expectation of surveillance has been that information is "disseminated" to those working in the public health system and to the general public. However, a fundamental concept is that the terms *dissemination* and *communication* should not be used interchangeably. Dissemination is a one-way process through which information is conveyed from one point to another. In comparison, communication is a process that involves at least two people in an effort to convey, receive, interpret, and agree on the meaning of data, information, or messages. The purpose of this process from the point of the "sender" might be to inform, influence, motivate, instruct, persuade, or some combination of these or other activities.

Communication should be considered as a loop—involving at least a sender and a receiver—a collaborative process. The sender's job is completed when the receiver of the information acknowledges receipt and comprehension of that information (7). This distinction between communication and dissemination is critical in planning, implementing, and evaluating programs that involve communication in public health practice (8).

Public health surveillance has been characterized as a process that provides "information for action." Public health programs must ensure more than the mere transmission or dissemination of surveillance results to others; rather, surveillance data should be presented in a manner that facilitates their use for public health action. These actions are directly related to the communication purposes of the surveillance system (7), as summarized below.

Detect and Control Outbreaks

When the purpose of a surveillance system is to detect outbreaks or other occurrences of disease in excess of predicted levels, the primary communication objective should be to inform two groups: *(a)* the population at risk of exposure or disease, and *(b)* persons and organizations responsible for immediate control measures and other interventions. These measures often have to be communicated rapidly and to a widespread audience. One recent example demonstrating the urgent need for effective communciation is the foodborne outbreak from *Salmonella*-contaminated peanut butter (*see* Box 7–1).

Determine the Etiology and Natural History of Disease

Public health surveillance of newly recognized or detected problems might be initiated to determine the epidemiology, etiology, and natural history of such conditions. In such circumstances, the communication objective might be simply to provide information sufficient to initiate surveillance. For example, when Eosinophilia-myalgia syndrome was recognized in the United States during the late 1980s, a case definition was developed and communicated to the public health community to enable the immediate implementation of national surveillance for the syndrome (9). This information was also communicated to the research community to help characterize the epidemiology and natural history of the syndrome and to assist in the development of hypotheses regarding its cause.

Box 7–1 Communicating Information about the Nationwide Peanut Butter Salmonella Outbreak

---

On November 25, 2008, an epidemiologic assessment began of a growing cluster of *Salmonella* serotype Typhimurium isolates that shared the same pulsed-field gel electrophoresis (PFGE) pattern in PulseNet, the national molecular subtyping network for foodborne disease surveillance (*10,11*). As of January 28, 2009, 529 persons from 43 states and one person from Canada had been reported infected with the outbreak strain. Epidemiologic and laboratory findings indicated that peanut butter and peanut paste produced at one plant are the source of the outbreak. These products also are ingredients in many foods produced and distributed by other companies.

The communication strategy was immediate and widespread, given the seriousness of Salmonella infection. Foods containing contaminated peanut butter were recalled and consumers were advised to discard and not eat any of these products. The U.S. Department of Health and Human Services, Food and Drug Administration (FDA), and Centers for Disease Control and Prevention (CDC) provided consumers and partners with social media tools to access information about the ongoing peanut butter and peanut-containing product recalls. Some products created for this response included podcasts for adults and children, widgets for web pages and social network profiles, mobile-accessible content at m.cdc.gov, Twitter messaging, promotion through social networks, and outreach to bloggers.

Evaluate Control Measures

For many public health conditions, surveillance is the principal means for assessing the impact of control measures. Epidemiologic trends and patterns that are based on surveillance findings must be conveyed to persons involved in control efforts to refine control activities and guide the allocation of resources in support of those activities.

For example, the incidence of measles in the United States surged in the mid-1980s, following a period of relative quiescence. When surveillance data indicated that vaccination coverage had declined substantially in some groups (e.g., children residing in inner-city locations), these important findings were communicated to and used by public health programs and primary care providers in targeting measles vaccination efforts.

Detect Changes in Disease Agents

In addition to monitoring trends in the occurrence of public health problems, surveillance systems are fundamental to the process of detecting changes in disease agents and the impact of these changes on public health. For example, in the late 1980s in the United States, surveillance documented an increase in the incidence of tuberculosis—an increase substantially in excess of predicted levels. In addition to this overall trend, transmission of multidrug-resistant tuberculosis (MDR-TB) was detected in health-care and prison settings (*12*). The public health implications of these findings are similar to the basic considerations outlined above for detecting and controlling outbreaks: specifically, there is need for timely and effective notification of populations at risk and of organizations responsible for control and prevention measures. Therefore, in the case of MDR-TB, the communication objectives would include immediate notification of the public health community about the problem with the intent of facilitating implementation of proper diagnostic, therapeutic, and preventive measures.

Detect Changes in Health Practices

Some surveillance systems monitor changes in health practices and behaviors in the population rather than changes in patterns of disease (*13*). This "lifestyle" information is particularly important for problems such as chronic disease, for which trends in risk behavior often precede changes in health outcome by years or even decades. The communication objective in this context is often to increase awareness regarding the role of behavior in causing disease or injury. In addition, this information might be used to identify high-risk groups in the population.

What is likely the most well-known example of an effective communication strategy involves the use of maps demonstrating the increasing prevalence of obesity in each state from 1990 to 2007 (*see* Box 7–2). Showing a slide presentation of these maps often leads to gasps of amazement from audiences.

Facilitate Planning of Health Policies

For some conditions, the most appropriate control measure is enactment of a public health policy. In this context, surveillance information about the public health impact of different conditions and problems must be effectively conveyed to legislators and makers of public health policy. For example, in California data about smoking-attributable mortality, morbidity, and economic costs helped enact Proposition 99 in 1988. This legislation provided for a 25-cent increase in the state cigarette tax, which funded statewide initiatives to prevent and control the use of tobacco. Subsequently, surveillance data regarding trends in prevalence of

---

Box 7–2 Communicating Information about the Increasing Prevalence of Obesity in the United States

Beginning in 1984, the Centers for Disease Control and Prevention instituted the Behavioral Risk Factor Surveillance System, using telephone surveys to assess the prevalence of behavioral risk factors (14). This surveillance system permitted for the first time ever, state-specific estimates of the leading risk factors for chronic diseases and injuries. Because the respondents are asked their height and weight, the prevalence of obesity (body mass index >30) can be reported for each state.

In 1999, Mokdad et al published a report in the *Journal of the American Medical Association* showing how the obesity epidemic spread across the nation (*15*). These "obesity maps" graphically communicated information that had been reported previously, but did so in a way that presented a clear and compelling case for the speed and impact of this epidemic.

Box 7–3 Communicating Surveillance Information about Breast Cancer Trends

A surveillance report from a state-based cancer reporting system revealed increasing breast cancer mortality rates among black women over the past 15 years, compared with stable and then declining death rates among white women in Wisconsin. The researchers posited that the trends are due to differences in breast cancer screening rates, as additional research in the same state had shown that black women were less likely to have received mammograms and were more likely to have been diagnosed at a late stage (16). Further research demonstrated that breast cancers had been detected at a later stage among women living in rural areas of a county in the state (17).

The information about disparities in breast cancer screening, early detection, and mortality could be communicated to the general public or to women specifically. This would increase awareness of the importance of mammography and early detection. It might also be targeted to policy makers, such as legislators considering developing a breast cancer detection program focused on reducing breast cancer deaths among minority women or women living in rural areas. Finally, the report could be given to an advocacy organization, such as a statewide minority health council, to use in their efforts to advocate for minority health programs, or programs for low income women, such as the National Breast and Cervical Cancer Early Detection Program (18).

---

smoking and the impact of this initiative assisted in ensuring the application of state funds to control tobacco use.

Similarly, findings of increasing breast cancer mortality among black women emphasize the need for effective breast cancer screening initiatives (*see* Box 7–3). Therefore, the intent of releasing this information might be to support a public health initiative, such as the National Breast and Cervical Cancer Early Detection Program (*18*).

COMMUNICATION MODELS AND FRAMEWORKS

Simple Communication Model

In the simplest communication model, a source (sender) sends a message to an audience (receiver) through a channel or channels (Fig. 7–1; refs. *19* and *20*). Note, however, that the arrows also go from audience to source and channel, indicating that individuals can seek information on their own. Sources are the institutions or individuals sending messages. Channels are typically considered interpersonal or mediated; channels that are mediated (e.g., mass media or small media) can reach large numbers of people.

Messages consist of symbols, words, or pictures used to transmit information. Audiences range in size from one person to entire populations. Context refers to many other factors, either at the individual or environmental level (e.g., emotions, absence of access to information sources), that can have some effect on whether audiences receive messages or how they interpret them (*19*).

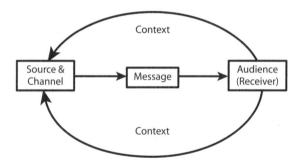

Figure 7–1 Basic communication model. *Source*: Nelson et al, 2009 (*19*).

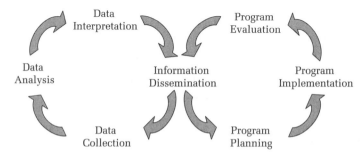

Figure 7–2 Integrating the "surveillance" and "program" loops in public health. *Source*: Adapted from Remington and Goodman, 1998 (*18*).

Communications: Integrating the "Surveillance Loop" With the "Program Loop"

Surveillance has been defined as a loop that includes data collection, analysis, interpretation, and dissemination—with the results of the information being used to reconsider and redesign the data collection methods. This "surveillance loop" is shown on the left side of Figure 7–2 (*18*). However, surveillance systems also include the capacity to communicate this information for use in planning, implementing, and evaluating programs and policy. This "program loop" is shown on the right side of Figure 7–2.

Showing a surveillance "system" with two interactive loops illustrates the distinct aspects of the type of work needed for an effective system. Work on the "left side" must consider the design of data collection systems, confidentiality, data quality, analytic approaches, and ways to report and disseminate information. These tasks are often accomplished by persons with formal training in epidemiology and statistics. In contrast, work on the "right side" must consider approaches to program planning, implementation, and evaluation. These tasks are often accomplished by persons with formal training in public health, health education, or community health.

Table 7–1 Framework for Communicating Surveillance Information

Step 1: Assess the quality of the surveillance information.
Step 2: Define the purpose of communicating the information.
Step 3: Define the audience.
Step 4: Develop the message.
Step 5: Select the channel.
Step 6: Market the information.
Step 7: Implement the communication plan.
Step 8: Evaluate the process and outcomes.

Source: Adapted from Parvanta et al. 2002 (*20*); Remington and Nelson 2006 (*2*).

The key to success of this model is the work at the communication interface between those involved in data collection and those involved in program planning and evaluation. Often these individuals work in different units in an organization or in different organizations. Epidemiologists focus on data quality and caution about overinterpretation of data. Program staff might want more resources allocated to programs instead of data collection and analysis. Without strong leadership in organizations, poor integration and communication between these two components leads to systems that fail to effectively communicate information for action.

Framework for Communicating Public Health Surveillance Information

Regardless of whether one is communicating surveillance information to one person, to public health officials, to the local media, or to millions of people as part of a national campaign, the chances that the information will be attended to—and potentially have an effect on audiences—is greatly enhanced by planning. Table 7–1 provides a useful planning framework for those who are communicating surveillance information to a variety of audiences (*2,20*).

Assess the Quality of the Surveillance Information

The first step in communicating surveillance information is to assess the quality of the data and interpretation of findings. This requires basic understanding of epidemiology and the principles and practice of surveillance, as outlined in the rest of this textbook. In particular, this requires a detailed understanding of the surveillance system, quality and representativeness of the data, and the potential that there results are influenced by bias, confounding, or chance. Details about approaches to understand the quality of data are beyond the scope of this chapter (*21*).

Define the Purpose of Communicating the Information

The second step is to clearly understand and define the purpose for communicating the surveillance information. The primary message or communication objective for the findings of any public health surveillance effort should reflect the basic purposes of the surveillance system (described above). For each of these purposes, the findings and interpretation of surveillance data might require a different type of public health response. The communication objectives should also dictate the delivery of the information to the relevant target groups and the stimulation of appropriate public health action.

Public agencies often report surveillance information without any specific goal, simply "because it is there." Other times, the purpose is to educate the public about a health issue. This is a worthy—but challenging—goal given the complexity of the message and the inability to shape the message for a specified audience.

The two basic purposes for communication include "informing" and "persuading." Communicators of surveillance information should be clear whether they are intending to inform or persuade audiences.

- *Informing* means to communicate information to increase an audience's knowledge with no intention of influencing a decision (although such information might inform people's decision-making process). This might occur, for example, when providing surveillance information about variation in disease or death rates in communities.
- *Persuading* refers to communicating surveillance information designed to change an audience's attitudes, beliefs, intentions, or behaviors. These data might be used to persuade individuals in the general population or public or private policymakers to support decisions about public health policies, programs, or resource allocation. For example, surveillance information about a specific foodborne outbreak might be communicated to persuade individuals not to eat a potentially contaminated product (9,10,22). Similar information might be presented to persuade policymakers to change policies regarding food inspection practices to prevent future outbreaks.

Much communication in public health is for the purpose of persuading people to do, or not do, something (23,24). As such, communicators of surveillance have an important ethical responsibility to be "honest brokers." Decisions about what surveillance data to select (or omit) and how to present them to audiences, can have a strong influence on conclusions reached by audiences (19). This means that the science underlying messages must be defensible, and practitioners must avoid overinterpreting, exaggerating, or suggesting greater certainty than can be justified, otherwise credibility can be lost.

Define the Audience

Once the objective for communicating the information has been established, identification of target groups is an essential next step in the process of developing strategies for communicating surveillance results.

Local health departments and health-care providers have been the long-standing audience of communicable disease surveillance information, because these professionals are responsible for implementing disease control strategies. In addition, health-care providers often provided data for these reports, and reporting information back to them shows the usefulness of the system and helps maintain their continued reporting (2).

The audience for public health surveillance information is much broader today and can include policymakers, news media representatives, health organizations, professional organizations, and the general public (3,25). Communication

Table 7–2 General Relationship Between the Purpose and the Audience in Communication Surveillance Information Effectively

Purpose (Why)	Audience (Who)	
	Individuals	Policymakers
Inform	Increase knowledge	Increase knowledge
	Facilitate informed decisions	Facilitate informed decisions
Persuade	Change attitude or behavior	Change or maintain program, policy, or law
	Learn new skill	Change or maintain resources

Source: Adapted from Parvanta et al., 2002 (20).

strategies can be developed to reach these audiences directly or indirectly. For example, surveillance information intended to influence policymakers might be communicated to voluntary organizations, who in turn use this information to communicate with and influence policymakers. Similarly, the media might be the direct audience for information from public health surveillance, but the intended audience is ultimately the general public or policymakers.

Audience segmentation is often necessary because people differ on a variety of demographic, cultural, personal, and psychological variables. Level of attention to health topics in general and level of interest in a specific public health topic play an overriding role in determining whether audiences attend to messages. Communicating epidemiologic information about sexual issues or domestic violence issues, for example, depends heavily on factors such as the age, gender, cultural background, and personal experience of the intended audience. A further challenge is that scientific and mathematical literacy is very low among most nonscientific audiences (2,19,26); most people will not understand common epidemiologic terms such as 95% confidence intervals or rates, necessitating explanations of basic epidemiologic and statistical principles and terms.

Table 7–2 shows the close relationship between the communication purpose (e.g., to inform vs. persuade) and the target audience (e.g., individuals vs. policymakers) (20). In this example, persuasive approaches will require that messages and communication channels be more closely matched to the characteristics of the audience than informational messages.

Develop the Message

The fourth step in communication is to develop the message concept and, if possible, test it on the intended audience. Message development involves condensing and translating surveillance information into simple and readily understood words or visual images. The important point is to clearly and simply state the most important findings (20). Creating a single overriding health communication objective can help translate complex scientific information into a few key statements (27). Pretesting depends on feasibility, resources, and timing and can be difficult in urgent situations or with policymakers. Even informal pretesting is valuable—for example, with staff members of policymakers.

The message should convey to the audience the following information: *(1)* what were the findings; *(2)* what do they mean (interpretation); and *(3)* what needs to be done *(19,28)*. Audiences will be most interested in the practical application (functionality) of health messages for themselves or other important persons in their lives *(19)*. Many public health messages can generate fear or other intense emotions (e.g., the number of cases of multidrug-resistant cases of tuberculosis tripled last year; the epidemic of "flesh-eating bacteria"). Before developing messages, it is helpful to recognize questions that audiences might have when processing information. If a message is likely to increase fear or anxiety, it is important that it also contain information about action(s) that people can take to effectively deal with the risk *(19)*. Examples might include providing a toll-free number to call for further information about the recall of a consumer product; steps to reduce the likelihood of contracting a sexually transmitted infection; types of equipment that can reduce occupational injury risk; or recommendations on how to increase physical activity.

The principal components of the message can be focused by selecting the most important point, then stating that point as a simple declarative sentence. This message, termed the *single overriding communication objective* (SOCO), should consider three questions:

- What is new?
- Who is affected?
- What works best?

For example, chronic disease surveillance information indicate that compared with younger women, older women are less likely to have received a Pap test in the past, are more likely to have cervical cancer diagnosed at a late stage, and have higher mortality rates resulting from cervical cancer. Traditionally, this information might be disseminated to health-care and public health providers through vital statistics reports and other published accounts about cervical cancer. However, if these findings are to be used as a basis for action, they first must be synthesized then communicated effectively. Thus, in addition to presenting these findings in detailed reports, they can be expressed through a single message, the SOCO: "All sexually active women need to get regular Pap smears."

Select the Channel

The fifth step is to choose the media and channels for delivering the message. Communication channels can be categorized broadly as interpersonal contact (e.g., face-to-face, small groups, oral presentations); written materials and audiovisuals such as correspondence, fact sheets, and scientific journal articles; mass media (e.g., television, newspapers, magazines); and electronic and other new media (e.g., the Internet) *(2)*.

Specification of the messages and audiences for surveillance results enable selection of the most suitable channels of communication for this information. Traditionally, surveillance information has been disseminated through published surveillance reports *(28)*. These reports are routinely sent to local public health agencies, physicians, health-care institutions, the media, and other interested individuals in the community or the state, either by e-mail or regular mail. A press release is occasionally used to increase the media interest in the story (*see* below for tips for writing a press release).

In addition to conventional means for communicating with traditional audiences, the advent of new methods and technologies have made possible improved communication with both old and new audiences. This spectrum of communication options includes professional and trade publications, electronic channels, broadcast media, print media, and public forums:

- Publications: government public health bulletins and surveillance reports, peer-reviewed public health and biomedical journals, newsletters
- Electronic: telecommunication systems, faxes and batch faxes, audioconferences, videoconferences, social media (e.g., Twitter, Facebook)
- Media: news releases, news conferences, fact sheets, video releases
- Public forums: briefings, hearings and testimony, conferences, and other planned meetings

The distinction between these categories has become blurred in recent years because of changes in technology—for example, e-mail listservs, Web sites, blogs, podcasts, RSS feeds, social networks, Twitter, and widgets. Increasingly, because of communication channel proliferation and fragmentation, multiple channels are being used to increase the likelihood that messages reach audiences. It is essential to know which communication channels your intended audiences prefer to use so that they are exposed to your messages (*2,19,29*)—for example, simply placing epidemiologic data on a website may not be as effective as "pushing" this information out to audiences through their preferred channels, such as public health blogs, RSS feeds, or Twitter.

"Market" the Information

Once the message has been defined and the target audience and channel selected, it is critical to ensure that the information is communicated using an active communication strategy, rather than relying solely on a passive strategy of simply placing surveillance data or other information in a report or on a Web site and hoping people will find it and take action (a "library" or "repository" model) (*19*). For some issues, such as an infectious disease outbreak, the public, news media, and policymakers are not only interested in the messages but might be seeking more information. In contrast, much surveillance information is routinely collected and reported, is not considered "newsworthy," and thus receives little interest by the news media and subsequently might not be noticed by the general public or policymakers. Those working to communicate public health surveillance information must seek ways to increase interest in these findings.

Marketing requires using an active communication strategy that attempts to gain the attention and interest of audiences. Active strategies can range from "word-of-mouth" approaches to activate social networks, to press releases, to extensive mass media campaigns. Increasingly, both active and passive communication strategies are used in combination (*19*). This can be considered as a "push–pull" approach: actively "pushing" messages, while having other materials available to interested seekers of information (e.g., at Web sites). To ensure that surveillance information is readily communicated to target audiences, public health agencies should use those techniques that are most effective for marketing information.

First, as a general principle, graphic formats and other visual displays are likely to be more effective in conveying information than conventional tabular presentations. Such formats include maps, bar graphs, histograms, diagrams, or other ways of visually depicting data that might not be comprehended readily through tabular presentation (*see* Chapter 6).

Techniques must be used to present (or "package") surveillance information in a manner that captures an audience's interest and focuses attention on a specific issue. Examples of these techniques are the use of introductory phrases such as: "A new study . . ."; "Recent findings . . ."; and "Information recently released. . . ." These terms are likely to appeal more to a target audience than a presentation that begins with a conventional preface, such as "Based on recent surveillance findings. . . ."

The method and forum of release of surveillance information is critical—particularly when a timely release is required or when the target audiences include the media, the public, or policymakers. Under such circumstances, news conferences or other news releases might be considered and should be held when they are likely to be attended. Foremost, the presenter should involve reporters in the public health surveillance process by "walking them through it" and should recognize opportunities to articulate the SOCO on camera or in print. Important adjuncts for presenting the information include readily available handouts and effective, but simple, visuals.

Finally, the communication should be timed to increase the chances of successfully achieving the communication objective. Sometimes this is obvious, such as when a new surveillance report or research study is published or during an acute outbreak situation. Timing might also be a consideration if a topic is receiving attention already, such as when a celebrity develops a preventable disease (*20*). It is especially important when policy decisions are imminent, such as town hall meetings or administrative hearings. There are times when communicating epidemiologic information should be avoided because audiences are distracted—for example, when there is a concurrent major news story. Each situation needs to be considered on a case-by-case basis.

Implement the Communication Plan

The seventh step is to implement and deliver the communication message(s). Although this is obvious, it is important to follow up to ensure that the communication activity or activities occurred.

Evaluate the Process and Outcomes

The final step in a communication plan is to evaluate how widely the information was disseminated (process evaluation) and whether the information led to the intended outcome (outcome evaluation) (*30*). News media tracking services will search for news stories in a defined geographic area (e.g., local or statewide newspapers) and provide electronic drafts of text with the selected "key words." These articles can be reviewed by the program staff to assess the geographic distribution and extent of the media coverage. In addition, the content of the clippings can be reviewed to assess both the accuracy and appropriateness of messages.

Determining outcomes of the communication effort on public audiences requires an evaluation of changes, such as knowledge, attitudes, behaviors, disease rates, and use of preventive services. This type of evaluation often requires establishing data collection systems or implementing surveys of the target population before and after the information has been disseminated to detect these changes.

CHALLENGES AND OPPORTUNITIES FOR COMMUNICATING PUBLIC HEALTH SURVEILLANCE DATA

Reporting Surveillance Information through the News Media

The news media play a central role in the communication of public health surveillance information. Public health agencies serve as a valuable source of health information for science and health writers, who can use this information to write stories of interest to the public. On the other hand, the news media meets the need of the public health agency by broadening the reach of their messages to the general public and secondarily to policymakers and other groups.

Communication can be helped or hindered by relations between the public health system and the news media. It is wise for public health agency staff members to remember at all times that they may not have common goals and objectives compared with the news media. Reporters view themselves as watchdogs for the public but also work in a competitive, entrepreneurial system (8). Reporters may want "the news regardless," whereas the approach of the public health system is often constrained by the dictum of "do no harm." The reporter must meet deadlines whereas the health scientist will work as long as necessary to try to find top-quality results. And the news media and public health often use a different set of terminology making collaboration between public health scientist and professional journalist challenging (8).

Fortunately, the tension created by these points of noncorrespondence between public health and news media can be used to good effect—and with the public as the ultimate beneficiary of the efforts of people in both categories. The interrelationships must be carefully cultivated, gently managed, and constantly reviewed and revised as needed. Table 7–3 lists practical tips for working with the media (8).

Public health practitioners should take a proactive approach when working with the media. It is important to study the patterns and type of reporting in the area and determine which media representatives appear to be most knowledgeable, most responsible, and most effective. It also helps if you have an existing relationship with them before the time that you have information to communicate.

Table 7–3 Checklist for Public Health Practitioners To Use in Dealing with Media Representatives

1. Prepare fact sheets (statements about problem to be discussed) for reporters about all problems to be covered. Keep them updated.
2. Avoid jargon.
3. Respect reporters' deadlines.
4. Always be polite and straightforward.
5. Always tell the truth. If information is not available or unreliable, say so.
6. Always set the single overriding communication objective (SOCO)—the message you need to convey—according to your own agenda, and stick to it. Answer the reporter's questions insofar as possible, but return to your own agenda.
7. If you are not sure about a question (the meaning of the question, or you simply do not hear it), ask the reporter to repeat it.
8. If you do not know an answer, but it is within your area of responsibility, try to find it. If it is outside your area, do not try to answer it. Admit that you do not know.
9. Stick to facts; do not offer your own opinions.
10. Explain the context and relevance of your message (e.g., public health significance).
11. Make notes (or a tape) of the meeting (interview).
12. Provide feedback to the reporter and his or her editor on the results of your interaction.

Source: Churchill, 2000 (*8*).

Practitioners should state clearly and concisely the facts and the desired messages and explain the relative importance of the issues and how they fit into the overall context of public health practice. This is accomplished by writing a press release that summarizes the main finding from the surveillance report and prepared in a standard format that is easily scanned by busy reporters (*see* Table 7–4).

Although communicating surveillance information through the media can reach a large audience, it can sometimes leave the public confused, bewildered, and in the state of "information overload." Organized strategies, with clearly defined communication objectives, are needed to improve the public's understanding of the information and increase the likelihood of achieving the intended outcome (*2*).

Crisis Communication

Surveillance data occasionally reveal public health hazards, such as by detecting infectious disease outbreaks or contaminations in the environment. During these times practitioners must have expertise in crisis communication (*19,31–34*). There are similarities between risk and crisis communication, especially when there has been a specific health condition identified (e.g., a cancer or birth defect cluster) or a specific health event that might result in a feared long-term health concern (e.g., exposure to dioxin resulting from a chemical spill) (*19,33*).

Several principles are key to having a successful experience in crisis communication. First, practitioners must have foresight and planning. In a crisis, the first 24 hours are critical. If you do not provide the facts and the implications of those facts, then the media and the public will speculate and form opinions on

Table 7–4 Tips for Writing Press Releases

1. Make sure the item is of sufficient interest, and scope to make it worthwhile for media representatives to use it.
2. Use the inverted pyramid style of writing: Most important items first, tapering down to detail. The title of the press release will often become the headline of the news story.
3. Open the press release with a summary lead: a paragraph in which you answer Who? What? When? Where? Who cares? and How?
4. Make the news release no longer than two pages. Use short, straightforward sentences. Avoid using jargon or specialized vocabulary.
5. Provide direct quotations, with the source and credentials of that source provided.
6. Consider providing audio or video segments to accompany the news release, if appropriate. If not feasible, supply appropriate still photographs and useful graphic material to illustrate or dramatize the message in the press release.

Source: Adapted from Churchill, 2000 (*8*).

their own (*8,33*). If there are delays in response on the part of the appropriate agency, the media and the public will define the problem for themselves—perhaps inaccurately. It is also important to anticipate or determine how (and when) the media will report the problem so your agency can react calmly or responsibly or make an appropriate announcement before the story appears in the popular media (*8,33*).

Second, agencies should name a primary person (and one who is experienced in media matters) to be the contact person for their organization. Multiple voices, even when delivering the same information, might be perceived as conveying different messages. This contact person should be in a key position (administration or public affairs), have experience in dealing with media, be responsible, remain calm, have a confident manner, and have the ability to speak clearly and convincingly (*8,33*).

Effective crisis communication involves centralized message development and control and the use of a trusted or strong authority figure (e.g., agency director, governor) as a spokesperson in many instances. Frequent communication with policymakers and the affected public, such as through frequent press releases or press conferences, is best because of the intense interest and need for information. The types of information communicated, especially initially, should be simple and short. They should involve a short description of the event, potential health effects, possible explanations (causes), actions being taken by health and other officials to address the problem, and specific actions or steps that affected people should take (*see* Table 7–5).

Politics and Partnerships

Information reported from public health surveillance systems often has political implications, and governmental agencies might be confronted with a potential conflict—between the duty to report the information and the responsibility to support the policies of the administration (*35*). For example, the Wisconsin Division of Public Health produced a minority health report in 2008 (*36*) that

Table 7–5 Guidelines for Dealing with a Health Crisis

The most frequently asked questions by media and public during a public health crisis include:
- What happened?
- When and where?
- Who was involved?
- What caused the situation?
- How was this allowed to happen?
- What are you doing (going to do) about it?
- How much (what kind) of damage is there?
- What safety measures are being (will be) taken?
- Who (what) is to blame?
- Do you (your agency) accept responsibility?
- Has this ever happened before? With what result?
- What do you have to say to those who were injured (endangered, inconvenienced, etc.)?
- How does (will) this problem affect your operations?

Some of the ways to channel the media's interest and efforts include:
- Assisting in pre-crisis education
- Conveying warnings
- Conveying instructions or other information to target audiences
- Reassuring the public
- Defusing inaccurate rumors
- Assisting in the response effort
- Providing health officials with updated information on conditions beyond the health agency
- Soliciting and obtaining help from the outside as needed

Source: Churchill, 2000 *(8)*; Reynolds, 2002 *(33)*

demonstrated significant health disparities among the states' minority populations. Such a report *could* imply that these health disparities were a result of ineffective programs and policies of the political party in power or that conversely that the party in power should be compelled to redirect existing resources to address this public health problem.

Theoretically, the decision to communicate results from a public health surveillance system should not be affected by politics. However, anyone who has worked in a governmental public health agency has experienced this conflict at some time in their career. In the example above, the Wisconsin Division of Public Health released the report but decided to omit any comments about the potential causes of these health disparities or recommended solutions—leaving this work for other organizations and individuals in the state. Public health workers are responsible to communicate public health information but must do so within the bureaucracy—often relying on others to interpret the findings and advocate for change *(35)*.

One strategy to address the political nature of governmental public health agencies is to develop partnerships in states or communities, so that they can help communicate this information effectively. Nongovernmental agencies, such as advocacy groups, health-care organizations, or private institutes, have played an important role in communicating information about the overall health of states and communities *(37)*.

CONCLUSIONS

Translating surveillance data into public health practice requires that information be communicated effectively to a wide variety of audiences. Strategies to communicate surveillance information range from the often chaotic media coverage of published research to well-organized, national public education campaigns. The approaches described above provide a brief introduction to this complex and rapidly evolving field. The challenge remains to use the most effective strategies to effectively communicate surveillance information, ultimately improving the public's health.

PUBLIC HEALTH COMMUNICATION RESOURCES

Centers for Disease Control and Prevention. *CDCynergy, Basic Edition 3.0.* Atlanta, Ga.: Centers for Disease Control and Prevention; 2004.

DHHS (U.S. Department of Health and Human Services). Making Health Communication Programs Work (NIH Pub. No. 02-5145). Bethesda, Md.: National Cancer Institutes, 2002.

Nelson DE, Brownson RC, Remington PL, Parvanta C, eds. Communicating Public Health Information Effectively. Washington D.C.: American Public Health Association, 2002.

Nelson DE, Hesse BW, Croyle RT. Making data talk: communicating public health data to the public, policy makers, and the press. New York: Oxford University Press, 2009.

Schiavo R. *Health Communication: From Theory to Practice.* San Francisco, CA: Jossey-Bass; 2007.

Siegel M, Doner L. *Marketing Public Health: Strategies to Promote Social Change.* 2nd ed. Sudbury, MA: Jones and Bartlett; 2007.

Thompson TL, Dorsey AM, Miller KI, Parrott R, eds. *Handbook of Health Communication.* Mahwah, NJ: Lawrence Erlbaum; 2003.

Witte K. The manipulative nature of health communication research: Ethical issues and guidelines. *Am Behav Sci.* 1994;38(2):285–293.

Wright KB, Sparks L, O'Hair D. *Health Communication in the 21st Century.* Malden, MA: Blackwell; 2008.

REFERENCES

1. Thacker SB, Berkelman RL. Public health surveillance in the United States. *Epidemiol Rev* 1988;10:164–190.

2. Remington PL, Nelson D. Communicating epidemiologic information. In: Brownson, Pettiti, eds. *Applied Epidemiology,* 2nd ed. New York: Oxford University Press; 2006.

3. Remington PL, Simoes E, Brownson RC, Siegel PZ. The role of epidemiology in chronic disease prevention and health promotion programs. *J Public Health Manag Prac* 2003;9(4):258–265.

4. Institute of Medicine, Committee on Health Literacy. *Health literacy: A Prescription to End Confusion.* Washington, DC: National Academy Press; 2004.

5. Association of Schools of Public Health. MPH Core Competency Development Project. http://www.asph.org/document.cfm?page=851. Accessed March 1, 2010.
6. Goodman RA, Foster KL, Gregg MB. Highlights in public health. *MMWR Suppl* 1999;48(LMRK):v–vi.
7. Goodman RA, Remington PL, Howard RJ. Communicating information for action within the public health system. In: Teutsch SM, Churchill RE, eds. *The Principles and Practice of Public Health Surveillance,* 2nd ed. New York: Oxford University Press; 2000.
8. Churchill RE. Using surveillance information in communications, marketing, and advocacy. In: Teutsch SM, Churchill RE, eds. *The Principles and Practice of Public Health Surveillance,* 2nd ed. New York: Oxford University Press; 2000.
9. Centers for Disease Control. Eosinophilia-myalgia syndrome—New Mexico. *MMWR* 1989;38:765–767.
10. Centers for Disease Control and Prevention. Multistate Outbreak of Salmonella Infections Associated with Peanut Butter and Peanut Butter-Containing Products, United States, 2008–2009. *MMWR* 2009;58(Early Release);1–6.
11. Centers for Disease Control and Prevention. Investigation Update: Outbreak of Salmonella Typhimurium Infections, 2008–2009. 2009. http://www.cdc.gov/salmonella/typhimurium/. Accessed March 1, 2010.
12. Centers for Disease Control. Nosocomial transmission of multidrug-resistant tuberculosis among HIV-infected persons—Florida and New York, 1988–1991. *MMWR* 1991;40:585–591.
13. Centers for Disease Control and Prevention. Surveillance of certain health behaviors and conditions among states and selected local areas—Behavioral Risk Factor Surveillance System (BRFSS), United States, 2006. *MMWR Surveill Summ* 2008;57(SS07):1–188.
14. Remington PL, Smith MY, Williamson DF, Anda RF, Gentry EM, Hogelin GC. Design, characteristics, and usefulness of state–based risk factor surveillance 1981–1986. *Public Health Rep* 1988;103(4):366–375.
15. Mokdad AH. Serdula MK, Dietz WH, Bowman BA, Marks JS, Koplan JP. The spread of the obesity epidemic in the United States, 1991–1998. *JAMA* 1999;282:1519–1522.
16. Russell A, Langlois T, Johnson G, Trentham-Dietz A, Remington P. Increasing gap in breast cancer mortality between white and black women. *WI Med J* 1999;98(8):37–39.
17. McElroy JA, Remington PL, Gangnon RE, Hariharan L, Andersen LD. Identifying geographic disparities in the early detection of breast cancer using a geographic information system. *Prev Chronic Dis* 2006;3(1):A10.
18. Remington PL, Goodman RA. Chronic disease surveillance. In: Brownson RC, Remington PL, Davis JR, eds. *Chronic Disease Epidemiology and Control,* 2nd ed. Washington, DC: American Public Health Association; 1998.
19. Nelson DE, Hesse BW, Croyle RT. *Making Data Talk: Communicating Public Health Data to the Public, Policy Makers, and the Press.* New York: Oxford University Press; 2009.
20. Parvanta C, Maibach E, Arkin E, Nelson DE, Woodward J. Public health communication: a planning framework. In: Nelson DE, Brownson RC, Remington PL, Parvanta C, eds. *Communicating Public Health Information Effectively: A Guide for Practitioners.* Washington, DC: American Public Health Association; 2002.
21. Riegelman RK. *Studying a Study and Testing a Test: How to Read the Medical Evidence,* 5th ed. Philadelphia: Lippincott Williams & Wilkins; 2005.

22. Centers for Disease Control and Prevention. Multistate outbreak of Salmonella Serotype Tennessee infections associated with peanut butter—United States, 2006—2007. *MMWR* 2007;56(21);521–524.

23. Higginson J, Chu F. Ethical consideration and responsibilities in communicating health risk information. *J Clin Epidemiol* 1991;44(Suppl 1):S51–S56.

24. Witte K. The manipulative nature of health communication research: ethical issues and guidelines. *Am Behav Sci* 1994;38(2):285–293.

25. Brownson RC, Malone BR. Communicating public health information to policy makers. In: Nelson DE, Brownson RC, Remington PL, Parvanta C, eds., *Communicating Public Health Information Effectively.* Washington, DC: American Public Health Association; 2002:97–114.

26. Kutner M, Greenberg E, Jin Y, *et al.* Literacy in Everyday Life: Results from the 2003 National Assessment of Adult Literacy. Report No. (NCES) 2007–480. Washington, DC: U.S. Department of Education; 2007.

27. Greenwell M. Communicating public health information to the news media. In: Nelson DE, Brownson RC, Remington PL, Parvanta C, eds. *Communicating Public Health Information Effectively.* Washington, DC: American Public Health Association; 2002:73–96.

28. Nelson DE. Translating public health data. In: Nelson DE, Brownson RC, Remington PL, Parvanta C, eds. *Communicating Public Health Information Effectively.* Washington, DC: American Public Health Association; 2002:33–45.

29. Hornik RC. *Public Health Communication: Evidence for Behavior Change.* Mahwah, NJ: L. Erlbaum Associates; 2002.

30. Rice RE, Atkin CK, eds. *Public Communication Campaigns*, 3rd ed. Thousand Oaks, CA: Sage; 2001.

31. Coombs WT. *Ongoing Crisis Communication: Planning, Managing, and Responding,* 2nd ed. Thousand Oaks, CA: Sage; 2007.

32. Fearn-Banks K. *Crisis Communications: A Casebook Approach,* 3rd ed. Mahwah, NJ: Erlbaum; 2007.

33. Centers for Disease Control and Prevention. Public health emergency response guide for state, local, and tribal public health directors. Version 1.0. Department of Health and Human Services. www.bt.cdc.gov/planning/pdf/cdcresponseguide.pdf. Accessed March 1, 2010.

34. Seeger MW, Sellnow MW, Ullmer RL. *Crisis Communication and the Public Health.* Cresskill, NJ: Hampton Press; 2008.

35. Regidor E, de la Fuente L, Gutiérrez-Fisac JL, *et al.* The role of the public health official in communicating public health information. *Am J Public Health* 2007;97(No. S1):S93–S97.

36. Wisconsin Division of Public Health. Minority Health Report, 2001–2005. Wisconsin Department of Health and Family Services, Madison, Wisconsin. January, 2008.

37. Remington P, Ahrens D. Communicating to private and voluntary health agencies. In: Nelson DE, Brownson RC, Remington PL, Parvanta C, eds. *Communicating Public Health Information Effectively.* Washington, DC: American Public Health Association; 2002:115–126.

8

Evaluating Public Health Surveillance

SAMUEL L. GROSECLOSE, ROBERT R. GERMAN, AND PETER NSUBUGA

> *There is nothing so terrible as activity without insight.*
> —Johann Wolfgang von Goethe

INTRODUCTION

As new outcomes of public health importance emerge and others become amenable to intervention, detection, and monitoring, the spectrum of health-related events considered for surveillance evolves. Typically, public health funding for surveillance and response has not grown to meet new information requirements. Therefore, the need to seek efficiencies in our surveillance efforts increases.

The purpose of evaluating public health surveillance systems is to ensure that problems of public health importance are being monitored efficiently and effectively. Public health surveillance systems should be evaluated periodically to determine how well they operate to meet their stated purposes and objectives. Evaluation findings should yield specific recommendations for improving surveillance quality, efficiency, and usefulness.

In addition to periodic evaluation, public health surveillance systems should be monitored routinely to ensure they continue to meet their objectives. Monitoring is done by ongoing measurement and tracking of progress toward achievement of the stated objectives of the surveillance system. Monitoring provides information that the evaluator can use to aid in decisions on improvements of the surveillance system. This chapter describes public health surveillance system monitoring and evaluation and the tasks involved in public health surveillance system evaluation, including:

- Engaging system stakeholders in the evaluation;
- Describing the surveillance system being evaluated;
- Focusing the evaluation design;
- Gathering credible evidence regarding surveillance system performance;
- Justifying and stating conclusions and recommendations; and
- Ensuring the use of evaluation findings (Table 8–1; ref. *1*).

Table 8–1 Checklist for Evaluating Public Health Surveillance Systems*

Task A. Engage the stakeholders in the evaluation

Task B. Describe the surveillance system to be evaluated
  1. Describe the public health importance of the health-related event under surveillance
     a. Indices of frequency
     b. Indices of severity
     c. Disparities or inequities associated with the health-related event
     d. Costs associated with the health-related event
     e. Preventability
     f. Potential future clinical course in the absence of an intervention
     g. Public interest

  2. Describe the purpose and operation of the surveillance system
     a. Purpose and objectives of the system
     b. Planned uses of the data from the system
     c. Health-related event under surveillance, including case definition
     d. Legal authority for data collection
     e. Organizational location of the system and system governance or management
     f. Level of organizational, informatics, or data integration with other systems
     g. Flow chart of system
           1) System inputs and outputs
           2) Stakeholder organizations and roles
           3) Information and technical architecture
     h. Components of system
           1) Population under surveillance
           2) Period of time of data collection
           3) Data collection methods
           4) Reporting sources of data
           5) Data management protocols
           6) Information technology(ies) used to support surveillance processes
           7) Data analysis and dissemination protocols
           8) Surveillance monitoring indicators and protocol
           9) Patient privacy, data confidentiality, and system security
          10) Records management and data release protocols

  3. Describe the resources used to operate the surveillance system
     a. Funding source(s)
     b. Personnel requirements
     c. Information technology resources
     d. Other resources

Task C. Focus the evaluation design
  1. Determine the specific purpose and scope of the evaluation
  2. Identify stakeholders who will receive the findings and implement recommendations of the evaluation
  3. Consider what will be done with the information generated from the evaluation
  4. Specify the questions that will be answered by the evaluation
  5. Determine standards for assessing the performance of the system

Task D. Gather credible evidence regarding the performance of the surveillance system
  1. Indicate the level of usefulness
  2. Describe each surveillance system attribute

(continued)

Table 8–1 (*continued*)

a. Simplicity
b. Flexibility
c. Data quality
d. Acceptability
e. Sensitivity
f. Predictive value positive
g. Representativeness
h. Timeliness
i. Stability
3. Describe informatics characteristics of surveillance information system
a. Information quality
b. System quality
c. User experience and service quality

Task E. Justify and state conclusions, and make recommendations
Task F. Ensure use of evaluation findings and share lessons learned

---

* Adapted from ref. *1*.

SURVEILLANCE MONITORING AND EVALUATION

Monitoring can be defined as the *routine* process of data collection and measurement of program or process changes over time using previously agreed-upon plans and schedules. Discrepancies between actual and planned implementation are identified and corrective actions are taken. In the case of a public health surveillance system, monitoring involves *routine* collection and analysis of indicators to measure how well the surveillance system is achieving its objectives (*2*). Evaluation, on the other hand, includes the use of specific study designs to assess *periodically* the relevance, effectiveness, and the impact of the surveillance system. Evaluations are often done in response to a change in the quality of the performance of the public health surveillance system, which is often observed during monitoring, or because there is a need to ensure that quality is maintained. In both monitoring and evaluation, the expected outcome is recommendations to improve surveillance activities. When the results of routine monitoring are used to track the effects or impact of the public health surveillance system, then monitoring can be referred to as *ongoing evaluation.*

Monitoring is performed using public health surveillance and response indicators that reflect surveillance performance (e.g., the timeliness and completeness of reports or timeliness and effectiveness of response [usefulness]) (*3*). Surveillance indicators generally depend on the type of health event that is under surveillance or the type of public health surveillance system that is being implemented (e.g., integrated [i.e., multiple outcomes concurrently monitored] or health event-specific) (*3–6*). To be useful, indicators, like good objectives, must be:

- specific in their scope,
- measurable by the operators of the system,

- achievable in the setting where the system is working,
- relevant to the setting in which the system operates, and
- obtainable in a timely manner.

Thus, the necessary changes can be made to improve system performance and data usefulness to yield improved health status. Indicators should have a defined performance target and a protocol or algorithm to identify and respond to causes of missed targets (*3,7*).

Indicators can be used to track and measure public health surveillance and response inputs, the processes, the immediate outputs, the eventual outcomes, and the impact of the systems on the condition under surveillance and the health of the public. Often, a few indicators are selected from each of the groups (i.e., inputs, processes, outputs, outcomes, impact) to track the progress on the "health" of a surveillance system (Table 8–2).

Public health surveillance is conducted within a broader public health system that requires the application of surveillance data for public health action within an infrastructure supporting prevention programs. Surveillance systems are supported by—and therefore their performance is influenced by—data providers, health-care providers, diagnostic laboratories, and organizational logistics. Functional public health surveillance systems support the following core activities: detection; confirmation and registration of case-patients; reporting or notification; data analysis and interpretation; and feedback and dissemination. These core activities, the associated response capacity and performance, and managerial and support functions can be evaluated together with the traditional surveillance system attributes (e.g., sensitivity, flexibility, timeliness, representativeness) (*2,8–12*).

Conceptualizing surveillance improvement as a process implies the need to measure changes in system performance indicators (routine monitoring) and surveillance attributes (episodic evaluation). Both surveillance monitoring and evaluation should be well-documented, systematic, and planned processes with measurable performance objectives. Each requires definition of outcomes and indicators and strategies to track and measure those outcomes over time. In the absence of routine monitoring, many surveillance evaluations are conducted with few quantitative data available to support assessment of key surveillance system attributes (e.g., sensitivity or timeliness [Epidemic Intelligence Service Officers' surveillance system evaluations, Centers for Disease Control and Prevention, October 2007, unpublished data]). Performance indicators are not static; they are often reformulated based on evaluation findings. Surveillance monitoring data or organizational priorities might indicate where more comprehensive evaluation is needed.

STAKEHOLDER INVOLVEMENT

Early in the evaluation planning process, the system stakeholders should be engaged in a discussion to ensure that the evaluation of a public health surveillance system addresses appropriate questions and assesses pertinent attributes and that its findings will be acceptable and useful. In that context, we define stakeholders as

Table 8–2 Examples of Surveillance Monitoring and Evaluation Indicators Used by Selected Surveillance Systems

Surveillance system	Surveillance indicator	Process or outcome indicator?
Integrated Disease Surveillance and Response (3)	Proportion of health facilities submitting weekly or monthly surveillance reports on time to the district level	Process
	Proportion of investigated outbreaks with laboratory confirmation	Process
	Attack rates for outbreaks of epidemic-prone diseases	Outcome
Human immunodeficiency virus/Acquired Immunodeficiency Syndrome surveillance (4)	Routine record linkage of HIV/AIDS case reports (all cases without minimum death information) and death certificate records (most recent year of deaths available), once a year (minimum)	Process
	≥85% of expected number of cases for a diagnosis year reported by 12 months after the diagnosis year	Outcome
	Risk factor ascertainment ≥85% of reported cases or a representative sample for a diagnosis year have an identified HIV risk factor within 12 months after the date of the initial HIV/AIDS case report, measured at 12 months after the diagnosis year	Outcome
Outbreak and early event detection systems (5)	Proportion of outbreaks with documentation of dates of selected outbreak detection and response processes (e.g., date of laboratory confirmation of diagnosis, date of report to public health authority) to support assessment of timeliness	Process
	Number of primary and secondary cases associated with the outbreak	Outcome
	Number of health-care workers infected during outbreak	Outcome
National measles, mumps, and rubella surveillance (6)	Proportion of confirmed cases reported to Nationally Notifiable Disease Surveillance System with complete information	Outcome
	Interval between date of symptom onset and date of public health notification	Outcome
	Proportion of confirmed cases that are laboratory-confirmed	Outcome

those persons or organizations who use data for the promotion of healthy lifestyles and the prevention and control of disease, injury, disability, or exposure to environmental hazards. Stakeholders who might be interested in defining questions to be addressed by the surveillance system evaluation and subsequently using the findings include public health practitioners; health-care providers; data providers and users; representatives of affected communities; governments at the local, state, and federal levels; and professional and private nonprofit organizations (1). Ideally, both surveillance system sponsors and other stakeholders participate as active partners in the evaluation process—motivated to champion evaluation activities and to improve their processes based on the findings.

As the public's demand for health information increases and as new health-related data become accessible, public health surveillance partnerships and networks might include new stakeholders expressing unique information needs (e.g., community health systems interested in supporting early public health response or pandemic preparedness (*13*), biologics and pharmaceutical manufacturers, and patient advocacy groups (*14*) . Regardless of stakeholders' information needs, however, the evaluation must first determine whether the surveillance system meets its primary objectives. Because of the collaborative nature of public health surveillance practice, stakeholders' needs and concerns must be taken into account during system design and evaluation. It might be feasible to investigate what it will take, in terms of process modification or resources, to address one or more stakeholders' new or unique information needs. In some situations, incremental, integrated efforts result in increased surveillance efficiency (e.g., pilot expansion of the National Electronic Injury Surveillance System in 2002 to support the monitoring of outpatient adverse drug events treated in emergency departments) (*15*).

SURVEILLANCE SYSTEM DESCRIPTION

Public Health Importance

The first step in evaluating a surveillance system is to answer the question, "Should this health event be under surveillance?" This question should be answered from a perspective external to the surveillance system itself (*see also* Chapters 2 and 3). It should also be asked when deciding whether to start a new system or before conducting a detailed evaluation of an existing one. This is done primarily to assess the public health importance of a health event. Once a health event is identified of high priority, it is important to consider both the options for data sources and surveillance methods, feasibility, and cost of conducting surveillance for that event. If this assessment leads to a decision to discontinue or not to start a surveillance system, a detailed evaluation of that system becomes superfluous.

The public health importance of a health event and the need for surveillance of that health event can be described in a variety of ways. Health events that affect many people or require large expenditures of resources are clearly important in a public health context. However, health events that affect relatively few persons might also be important, especially if the events cluster in time and place (e.g., a limited outbreak of a severe disease). At other times, public concerns might focus attention on a particular health event, creating or heightening the sense of importance associated with it (e.g., enhanced surveillance during high-profile community events) (*16,17*). In addition, the public health importance of a health event is influenced by its preventability and the ability of public health action to prevent or control the event.

Efforts have been made to quantify the public health importance of health conditions and to prioritize public health interventions (*18–20*). Parameters for measuring the importance of a health-related event—and therefore the public health surveillance system with which it is monitored—can include:

- indices of frequency (e.g., the total number of cases and/or deaths; incidence rates, prevalence, or mortality rates);
- summary measures of population health status (e.g., disability-adjusted life years [DALYS]) (20,21);
- indices of severity (e.g., case-fatality rates, hospitalization rates, disability rates) (22);
- disparities or inequities associated with the health-related event (23);
- costs associated with the health-related event;
- preventability (24);
- beneficial health effects of programs that must be sustained to protect health (e.g., immunization programs) (25); and
- public interest.

Measures of importance used should account for the effect of previously implemented prevention strategies on the occurrence of the health event. For example, in the United States, the number of cases of vaccine-preventable illness has declined following the implementation of school immunization laws, and the public health importance of vaccine-preventable diseases in jurisdictions with adequate vaccine coverage is underestimated by case counts alone (18). In such instances, it might be possible to estimate the number of cases that would be expected in the absence of control programs.

Preventability can be defined at several levels, including primary prevention (i.e., preventing the occurrence of disease or other health-related event), secondary prevention (i.e., early detection and intervention with the aim of reversing, halting, or at least retarding the progress of a condition), and tertiary prevention (i.e., minimizing the effects of disease and disability among persons already ill). For infectious diseases, preventability can also be described as reducing the secondary attack rate or the number of cases transmitted to contacts of the primary case. From the perspective of surveillance, preventability reflects the potential for effective interventions at any of these levels.

The need for surveillance might also be affected by factors other than those mentioned above. Political and public pressure might affect whether surveillance is undertaken—or, at the other extreme, forbidden—for a specific health event. Regulations, laws, and public health programs might be implemented on the basis of considerations other than those listed above. However, it is still important to make the surveillance objectives and scientific criteria for evaluation as clear and explicit as possible. Even when using quantitative measures, judgment is necessary to decide which criteria are most relevant for assessing the importance of each condition. It is important to make these judgments as explicit—and as early—as possible.

Purpose and Objectives

The purpose of the surveillance system indicates why the system exists; its objectives relate to how the data are used for public health action. For example, data from a public health surveillance system can be used to:

- guide immediate action for cases of public health importance;
- measure the burden of a disease (or other health-related event), including changes in related factors, the identification of populations at high risk, and the identification of new or emerging health concerns;
- monitor trends in the burden of a disease or other health-related event;
- support early detection and response to outbreaks or emerging threats;
- guide the planning, implementation, and evaluation of programs to prevent and control disease, injury, disability, or exposure to environmental hazards;
- inform risk management and decision making by contributing health, hazard, and threat data to support an integrated picture of a community's health and threat environment (situation awareness) (26);
- provide reassurance during periods of perceived increased risk that incidence of a health condition is not increasing (26,27);
- evaluate public policy;
- detect changes in health practices and the effects of these changes;
- prioritize the allocation of health resources;
- describe the clinical course of disease; and
- provide a basis for epidemiologic research.

The purpose and objectives of the system, including the planned uses of its data, establish a frame of reference for evaluating specific components. However, during evaluation of an established surveillance system, clearly documented purposes and objectives for the system might not be found. In this situation, one group of investigators identified objectives by observing the current outputs from the system and validated the candidate objectives by getting input from stakeholders (28).

Each public health surveillance system requires a clear case definition for the health-related event or exposure under surveillance (see Chapter 4). The case definition of a health-related event can include clinical manifestations (i.e., symptoms and signs); laboratory, radiologic, or other diagnostic clinical findings; and epidemiologic information (e.g., person, place, and time). Case definitions may also be further specified based on level of certainty (e.g., confirmed/definite, probable/presumptive, or possible/suspected). The specification and use of a standard case definition increases the specificity of reporting and improves the comparability of the health-related event reported from different sources of data and from different geographic areas. When the health event can be monitored using different data sources, case definitions should be specified for each data source to categorize the health event using each source's information data type (e.g., by ICD-9-CM code representation, self-reported survey question responses, or reported clinical and laboratory information, as illustrated by the asthma surveillance case definitions outlined in Table 8–3) (29).

Surveillance case definitions exist for a variety of health-related events, including diseases, injuries, adverse exposures, and risk or protective behaviors. For example, in the United States, the Centers for Disease Control and Prevention and the Council of State and Territorial Epidemiologists have agreed on standard definitions for selected occupational health and chronic disease indicators and infectious conditions and periodically update them (30–32).

Table 8–3 Sample Case Definition: Asthma Surveillance Case Definitions by Data Source

Data source	Surveillance case definition categories			Recommendations
	Confirmed	Probable	Suspect/Possible	
Vital statistics and administrative data: mortality and hospital discharge classification	Not applicable.	Mortality: ICD-9/-10* diagnostic code for asthma as *underlying* cause of death. Hospital records: ICD-9-CM** diagnostic code for asthma as *primary diagnosis*.	Mortality: ICD-9/-10 diagnostic code for asthma as *contributing* cause of death. Hospital records: ICD-9-CM diagnostic code for asthma as *secondary diagnosis*. In children <12 years, include diagnostic codes for bronchiolitis and chronic bronchitis.	For data sources using ICD-coded data, periodically review additional ICD codes that might represent misdiagnoses to assess potential changes in diagnostic code distributions over time. To validate surveillance findings, programs are encouraged to periodically review clinical record data. Where applicable, confirmed and probable cases should be combined for asthma case counts. Physician reporting and asthma registries are not recommended surveillance methods.
Survey self-response: prevalence classification	Not applicable.	Lifetime asthma: If "Yes" to "Did a doctor ever tell you that you had asthma?" Current asthma: If "Yes" to "Did a doctor ever tell you that you had asthma?" AND "Do you still have asthma?"	Reports taking prescription or over-the-counter medication for asthma in past year OR wheezing episodes in past year?	

| Clinical records: medical and laboratory classification | Meets clinical criteria three (3) times in past year and at least one laboratory criterion. | Meets one of the following: if no lab information available, evidence of clinical criteria three (3) times in past year OR if no clinical information, meets at least one laboratory criterion OR, if no clinical or lab information available, reports taking prescription medication for asthma in past year. | Suggestive laboratory criteria OR suggestive clinical criteria. |

* ICD-9/-10: International Classification of Diseases, Ninth Revision; International Classification of Diseases, Tenth Revision

** ICD-9-CM: International Classification of Diseases, Ninth Revision, Clinical Modification

When possible, a public health surveillance system should use an established surveillance case definition, and if it does not, an explanation should be provided. Case definitions should be modified whenever new knowledge on the epidemiology, pathogenesis, or other relevant factors becomes available.

Operation and Components of the System

The evaluation of the public health surveillance system needs to include an accurate and reliable description of the system's operation and the business processes conducted to accomplish its purpose and objectives. Understanding how well the system is meeting its objectives is important to provide evidence for prevention and control efforts, including policy decisions. The description of the system should discuss its organizational location and governance, its linkages to or dependence on other information systems or processes, and its processes and functions supporting public health action.

In addition to the surveillance system characteristics described above, the system description should:

- Cite any legal authority for the data collection.
- Describe the organization(s) sponsoring and contributing to the system, including the political, administrative, geographic, or social context in which the system evaluation will be done.
- Describe the level of organizational, informatics, or data integration with other systems (*33*). Organizational integration refers to the structures and policies that govern information management and those system features that promote a public health enterprise- or systems-wide perspective to align, streamline, and improve surveillance and monitoring processes within the organization (*34*). Informatics integration refers to the system's use of information technologies and other informatics standards and best practices that promote interoperability, improve data quality or timeliness, support surveillance processes, and enhance surveillance efficiency. Data integration refers to the system's use of data standards or data mapping, transformation, or linkage methods to support sharing of data between surveillance information systems to create new knowledge.
- Describe system inputs and outputs, data flow, and surveillance processes and associated stakeholders' roles through use of a system flow chart (e.g., Fig. 8–1). A description of system inputs might include specification of types of data reported, surveillance data sources, or data variables and formats; outputs include indicator monitoring, data quality, or descriptive epidemiology reports. If one is evaluating the informatics aspects of the surveillance system, then a more detailed description of surveillance tasks, roles and responsibilities, and system functionality should be provided to allow identification of business processes amenable to performance improvement (*see* below). A surveillance business process is a set of related work tasks designed to address a desired surveillance objective or support a required surveillance process or activity (*35*).

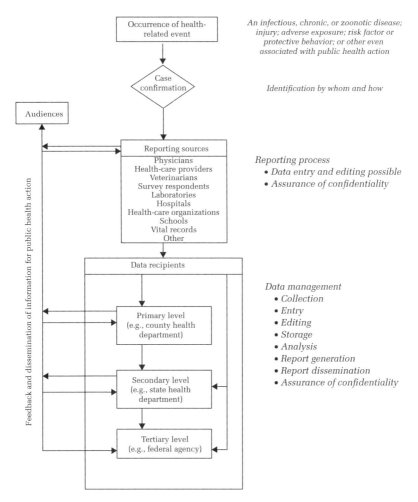

Figure 8–1 Simplified flow chart for a generic surveillance system.

The evaluation should address the following questions:

- What is the population under surveillance? What subgroups, if any, are excluded?
- What is the period of data collection?
- What data are collected and how are they collected?
- What are the reporting sources of data for the system?
- How are the system's data managed (e.g., the transfer, entry, editing, transformation, storage, and back-up of data)? Does the system comply with applicable standards for data formats and coding schemes? If not, why?
- What information technologies are used to support surveillance data collection, reporting, analysis, interpretation, and dissemination?
- How are the system's data analyzed and disseminated? How frequently? To whom? For what purpose?

- What policies and procedures are in place to ensure patient privacy, data confidentiality, and system security?
- What is the policy and procedure for releasing data? Do these procedures comply with applicable laws, statutes, and regulations? If not, why?
- Does the system comply with an applicable records management program? For example, are the system's records properly audited, archived, and/or disposed of?

Listing the discrete steps that are taken in processing the health event reports by the system and then depicting these steps in a flow chart is often useful (e.g., Fig. 8–1). The roles and surveillance process responsibilities of the stakeholders that support the system could be included in this chart (e.g., What is the workflow? What tasks are performed and by whom?) (36). The depiction of the system's information architecture and data flow should be detailed sufficiently to explain all of the system's operational characteristics, including average times between process steps and data transfers.

The influence of information technology on system performance should be described, including the hardware environment, software tools, user interface, data security, and use of standard data formats and coding to facilitate efficient data interchange, linkage, or de-duplication within the system or to other systems. Additional considerations for evaluation of informatics attributes of the system are discussed in the next section.

The data analysis description might indicate who analyzes and interprets the data, how often analyses are performed, the objective(s) of the analysis (e.g., burden assessment, trend monitoring, outbreak detection, or identification of high-risk subpopulations), and the types of data output generated. This description could also address the data analysis and visualization methods used and how the system ensures that appropriate methods are used to analyze the data (see Chapter 6).

The public health surveillance system should operate in a manner that allows effective dissemination of health data so that decision makers at all levels can readily understand the implications of the information (see Chapter 7). Audiences for public health surveillance data and information include public health practitioners, health-care providers, members of affected communities, professional and voluntary organizations, policymakers, the press, and the general public. Dependent on the audience, options for disseminating data or information from the system include electronic data interchange; public-use data files; the Internet; press releases; newsletters; bulletins; routine and special-focus surveillance reports; secure peer-to-peer collaboration networks; publication in scientific, peer-reviewed journals; and poster and oral presentations, including those at individual, community, and professional meetings. Periodic surveys of users of the system's data and information products can assess how and by whom they are being used and might identify additional information requirements.

Public health agencies are authorized to collect personal health data about individuals to support public health prevention and control and thus have an ethical obligation to protect against inappropriate use or release of that data (see chapter 9).

The protection of patient privacy (recognition of a person's right not to share information about him or herself), data confidentiality (assurance of authorized data sharing), and system security (assurance of authorized system access) are essential to maintaining the credibility of any surveillance system. Physical, administrative, operational, and computer safeguards for securing the system and protecting and releasing its data must allow authorized access while denying access by unauthorized users. Such safeguards and associated policies should be reviewed as part of the evaluation and judged for adequacy. To ensure that data are used to their full potential, that work is not duplicated, and that funds are not spent unnecessarily, surveillance data should be released or shared in accordance with the objectives and conditions under which the data were collected or obtained. The surveillance system's policies and procedures for data release should be obtained and reviewed.

Resources Used to Operate the System

With limited public health funding for detection and response, assessment of resources devoted to surveillance is critical. Different types of costs might be determined during a surveillance evaluation depending on the evaluation design and purpose and include:

- *Direct costs*: those personnel and material resources required for operation of surveillance (e.g., data provider or public health system person-time expended per year of operation [by discipline and associated salary and benefits cost], travel, training, information dissemination, information technology hardware, software, and support);
- *Indirect costs*: those costs that result from preparedness and response to surveillance findings (e.g., follow-up diagnostic laboratory tests; community information, education, and communication activities; case management; and outbreak response) (*37*); and
- *Prevention benefits or costs from societal perspective*: cost estimates of the effect of the system and the information generated on decision making, treatment, care, prevention, education, or research (e.g., cost of responding to false alarms; cost of missing outbreaks; and productivity losses averted) (*38*).

The assessment of the system's operational resources should not be done in isolation of the program or initiative that relies on the public health surveillance system. A more formal economic evaluation of the system (e.g., judging costs relative to benefits) could be included with the resource description. For example, investigators have modeled the expected future costs of different strategies for continued vaccination, surveillance, and other activities supporting polio risk management after eradication to provide information for policy formulation (*39*). However, because of the complexity of the public health surveillance and response processes, it is usually difficult to define indirect costs attributable to surveillance activities or to model cost-savings in the presence (or absence) of surveillance programs. Therefore, assessment of surveillance resources typically focuses on only those personnel and material resources required for the operation of the system (i.e., direct costs).

If evaluating a system early in its developmental lifecycle, it is useful to differentiate direct costs associated with the system development and implementation phases from ongoing operating costs to provide insight into system feasibility and sustainability (40). When considering the cost or acceptability of surveillance systems, it is also relevant to consider whether the system serves more than one function—does it allow the monitoring of multiple health outcomes (i.e., marginal cost perspective), or can it be used for both routine notifiable disease surveillance and outbreak detection (i.e., dual-use systems) (41,42). To monitor investment and implementation costs of the World Health Organization's Integrated Disease Surveillance and Response (IDSR) strategy, task force members developed a spreadsheet tool, SurvCost, for measuring the incremental or additional costs of establishing and subsequently operating IDSR-related activities (37). The tool follows a cost analysis method to gather and structure information about the existing program costs, including direct costs for surveillance. Structured cost data for surveillance system processes can be used to identify more cost-effective program strategies and to forecast future program resource needs.

FOCUSING THE EVALUATION DESIGN

An evaluation of a public health surveillance system is often done by a small team consisting of a field epidemiologist and a few other public health workers, many times as part of a training activity. This small team might engage other stakeholders in the course of the evaluation, especially if there is need to evaluate activities across different levels of the health system. However, in some situations the surveillance evaluation is a major event with several public health personnel with different skills (e.g., field epidemiology, public health laboratory practice, data analysis, informatics, and program management) working together in teams to obtain a representative estimate of the performance of the public health surveillance system or systems in a jurisdiction often as the precursor to major surveillance and response reform (11). Whether the evaluation is a part of a large reform effort or it is a small undertaking, stakeholders should be engaged and the following steps should be followed to obtain credible results:

- planning for the evaluation (including assembling and reviewing existing information and developing surveillance attribute performance measures and key questions, clear terms of reference, and an evaluation protocol);
- conducting the evaluation (including developing or adapting and pretesting evaluation tools and formats, collecting, and analyzing and interpreting data);
- creating a plan for change based on the results of the evaluation (including disseminating the plan appropriately); and
- following-up that plan to ensure that change happens with a robust monitoring plan, routine monitoring activities, and interim evaluations.

Recent public health surveillance evaluation guidance (*1,2,27*) has described evaluation of core surveillance processes, support functions, and system attributes within the public health system. Although comprehensive evaluation requires consideration of each of these domains, each evaluation should be individually tailored because surveillance systems vary in scope, methods, and objectives. Few evaluations address fully all of the metrics outlined in this chapter, and many profitably focus on only one or two major attributes, such as sensitivity and timeliness (*42–48*).

Depending on the specific purpose of the evaluation, its design could be straightforward or complex. An effective evaluation design is contingent on *(1)* its specific purpose being understood by all of the stakeholders in the evaluation; *(2)* detailed knowledge of the information needs of stakeholders and surveillance business processes that must be supported; and *(3)* the commitment of stakeholders to use the information generated from it. In addition, when multiple stakeholders are involved, agreements that clarify their roles and responsibilities prior to and following the evaluation might need to be established among those who are implementing the evaluation.

Standards for assessing how the public health surveillance system performs establish what the system must accomplish to be considered successful in meeting its objectives. Ideally, system users specify the target performance standards for the system's attributes during system design (e.g., what levels of timeliness or representativeness are relevant for the system, given its objectives?). If target performance standards are not available, define them before initiating the evaluation. Information useful for defining relevant standards for assessment of the surveillance system's performance can be derived from a review of the current scientific literature on the health-related event under surveillance or via interview of system stakeholders to define systematically the key surveillance tasks, information needs, and required system functionality (*41*). Evaluation data might be obtained by the evaluation team using a mix of qualitative approaches (e.g., key informant interviews and observations) and quantitative methods (e.g., measuring the average elapsed time in surveillance processes to determine timeliness). As surveillance practice evolves, so do evaluation methods. For example, to assess quantitatively the effectiveness of a syndromic surveillance system's alerting algorithm for early detection, some investigators have used simulated outbreak data superimposed onto real surveillance data as data from real outbreaks are typically not in the form or quantity needed (*26,27*). Such approaches enable efficient evaluation of the algorithm's performance across a range of types of outbreak signals.

ASSESSING THE SURVEILLANCE ATTRIBUTES OF THE SYSTEM

A public health surveillance system has attributes that characterize its role in public health action. Credible evidence of the system's performance includes quantitative and qualitative indicator data that determine strengths and weaknesses. The interdependence of the system's attributes reflect the public health mission of the system, and some attributes might be more important than others. For example, some systems might require rapid responses to prevent death and disability (*49*). Many potential sources of evidence regarding the system's performance exist, including consultations with professionals associated with the system and reports on its performance.

Surveillance system attributes can include simplicity, flexibility, data quality, acceptability, sensitivity (also referred to as completeness), predictive value positive (PVP), representativeness, timeliness, and stability. Table 8–4 summarizes definitions of these attributes and methods to compute them (*1*).

A complex system in public health action can involve several attributes, plus any system-specific attributes not listed here, making their combined assessment more involved than a simpler system, which is often more flexible. A literature review can be helpful in determining which attributes are relevant in evaluating the system. Yet, attributes must be measured in context, such as using the relevant gold standard or referent (e.g., review of medical records or registry data) in determining what is timely or acceptable when calculating sensitivity and PVP (Table 8–5). Qualitative measurement of some attributes (e.g., acceptability, flexibility, or simplicity) might be necessary.

The calculation of sensitivity and PVP typically requires the collection of, or access to, data external to the surveillance system (*1*). Yet the measurement of these attributes is often based on the best available data from the system. Examples of data types used as gold standards for estimating surveillance information sensitivities and PVPs include data from medical records, health claims logs, other health registries, vital statistics records, unduplicated databases from merging multiple data sources, telephone interviews, enhanced surveillance (such as follow-up of cases), and physical examinations (*50*). For a variety of health events under surveillance (e.g., birth defects, injuries, poliomyelitis, sexually transmitted diseases, and tetanus) total cases have been estimated, for example, using capture–recapture methods (*50,51*).

System attributes are related to each other. Data of poor quality make the system less acceptable and its data less representative of the population under surveillance. Strengthening one system attribute could adversely affect another attribute of a higher priority. The points at which bias can enter a surveillance system and decrease representativeness are illustrated in Figure 8–2. Efforts to improve sensitivity, PVP, representativeness, timeliness, and stability can increase the cost of a surveillance system, although savings in efficiency through use of information technology (e.g., electronic reporting) might offset some of these costs. As sensitivity and PVP approach 100%, a system is more likely to be representative of the population with the event under surveillance. However, as sensitivity increases, PVP might decrease.

ASSESSING THE INFORMATICS ATTRIBUTES OF THE SYSTEM

As information technologies are increasingly used to support public health surveillance, one must consider the impact of informatics and information technology

Table 8–4 Summary of Surveillance System Attributes*

Attribute	Definition	Methods
Simplicity	Refers to the system's structure and ease of operation. Systems should be as simple as possible.	Measures for determining simplicity include but are not limited to: Amount and type of data necessary to establish occurrence of the health-related event; amount and type of other data on cases; number of organizations involved in receiving case reports; integration with other systems; data collection, management, analysis, and dissemination procedures; amount of follow-up to update case data; staff training requirements; and time spent on maintaining the system.
Flexibility	Ability to adapt to changing information needs or technological operating conditions with little additional time, personnel, or allocated funds.	Probably best evaluated retrospectively by observing how a system has responded to new demand, such as changes in case definitions, information technology, funding, or reporting sources.
Data quality	Refers to the completeness and validity of the data recorded in the system.	Measures for determining data quality include percentages of "unknown," invalid, and missing responses to items on data collection forms. In addition, data quality can be measured by applying edits for consistency in the data. However, a full assessment may require a special study.
Acceptability	Reflects the willingness of persons and organizations to participate in the system.	Measures for determining acceptability include: Subject or agency participation rate; interview completion rates and question refusal rates; completeness of reporting forms; physician, laboratory, or hospital/facility reporting rate; and timeliness of data reporting. A special study or survey may be required to obtain quantitative and qualitative data.
Sensitivity	Can be considered on at least two levels. At the level of case reporting, sensitivity refers to the proportion of cases of a disease (or event) detected by the system. On another level, it can refer to the ability to detect outbreaks over time. In evaluation of surveillance systems, "completeness" is often synonymous with sensitivity.	Assuming that reported cases are correctly classified, the primary emphasis in assessing sensitivity is to estimate the proportion of the total number of cases in the population under surveillance being detected by the system, represented by $A / (A + C)$ in Table 8–5. The capacity for a system to detect outbreaks might be enhanced if detailed diagnostic tests are used. The measurement of sensitivity requires collection of or access to data usually external to the system to determine the true frequency of the condition and validation of data collected by the system. Also, the calculation of more than one measurement of the attribute might be necessary.

(*continued*)

Table 8–4 (*continued*)

Attribute	Definition	Methods
Predictive value positive	The proportion of reported cases that actually have the event under surveillance.	Sensitivity and predictive value positive provide different perspectives regarding how well the system is operating. Assessing predictive value positive whenever sensitivity has been assessed might be necessary. In Table 8–5, predictive value positive is represented by A / (A + B). In assessing this attribute, primary emphasis is placed on case confirmation, and records might be kept of investigations prompted by information obtained form the system. More than one measurement of predictive value positive might be necessary.
Representativeness	Ability to accurately describe the occurrence of a health-related event over time and its distribution in the population by place and person.	Representativeness is assessed by comparing the characteristics of the reported events to all such actual events. Although the latter information is generally not known, knowledge of the characteristics of the general population, clinical course of the disease or event, and prevailing medical practices, as well as collection of data from multiple sources, can be used to assess this attribute. Special studies based on samples of cases might be used. Also, the choice of an appropriate denominator for rate calculations should be given careful consideration.
Timeliness	Reflects the speed between steps in a system.	The time interval linking any of the steps in a system can be examined; these steps can include event occurrence, event recognition by reporting source, event reported to surveillance system, and control and prevention activities with feedback to stakeholders. The most relevant time interval might vary with the type of event under surveillance.
Stability	Refers to the system's reliability (ability to collect, manage, and provide data without failure) and availability (ability to be operational when needed). (*See also* informatics-based attributes Table 8–6.)	Measures for determining stability can include the number of unscheduled outages and down times for computer system; the costs involved with any computer repair; the percentage of time the system is operating fully; and the desired and actual amount of time required for the system to collect, manage, and release data.

* Reference *1*.

Table 8–5 Calculation of Sensitivity* and Predictive Value Positive** for a
Surveillance System

Detected by surveillance?	Condition present?		
	Yes	*No*	
Yes	True-positive (A)	False-positive (B)	A + B
No	False-negative (C)	True-negative (D)	C + D
	A + C	B + D	

* Sensitivity = A / (A + C)
** Predictive value positive (PVP) = A / (A + B)

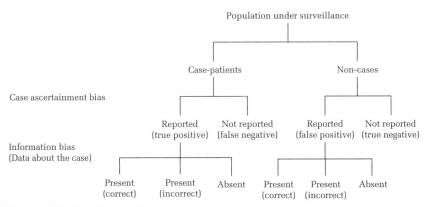

Figure 8–2 Biases in surveillance.

on surveillance processes and public health practice. Public health informatics
is defined as the systematic application of information and computer science
and technology to public health practice, research, and learning (52). It follows
then that information science and technology attributes relevant for surveillance
information collection, management, interchange, and use can be defined and
described in addition to more traditional surveillance evaluation attributes, such
as timeliness or sensitivity.

As in a traditional surveillance system evaluation, an informatics-focused evaluation of surveillance systems requires consideration of the population under surveillance, the public health importance and epidemiology of the condition under
surveillance, and the ethical, legal, organizational, fiscal, and political context
(53). In addition, surveillance evaluations that include an informatics perspective
must consider the range of feasible information technology options that can support surveillance processes and enhance system performance.

Informatics attributes of surveillance systems can be considered across the
range of information technologies—from pencil-and-paper systems to computerized systems supporting remote data collection, real-time electronic data
interchange, and data integration. Introducing information technologies within
public health systems almost invariably results in a variety of impacts on the

design of the public health surveillance system (*54*). For example, use of information technology provides opportunities to automate surveillance processes currently performed manually (e.g., record de-duplication, statistical analysis to identify unusual data patterns requiring further investigation), to support the public health workforce (e.g., providing up-to-date data that can be manipulated electronically), and to increase the efficiency and quality of surveillance processes and information (e.g., improved timeliness and increased data accuracy).

Numerous information system evaluation frameworks relevant for surveillance systems have been described (*26,41,55–57*). Key informatics-focused evaluation domains for surveillance information systems are: information quality, system quality, and user experience and service quality (*56*). Table 8–6 presents selected attributes for each domain and example evaluation criteria (refs. *26,55,* and *56*; R. Chapman, Centers for Disease Control and Prevention, written communication, December 2003). Once the current surveillance tasks and attributes are defined and organized, those evaluating the system and system stakeholders should identify collaboratively the inefficiencies and the processes, ideally repeatable or automated, to address those inefficiencies (*35*).

The evaluation should assess how well the public health surveillance system is integrated with other surveillance and health information systems (e.g., does the surveillance system rely on primary data collection or use protocols for data transformation and interchange to allow use of data that might be collected for other appropriate public health purposes [i.e., data re-use]?; is the system's information content represented using standard codes to support data interchange?). Evaluation of the processes of data collection and reporting might identify related information system protocols and surveillance processes that can be shared or standardized as the public health surveillance environment moves toward system interoperability and data integration (*58,59*). Although individual systems need to meet specific surveillance objectives, linkage of surveillance processes avoids the duplication of effort and lack of standardization that can arise from independent systems. Additionally, linkage of multiple-source public health data in an integrated public health surveillance environment can address comorbidity monitoring (e.g., persons infected with both HIV and *Mycobacterium tuberculosis*); identify previously unrecognized risk factors; provide the means for monitoring additional outcomes associated with a health-related event; and improve efficiency of surveillance processes and resource utilization.

Evaluation of the informatics aspects of surveillance information systems should identify the human and organization changes required to maximize the public health benefits afforded by information technology. When new information technology is introduced, its impact on system processes should be monitored to determine if proposed benefits have been realized. In communities with fixed public health funding, the costs of implementing new information and communication technologies must be weighed against the benefits of direct support for public health preparedness and response activities. Additionally, failure of new information technologies (e.g., inability to access or analyze key data elements) can lead to negative effects on the community and staff (*57*).

Table 8–6 Selected Informatics-Based Surveillance Information System Attributes and Evaluation Criteria by Evaluation Domain*

Evaluation domain	Informatics-based attribute	Example evaluation criteria
Information quality	Accuracy	Do the data express meaning clearly and unambiguously?
		Does the coding system selected for each data element express the intended domain of meaning?
		Is the information captured at a specific-enough level of detail to support all needed analysis?
	Completeness	Are all required surveillance or information system data elements collected?
		How complete are the valid responses for required data elements?
	Relevance	Are data available to system users when needed for surveillance purposes?
		Has the system been assessed to eliminate the collection or storage of unnecessary or redundant data elements?
	Consistency	Are data unchanged when replicated or interchanged between surveillance partners? Are data transformations well-documented?
System quality	Usability	Is the system understandable and useable by the intended user community?
		How much user training is required prior to system use?
		Is the sequence of actions involved in operation of the system sensible and understandable to the user community?
		Does the system mirror common workflow?
	Availability**	Is the system available at all needed times? From all needed locations? For all intended users?
		Can the system be accessed in multiple ways using various technologies?
	Adaptability	Can the system be modified in response to changing information needs, data structures, functional requirements, or changes in workload?
		Is the system able to add new connectivity or interfaces to support system or information integration?
	Response time	What is the desired and actual amount of time required for the system to generate data for public health action?
		Is the system able to provide its indicated services in a timely manner?
		Can the system handle the workload with sufficient throughput for data processing, analysis, report generation, or data interchange?
	Functionality	Does the system support users in accomplishment of their various tasks and responsibilities?
		Is the system configured or architected to support introduction of changes in functionality (e.g., creation of new data views to support emerging analytic needs, or receipt, de-duplication, linkage, and translation of new data types)?
		Does the system have sufficient storage capacity?
	Data quality	Do the data take only defined values?
		Are data elements cross-checked (e.g., zip codes correspond to counties, males are not coded as "pregnant = yes")?

(*continued*)

Table 8–6 (*continued*)

Evaluation domain	Informatics-based attribute	Example evaluation criteria
	Portability	Are the system's technical architecture, hardware configuration, or software adaptable for use by other jurisdictions?
		Can components of the system be re-used elsewhere (e.g., by other surveillance systems managed within the organization's information architecture)?
	Improved data capture	Based on context of surveillance system, does the system use best available technology (whether electronic or hardcopy) for data collection to avoid duplicate data entry and to reduce data entry error?
		Does system support multiple modalities for data collection, importing, or interchange?
		Do procedures exist for validating timeliness, completeness, and accuracy of all data entry?
	Error reduction	Can the system operate despite adverse conditions such as operator error, bad data, device failure, or partial network outages?
		Is the system free of internal defects that cause it to cease operation?
	Use of standards	Are data standards used to represent data elements (e.g., Logical Observation Identifiers Names and Codes [LOINC]) for representing lab test type?
		Are data interchanged electronically using standard data interchange protocols (e.g., Health Level 7)?
	Security	Are security levels and procedures for data or system access defined and enforced?
		Is a data use and release policy and protocol available?
		Is access to the application to perform specific functions (e.g., to read or modify the data) controlled?
User experience and service quality	Reliability**	Does the system perform the intended surveillance support functions under the conditions defined by system users?
		Is the information system dependable?
	Responsiveness	Do users receive prompt service when requesting assistance on the system?
		Do users report that system support staff are willing to respond to user questions and to provide support services?
	Assurance	Are surveillance information system support staff knowledgable?
		Is all required training provided to enable effective use of system?
		Are support staff able to inspire trust and confidence in system users?
	Empathy	Are system change requests derived from user feedback managed in a responsive manner?
		To what degree do the system designers, developers, or implementers base technological solutions and approaches on the business needs of public health surveillance and of the system stakeholders (e.g., achieving objectives or improving surveillance attribute performance)?

* References *26,55,56*; R. Chapman, Centers for Disease Control and Prevention, written communication, December 2003.
** *See* surveillance system attribute, stability, Table 8–4.

CONCLUSIONS, RECOMMENDATIONS, AND USE OF EVALUATION FINDINGS

Conclusions from the evaluation can be justified through appropriate analysis, synthesis, interpretation, and judgment of the gathered evidence regarding the performance of the public health surveillance system (Table 8–7). The conclusions should state whether the surveillance system is addressing an important public health problem and is meeting its objectives. The qualitative and quantitative findings should be linked to the system's defined evaluation metrics and interpreted in collaboration with system stakeholders. Involvement of stakeholders in the review of evaluation findings and definition of recommendations should increase the likelihood of their participation in surveillance performance improvement.

Recommendations should address the modification or continuation of the public health surveillance system. Before recommending modifications to a system, the evaluation should consider the interdependence of the system's costs and attributes (*49*). If a system is to be integrated into an organization or existing information environment, the readiness for change and attitudes of people affected by the introduction of the system should be assessed. Evaluation findings might require articulation of recommendations regarding ethical obligations in operating the system, (e.g., modifying procedures to ensure personal privacy (*see also* Chapter 9) or more timely and effective use of data for preparedness and response).

In some instances, conclusions from the evaluation indicate that the most appropriate recommendation is to discontinue the public health surveillance system. An evaluation of the acceptability of an enhanced sexually transmitted infection (STI) surveillance system found that the system was not meeting its objectives (*60*). In response, system stewards and stakeholders discontinued the enhanced system and modified another existing STI surveillance system to improve surveillance efficiency while still achieving their priority objectives. However, this type of recommendation should be considered carefully before it is issued. The cost of re-initiating a system that has been discontinued could be substantially greater than the cost of maintaining it. Therefore, the stakeholders in the evaluation should consider relevant public health and other consequences of discontinuing a surveillance system.

Regardless of the evaluation strategy and methods used, an evaluator's comments will be of little use if they are not communicated in a clear, focused, credible evaluation report that directly addresses the purpose of the evaluation. Deliberate effort is needed to ensure that the evaluation findings are used and disseminated appropriately. During the implementation of the evaluation, considering political sensitivities and how potential findings (particularly negative findings) could affect decisions made about the surveillance system is often necessary. When conclusions from the evaluation and recommendations are made, follow-up is necessary to prevent lessons learned from being lost or ignored. If timeliness and completeness require improvement, for example, introducing routine monitoring of reporting timeliness and completeness and ensuring responsive technical assistance might be required to bring about performance improvement.

Table 8–7 Example of a Surveillance System Evaluation: National Electronic Injury Surveillance System-Cooperative Adverse Drug Event Surveillance Project (NEISS-CADES)*

System characteristic	Finding	How defined or measured?
Public health importance	Public health impact of adverse drug events (ADEs) substantial: In 2004, ADEs were noted in 1,211,100 hospital stays, (~3.1 percent of all stays); Many ADEs preventable; National ADE surveillance inadequate.	Literature review
Purpose	To evaluate feasibility of modifying existing surveillance system to conduct enhanced, nationally representative surveillance of ADEs treated in hospital-based emergency departments (EDs)	In 2000, U.S. Government Accountability Office found national ADE surveillance, particularly surveillance for outpatient ADEs to be insufficient. System sponsors sought to characterize the public health burden of outpatient ADEs treated in EDs to supplement existing data on hospitalized patients.
Objectives	Can the surveillance system: *(1)* detect ADEs in timely way to permit control and prevention; *(2)* estimate magnitude of morbidity and identify associated risk factors; *(3)* stimulate research leading to prevention; *(4)* detect trends in ADEs over time; *(5)* permit assessment of prevention measures, or *(6)* lead to improved clinical, social, or policy practice that mitigates or prevents ADEs?	Evaluators reviewed application of NEISS-CADES surveillance data to issues of public health importance from 2004 to 2006 for evidence that system could address these questions
Case definition	An ED visit for a condition that the treating physician explicitly attributes to the use of a drug or a drug-specific effect. Inclusions/exclusions described.	System sponsors defined an ADE case by specifying eligible events (e.g., adverse effects of medications at recommended doses) and drugs (e.g., prescription and over-the-counter medications)
Sponsoring organizations	Consumer Product Safety Commission (CPSC); Centers for Disease Control and Prevention (CDC); Food and Drug Administration (FDA)	Agency roles, responsibilities, and expertise defined the critical system sponsors
Operational resources	System cost data not presented.	Not applicable

(continued)

Table 8–7 (*continued*)

System characteristic	Finding	How defined or measured?
Representativeness	Surveillance data are derived from nationally representative sample to yield national estimates. Wide-spectrum of ADEs monitored. Limited to persons seeking care in hospital EDs.	Review of hospital sample selection protocol
Predictive value positive	0.92 (0.85–1.0 95% confidence interval; weighted estimate)	From randomly selected days in convenience sample of participating hospitals, calculated the proportion of ADEs identified by NEISS-CADES that are true ADEs as determined by expert review of reported cases and corresponding ED medical records to determine if they met case definition
Acceptability	Minimal administrative requirements and resource expenditures for participating hospitals. No enrolled hospitals have revoked their participation in the surveillance system. Outcomes achieved via integration with existing NEISS surveillance infrastructure imply limited marginal costs.	Review of surveillance processes and enrolled hospital participation
Data quality	*(1)* 82%–100% completeness of data element reporting for selected data elements; *(2)* 0.93 agreement for drug identity and patient diagnosis between information in the NEISS report and data abstracted during expert review of ED medical charts.	Reviewed: *(1)* completeness of reporting of key data elements, and *(2)* agreement between abstractors and expert reviewers for "important" data elements (e.g., drug identity, patient diagnosis)
Flexibility	Noted use of standard vocabularies for medical and drug coding that provide robust and flexible code structure to support changing information needs over time. Because NEISS-CADES is a subsystem of NEISS, requested modifications are subject to CSPS priorities and constraints.	Review of surveillance protocol
Timeliness	67% of cases reported within 7 days of ED visit; 93% reported within 30 days. Final annual analysis occurs at least 6 months after end of each calendar year, following data quality review, data coding, and assignment of sample weights.	Review of surveillance data and protocol

(*continued*)

Table 8–7 (continued)

System characteristic	Finding	How defined or measured?
Sensitivity	0.33 (0.23–0.44 95% confidence interval; weighted estimate)	Compared ADEs identified by NEISS and ADEs identified via expert review of all ED medical records from randomly selected days in convenience sample of participating hospitals
Simplicity	Extensive amount of data abstracted by professional abstractors for each case, but it is derived from single data source. Multi-agency collaboration on data management and analysis complicates system. Modifications to protocol require training of data coders and project managers increasing complexity.	Review of surveillance protocol and processes
Stability	NEISS has been operational since 1971 and numerous enhancements have been implemented successfully during that time. Funded on a year-to-year basis.	Review of surveillance protocol and processes
Usefulness	Between 2003 and 2006, system demonstrated: (1) ability to detect ADEs in time to implement prevention efforts (i.e., surveillance data quantified percentage of potentially preventable overdoses in children associated with treatment of attention deficit hyperactivity disorder (ADHD) with publication of data within 3 months after the first FDA Advisory Panel meeting to address safety of ADHD therapy), and (2) ability to estimate morbidity and identify ADE-associated risk factors. With longer use, may be able to address other objectives (above).	Reviewed uses of system's data from 2004 to 2006. Since 2006, data from the surveillance system have contributed to new labeling of children's cough and cold medicines (61); new messages to promote appropriate antibiotic use (62); and reassessment of quality measures to improve prescribing for older adults (63).

* Reference 15.

Strategies for communicating the evaluation findings, recommendations, and response activities should be tailored to relevant audiences, including persons who provided data used for the evaluation. For example, in the public health community, oral presentations, formal written reports, and peer-reviewed journal articles have been used to communicate findings and recommendations from the evaluation to relevant audiences (15,28,42,64–67).

CONCLUSIONS

To promote the best use of public health resources, all public health surveillance systems should be monitored routinely and evaluated periodically. No perfect system exists, however, and trade-offs must always be made. Each system is unique and must balance public health benefit with personnel, resources, and cost allocated to each of its components if the system is to achieve its intended purpose and objectives.

The approach to evaluation of public health surveillance systems described in this chapter can be applied to a variety of systems, including health information systems used for public health action, proposed surveillance systems that are being pilot-tested, integrated surveillance systems monitoring multiple outcomes, and information systems at individual health-care organizations or facilities. Regardless of the system type or its stage of implementation, stakeholder input during evaluation design and implementation of evaluation recommendations is essential. The appropriate evaluation design becomes paramount as these systems adapt to revised case definitions, emerging information needs, new health-related events, new data sources and types, new information technology, and changing requirements for protecting patient privacy, data confidentiality, and system security. Progress in surveillance theory, technology, and practice continues, and guidance for evaluating a surveillance system will necessarily evolve.

REFERENCES

1. Centers for Disease Control and Prevention. Updated guidelines for evaluating public health surveillance systems: recommendations from the guidelines working group. *MMWR Recomm Rep* 2001;50(RR-13):1–35. http://www.cdc.gov/mmwr/PDF/rr/rr5013.pdf. Accessed January 30, 2009.
2. World Health Organization. Communicable disease surveillance and response systems: guide to monitoring and evaluating. 2006. WHO/CDS/EPR/LYO/2006.2. http://www.who.int/csr/resources/publications/surveillance/WHO_CDS_EPR_LYO_2006_2/en/. Accessed January 30, 2009.
3. World Health Organization Regional Office for Africa, Division of Communicable Disease Prevention and Control. *Guide for the Use of Core Integrated Disease Surveillance and Response Indicators in the African Region.* June 2005. http://www.cdc.gov/idsr/files/guide.pdf. Accessed January 30, 2009.
4. Hall HI, Mokotoff ED, Advisory Group for Technical Guidance on HIV/AIDS Surveillance. Setting standards and an evaluation framework for human immunodeficiency virus/acquired immunodeficiency syndrome surveillance. *J Public Health Manag Pract* 2007;13:519–523.
5. Potter MA, Sweeney P, Iuliano AD, Allswede MP. Performance indicators for response to selected infectious disease outbreaks: a review of the published record. *J Public Health Manag Pract* 2007;13:510–518.
6. Roush SW, Wharton M. Surveillance indicators. In: Roush SW, McIntyre L, Baldy LM, eds. *Manual for the Surveillance of Vaccine-Preventable Diseases,* 4th ed. Atlanta, GA: Centers for Disease Control and Prevention; 2008. http://www.cdc.gov/vaccines/pubs/surv-manual/default.htm. Accessed January 30, 2009.

7. Wilkins K, Nsubuga P, Mendlein J, Mercer D, Pappaioanou M. The Data for Decision Making project: assessment of surveillance systems in developing countries to improve access to public health information. *Public Health* 2007;doi:10.1016/j.puhe.2007.11.002.

8. McNabb SJN, Surdo AM, Redmond A, *et al.* Applying a new conceptual framework to evaluate tuberculosis surveillance and action performance and measure the costs, Hillsborough County, Florida, 2002. *Ann Epidemiol* 2004;14:640–645.

9. World Health Organization. Protocol for the evaluation of epidemiological surveillance systems. 1997. WHO/EMC/DIS/97.2. http://whqlibdoc.who.int/hq/1997/WHO_EMC_DIS_97.2.pdf. Accessed January 30, 2009.

10. World Health Organization. An integrated approach to communicable disease surveillance. *Wkly Epidemiol Rec* 2000;75:1–8.

11. Nsubuga P, Eseko N, Wuhib T, Chungong S, Ndayimirije N, McNabb S. Structure and performance of infectious disease surveillance, Tanzania 1998. *Bull World Health Organ* 2002;80:196–203.

12. Centers for Disease Control and Prevention. Assessment of infectious disease surveillance—Uganda, 2000. *MMWR* 2000;49;687–691.

13. Wu TSJ, Shih FYF, Yen MY, *et al.* Establishing a nationwide emergency department-based syndromic surveillance system for better public health responses in Taiwan. *BMC Public Health* 2008;8:18.

14. Shannon JJ, Catrambone CD, Coover L. Targeting improvements in asthma morbidity in Chicago: a 10-year retrospective of community action. *Chest* 2007;132:866–873.

15. Jhung MA, Budnitz DS, Mendelsohn AB, Weidenbach KN, Nelson TD, Pollock DA. Evaluation and overview of the National Electronic Injury Surveillance System—Cooperative Adverse Drug Event Surveillance Project (NEISS-CADES). *Med Care* 2007;45:S96–S102.

16. Meyer N, McMenamin J, Robertson C, Donaghy M, Allardice G, Cooper D. A multi-data source surveillance system to detect a bioterrorism attack during the G8 Summit in Scotland. *Epidemiol Infect* 2008;136:876–885.

17. Schenkel K, Williams C, Eckmanns T, et al. Enhanced surveillance of infectious diseases: the 2006 FIFA World Cup Experience, Germany. *Euro Surveill* 2006;11:ii–670.

18. Thacker SD, Stroup DF, Carande-Kulis V, Marks JS, Roy K, Gerberding JL. Measuring the public's health. *Public Health Rep* 2006;121:14–22.

19. Murray CJL, Salomon J, Mathers DC, Lopez AD, Lozano R, eds. *Summary Measures of Population Health: Concepts, Ethics, Measurement and Applications.* Geneva: World Health Organization, 2002. http://whqlibdoc.who.int/publications/2002/9241545518.pdf. Accessed January 30, 2009.

20. Michaud CM, McKenna MT, Gegg S, *et al.* The burden of disease and injury in the United States, 1996. *Popul Health Metr* 2006;4:11. http://www.pophealthmetrics.com/content/4/1/11. Accessed January 30, 2009.

21. Mather CD, Loncar D. Projections of global mortality and burden of disease from 2002 to 2030. *PLoS Med.* 2006;3:e42–e442. http://medicine.plosjournals.org/archive/1549-1676/3/11/pdf/10.1371_journal.pmed.0030442-L.pdf. Accessed January 30, 2009.

22. Curry CW, De AK, Ikeda RM, Thacker SB. Health burden and funding at the Centers for Disease Control and Prevention. *Am J Prev Med* 2006;30:269–276.

23. Keppel KG. Ten largest racial and ethnic health disparities in the United States based on Healthy People 2010 Objectives. *Am J Epidemiol* 2007;166:97–103.

24. Haddix A, Teutsch S, Corso P, eds. *Prevention Effectiveness: A Guide to Decision Analysis and Economic Evaluation*, 2nd ed. New York: Oxford University Press; 2002.

25. Kimmel SR. Addressing immunization barriers, benefits, and risks. *J Fam Pract* 2007;56:S51–S69.

26. Buckeridge DL, Thompson MW, Babin S, Sikes ML. Evaluating automated surveillance systems. In: Lombardo JS, Buckeridge DL, eds. *Disease Surveillance: a Public Health Informatics Approach*. Hoboken, NJ: John Wiley & Sons;. 2007:399–424.

27. Centers for Disease Control and Prevention. Framework for evaluating public health surveillance systems for early detection of outbreaks; recommendations from the CDC Working Group. *MMWR Recomm Rep* 2004;53(RR-5):1–13.

28. Miller M, Roche P, Spencer J, Deeble M. Evaluation of Australia's National Notifiable Disease Surveillance System. *Commun Dis Intell* 2004;28:311–323.

29. Council of State and Territorial Epidemiologists. Asthma Surveillance and Case Definition. Position Statement 1998-EH/CD 1. http://www.cste.org/ps/1998/1998-eh-cd-01.htm. Accessed January 30, 2009.

30. Thomsen C, McClain J, Rosenman K, Davis L. Indicators for occupational health surveillance. *MMWR Recomm Rep* 2007;56(RR-1):1–7.

31. Centers for Disease Control and Prevention. Case definitions for infectious conditions under public health surveillance. http://www.cdc.gov/ncphi/disss/nndss/casedef/case_definitions.htm. Accessed January 30, 2009.

32. Centers for Disease Control and Prevention, Council of State and Territorial Epidemiologists, Association of State and Territorial Chronic Disease Program Directors. Indicators for Chronic Disease Surveillance. *MMWR Recomm Rep.* 2004;53(RR11);1–6. http://www.cdc.gov/mmwr/preview/mmwrhtml/rr5311a1.htm. Accessed January 30, 2009.

33. Wild EL, Hastings TM, Gubernick R, Ross DA, Fehrenbach SN. Key elements for successful integrated health information systems: lessons from the states. *J Public Health Manag Pract* 2004;11(Suppl):S36–S47.

34. Williams W, Lyalin D, Wingo PA. Systems thinking: what business modeling can do for public health. *J Public Health Manag Pract* 2005;11:550–553.

35. Public Health Informatics Institute. *Taking Care of Business: A Collaboration to Define Local Health Department Business Processes*. Decatur, GA: Public Health Informatics Institute; 2006.

36. Kitch P, Yasnoff WA. Assessing the value of information systems. In: O'Carroll PW, Yasnoff WA, Ward ME, Ripp LH, Martin EL, eds. *Public Health Informatics and Information Systems*. New York: Springer-Verlag; 2003:114–158.

37. Somda ZC, Meltzer MI, Perry HN. *SurvCost 1.0: A Manual to Assist Country and District Public Health Officials in Estimating the Cost of the Implementation of Integrated Disease Surveillance and Response Systems (Beta Test Version)*. Atlanta, GA: Centers for Disease Control and Prevention, U.S. Department of Health and Human Services; 2007. http://www.cdc.gov/idsr/survcost.htm. Accessed January 30, 2009.

38. Morris S, Gray A, Noone A, Wiseman M, Jathanna S. The costs and effectiveness of surveillance of communicable disease: a case study of HIV and AIDS in England and Wales. *J Public Health Med* 1996;18:415–422.

39. Tebbens RJD, Sangrujee N, Thompson KM. The costs of future polio risk management policies. *Risk Anal* 2006;26:1507–1531.

40. Kirkwood A, Fleishchauer AT, Gunn J, Hutwagner L, Barry MA. Direct cost associated with the development and implementation of a local syndromic surveillance system. *J Public Health Manag Pract* 2007;13:194–199.

41. Bravata DM, McDonald KM, Szeto H, Smith WK, Rydzak C, Owens DK. A conceptual framework for evaluating information technologies and decision support systems for bioterrorism preparedness and response. *Med Decis Making* 2004;24:192–206.

42. Doroshenko A, Cooper D, Smith G, *et al.* Evaluation of syndromic surveillance based on National Health Service Direct derived data—England and Wales. *MMWR* 2005;54(Suppl.):117–122.

43. Bravata DM, McDonald KM, Smith WM, *et al.* Systematic review: Surveillance systems for early detection of bioterrorism-related diseases. *Ann Intern Med* 2004;140:910–922.

44. Overhage JM, Grannis S, McDonald CJ. A comparison of the completeness and timeliness of automated electronic laboratory reporting and spontaneous reporting of notifiable conditions. *Am J Public Health* 2006;98:344–350.

45. Dailey L, Watkins RE, Plant AJ. Timeliness of data sources used for influenza surveillance. *J Am Med Inform Assoc* 2007;14:626–631.

46. Hedberg CW, Greenblatt JF, Matyas BT, *et al.* Timeliness of enteric disease surveillance in 6 US states. *Emerg Infec Dis* 2008;14:311–313.

47. Vogt RL, Spittle R, Cronquist A, Patnaik JL. Evaluation of timeliness and completeness of a web-based notifiable disease reporting system by a local health department. *J Public Health Manag Pract* 2006;12:540–544.

48. Ihekweazu C, Maxwell N, Organ S, Oliver I. Is STI surveillance in England meeting the requirements of the 21st century? An evaluation of data from the Southwest Region. *Euro Surveill* 2007;12(5):ii–708.

49. Hopkins RS. Design and operation of state and local infectious disease surveillance systems. *J Public Health Manag Pract* 2005;11:184–190.

50. German RR. Sensitivity and predictive value positive measurements for public health surveillance systems. *Epidemiology* 2000;11:720–727.

51. Hook EB, Regal RR. Capture-recapture methods in epidemiology: methods and limitations. *Epidemiol Rev* 1995;17:243–264.

52. O'Carroll PW. Introduction to public health informatics. In: O'Carroll PW, Yasnoff WA, Ward ME, Ripp LH, Martin EL, eds. *Public Health Informatics and Information Systems.* New York: Springer-Verlag; 2003:3–15.

53. Lewis D. Evaluation for public health informatics. In: O'Carroll PW, Yasnoff WA, Ward ME, Ripp LH, Martin EL, eds. *Public Health Informatics and Information Systems.* New York: Springer-Verlag; 2003:239–250.

54. Ashurst C, Doherty NF. Towards the formulation of a 'best practice' framework for benefits realisation in IT projects. *Electronic J Information Systems Evaluation.* 2003;6:1–10.

55. DeLone WH, McLean ER. The DeLone and McLean model of information systems success: a ten-year update. *J Manag Information Systems* 2003;19:9–30.

56. Public Health Informatics Institute. *Towards Measuring Value: An Evaluation Framework for Public Health Information Systems.* Decatur, GA: Public Health Informatics Institute Technical Report; April 2005.

57. Ammenwerth E, Graber S, Herrmann G, Burkle T, Konig J. Evaluation of health information systems—problems and challenges. *Int J Med Inform* 2003;71:125–135.

58. Amato-Gauci A, Ammon A. The surveillance of communicable diseases in the European Union – a long-term strategy (2008–2013). *Euro Surveill* 2008;13(26):ii–18912. http://www.eurosurveillance.org/ViewArticle.aspx?ArticleId=18912. Accessed January 30, 2009.

59. Centers for Disease Control and Prevention. Progress in improving state and local disease surveillance—United States, 2000–2005. *MMWR* 2005;54;822–825.

60. Kivi M, Koedijk FDH, van der Sande M, van de Laar MJ. Evaluation prompting transition from enhanced to routine surveillance of lymphogranuloma venereum (LGV) in the Netherlands. *Euro Surveill* 2008;13(14):ii–8087.

61. Schaefer MK, Shehab N, Cohen AL, Budnitz DS. Adverse events from cough and cold medications in children. *Pediatrics* 2008;121:783–787.

62. Shehab N, Patel PR, Srinivasan A, Budnitz DS. Emergency department visits for antibiotic-associated adverse events. *Clin Infect Dis* 2008;47:735–743.

63. Budnitz DS, Shehab N, Kegler SR, Richards CL. Medication use leading to emergency department visits for adverse drug events in older adults. *Ann Intern Med* 2007;147:755–765.

64. Bingle CL, Picard L, Holowaty PH, Stewart PJ, Koren IE, Feltis SL. An evaluation of the Ontario Rapid Risk Factor Surveillance System. *Can J Public Health* 2005;96:145–150.

65. Wolkin AF, Patel M, Watson W, *et al.* Early detection of illness associate with poisoning of public health significance. *Ann Emerg Med* 2006;47:170–176.

66. Meynard JB, Chaudet H, Green AD, *et al.* Proposal of a framework for evaluating military surveillance systems for early detection of outbreaks on duty areas. *BMC Public Health* 2008;8:146.

67. Braun KVN, Pettygrove S, Daniels J, *et al.* Evaluation of a methodology for a collaborative multiple source surveillance network for autism spectrum disorders—Autism and developmental disabilities monitoring network, 14 sites, United States, 2002. *MMWR Surveill Summ* 2007;56(SS-1):29–40.

9

Ethics in Public Health Surveillance

CHARLES M. HEILIG AND PATRICIA SWEENEY

Most people say that it is the intellect which makes a great scientist. They are wrong: It is character.

—Albert Einstein

Public health surveillance both supports conditions for human health and risks breaching individual liberty and privacy. In this chapter, we approach this apparent conflict by reflecting on appropriate norms for public health surveillance and then presenting pragmatic guidelines for ethics in public health surveillance. The moral foundation is set in public health as a collective effort to achieve a public good, and government's fundamental duty to promote and protect the health of the public. The systematic measurement of the public's health is necessary for identifying conditions that support individual and population health, informing appropriate actions to assure these conditions, and guiding those who take action on behalf of society. But what are the proper limits on accumulating information about individuals in serving the common good?

In the first part of this chapter, we establish a broad context for ethics in surveillance by reviewing recent developments in public health ethics and more firmly established principles from biomedical ethics. In the second part of the chapter, we discuss specific formulations of ethics for collecting, using, disclosing, and storing personal, health-related information and relate them to pragmatic tools for public health practitioners.

PUBLIC HEALTH

As formulated by the Institute of Medicine (IOM), "Public health is what we, as a society, do collectively, to assure the conditions in which people can be healthy" (*1*). The IOM supplemented this formulation by affirming that "[h]ealth is a primary public good because many aspects of human potential such as employment, social relationships, and political partnerships are contingent on it" (*2,3*).

Because government has a unique role in promoting and protecting public health, our treatment focuses in particular on the role of public health officials, defined as "any officer, employee, private contractor or agent, intern, or volunteer of a public health agency with authorization from the agency or pursuant to law to acquire, use, disclose, or store protected health information" (*4*). Public health surveillance falls squarely within the core public health function of assessment:

> The [IOM] committee recommends that every public health agency regularly and systematically collect, assemble, analyze, and make available information on the health of the community, including statistics on health status, community health needs, and epidemiologic and other studies of health problems (*1*).

This charge extends through the local, tribal, state, and federal levels of government. Although the IOM noted that private organizations and individuals share in the mission of public health, we focus on the role of government agencies and their direct partners and agents.

Public health ethics has emerged as a new field over the past decade. Many details remain to be worked out and consensus continues being built around specific principles (*5–9*). Here, we highlight how the current state of dialog about ethics in public health is related to the dialog of ethics in public health surveillance. We start with commonly invoked principles of bioethics: beneficence, respect for persons, and justice. These principles might be inadequate in consideration of differences between public health and biomedical ethics. Key points from human rights, social justice, and paternalism supplement the discussion. We also take guidance from model legislation while highlighting the important distinction between compliance with regulations on one hand and ethical practice on the other; this portion of the discussion is especially relevant for thinking about the difference between research and the practice of public health.

PRINCIPLES AND OTHER MORAL CONSIDERATIONS

The field of public health ethics often uses as its touchstone the prevailing set of principles of biomedical ethics. The *Belmont Report* (*10*) presents the predominant framework for analyzing ethics in human research. Beauchamp and Childress also present a set of principles for systematically analyzing ethics of activities in a biomedical context (*11,12*). Although the pointedly concise *Belmont Report* addresses the boundary between medical research and practice, it focuses on analyzing ethics of human research. Beauchamp and Childress take a much broader view of the range of activity that is subject to ethical analysis. As Mann (*13*) reflected, "The fundamental difference [between medicine and public health] involves the population emphasis of public health, which contrasts with the essentially individual focus of medical care." Insights from biomedical ethics inform but might not directly carry over to public health practice or research.

To guide the ethics of human research, the National Commission for the Protection of Human Subjects of Biomedical and Behavioral Research formulated three principles, "general judgments that serve as a basic justification for the many particular ethical prescriptions and evaluations of human actions":

> Beneficence: One ought not inflict harm. One ought to maximize possible benefits and minimize possible harms.

Respect for persons: One ought to treat individuals as autonomous agents and protect persons with diminished autonomy.

Justice: One ought to ensure that burdens and benefits are distributed fairly.

The *Belmont Report* advances these three principles as a comprehensive aid to those who would review human research, although they will not resolve every dispute. As Childress et al. (*6*) explain, moral considerations must be further delineated in their scope and relative weight. What benefits are relevant to the ethics of public health? Under what circumstances might considerations of justice outweigh considerations of individual autonomy?

Beneficence

Beauchamp and Childress (*11,12*) formulate two separate principles—nonmaleficence and beneficence—related to the National Commission's single principle of beneficence. Nonmaleficence requires intentionally refraining from actions that cause harm; its prohibitions must be followed impartially and imply sanctions for prohibited actions. Beneficence entails an obligation to act for the benefit of others by helping them further their important and legitimate interests; it concerns positive norms for actions that ought to be conducted but generally does not imply moral sanctions for not acting accordingly. The subsidiary principle of utility or proportionality requires efforts to balance harms, benefits, or costs against benefits.

In public health surveillance, the positive duty to promote health depends on collecting, analyzing, and using data as empirical evidence that informs programmatic public health efforts. Because data are often collected in a format that might directly identify individuals and thereby expose them to social harm, public health officials have a duty to refrain from disclosing private information. Circumstances might exist, however, in which it is both appropriate and necessary to disclose private information—for example, to prevent harm to others. Where disparate interests or ethical norms conflict, additional effort is needed to moderate and perhaps resolve that conflict.

The principle of beneficence might need to be adapted or reformulated for public health, motivated by differences between research and practice and between biomedical and public health contexts. The National Commission distinguished research and practice specifically in terms of intended benefits:

> For the most part, the term "practice" refers to interventions that are designed solely to enhance the well-being of an individual patient or client and that have a reasonable expectation of success. The purpose of medical or behavioral practice is to provide diagnosis, preventive treatment or therapy to particular individuals. Even when a procedure applied in practice may benefit some other person, it remains an intervention designed to enhance the well-being of a particular individual or groups of individuals; thus, it is practice and need not be reviewed as research. By contrast, the term "research" designates an activity designed to test an hypothesis, permit conclusions to be drawn, and thereby to develop or contribute to generalizable knowledge (expressed, for example, in theories, principles, and statements of relationships) (*10*).

Thus, the *Belmont Report* ties the distinction between research and nonresearch activities to the principle of beneficence. The National Bioethics Advisory Commission (*14*) noted that the National Commission's operational definition of research does not translate readily from the clinical setting to other areas such as public health surveillance.

The U.S. Federal Policy for the Protection of Human Subjects defines *research* as "a systematic investigation … designed to develop or contribute to generalizable knowledge" (*15*). Unlike the *Belmont Report*, the regulation does not define *research* in explicit contrast to *practice* and thereby obscures the link to the principle of beneficence. Prominent national discussions bear out the difficulties in translating the regulatory definition of *research* to public health. Guidelines from the Centers for Disease Control and Prevention (CDC) identified surveillance, emergency responses, and evaluation as activities at the boundary between research and nonresearch (*16*), which poses difficulty in deciding the appropriate standards for review and oversight. CDC's analysis emphasizes the regulation's word *designed* as the key concept for deciding whether a public health activity constitutes research: "The primary intent of research is to generate or contribute to generalizable knowledge. The primary intent of non-research [sic] in public health is to prevent or control disease or injury and improve health, or to improve a public health program or service." According to guidance from the Council of State and Territorial Epidemiologists (*17,18*), public health practice can be characterized in part by specific legal authorization for conducting the activity as public health practice; a corresponding governmental duty to perform the activity to protect the public's health; and direct performance or oversight by a governmental public health authority (or its authorized partner) and accountability to the public for its performance.

These efforts to operationalize the regulatory definition of *research* focus less on explicit moral considerations than on regulatory concerns. The ethical dimension of this inquiry comes through the implied appeals to the principle of beneficence, reformulated for public health. Under CDC's 1999 guidelines, public health beneficence entails preventing or controlling disease or injury. In CSTE's 2004 analysis, beneficence is predicated on governmental duty and authorization to protect the public's health, and potential harms are restrained by accountability to the public. The calculus for justifying possible benefits and harms changes with the understanding of beneficence. The first question in the ethical (rather than regulatory) analysis of an activity should be, "To whom are the benefits intended to accrue?" rather than, "Is it research?" The intended-benefits question, however, requires a great deal of care, because it would be too easy to misclassify intended beneficiaries and careen toward exploiting some individuals for the benefit of others. The problem of specifying a principle of beneficence appropriate to public health surveillance remains only partially resolved.

Respect for Persons

The principle of respect for persons asserts both positive and negative obligations. The positive obligation, under the rubric of autonomy, calls for giving due weight to autonomous individuals' ability to take their own decisions and to act on them.

The negative obligation, under the rubric of liberty, requires that one refrain from interfering with autonomous decision making, at least to the extent that it does not harm others. The principle of respect for persons further accords special protections for persons with limited capacity to act autonomously, such as children and adults with limited or transient decision-making abilities. These protections might range from enhanced efforts to assure informed, autonomous decisions to proxy decision making or even exclusion from some activities.

In research, respect for persons underlies the general requirement to seek free and informed consent for participation by prospective subjects. In the context of surveillance, the obligations of the government might directly conflict with individual autonomy and freedom (19). Public health surveillance has historically imposed specific limits on personal privacy in service of monitoring public health (20). A patient seeking care often does not have the right to prevent personal information from being reported to the state for mandatory public health surveillance activities.

Privacy concerns became particularly pointed with the emergence of HIV surveillance and the prospect of name-based reporting, as the principles of beneficence and respect for persons could be seen to conflict with each other. The state has an interest in quality monitoring of public health to manage delivery of HIV-related services. If an individual perceives the only choices as name-based reporting and avoiding care, then it appears that autonomy is curtailed. Burris (21) analyzes name-based reporting through the concept of social risk by differentiating between the actual threat to confidentiality (which historically is low) and the *perception* of risk. Although legal protections exist to mitigate real risks, Burris argues that public health workers might address more appropriately the perceived risks by helping patients address those perceptions of risk and make sensible choices for themselves. In this instance, honoring the principle of respect for persons might help honor the principle of beneficence rather than conflict with it.

The literature on public health ethics has highlighted and parsed the potential value of paternalism (22), defined as "the intentional overriding of one person's preferences or actions by another person [for] benefiting or avoiding harm to the person whose preferences or actions are overridden" (12). This discussion has emerged largely as a reaction to individual-focused autonomy in biomedical ethics, which is portrayed as clashing with needs in public health:

> "[A] focus on population-based health requires a population-based analysis and a willingness to recognize that the ethics of collective health might require far more extensive limitations on privacy, as in the case of public health surveillance, and on liberty, as in the case of isolation and quarantine, than would be justified from the perspective of the autonomy-focused orientation of the dominant current in bioethics. … [W]hile a public health perspective will not privilege liberty and privacy, it does not follow that it should be insensitive to the importance of protecting individual rights" (20).

In contrast, it has been argued (23) that an imbalanced focus on paternalism could be redirected instead to a proper reframing of the principle of justice, as discussed in the next section.

Justice

The principle of justice concerns how social burdens and benefits ought to be distributed. Under the concept of fair opportunity (*12*), "no persons should receive social benefits on the basis of undeserved advantageous properties ... [and] no persons should be denied social benefits on the basis of undeserved disadvantageous properties." This conception of justice has led to critical analysis of structural contributors to morbidity and to calls to eliminate health disparities (*24,25*). Mann (*13*) and Buchanan (*23*) observed that the IOM's definition of public health embeds an implicit appeal to justice: "what we, as a society, do collectively, to assure the conditions in which people can be healthy." Mann argued further that the framework of human rights provides a better schema than bioethics for analyzing, discussing, and addressing the societal preconditions for human well-being and dignity (*26–28*).

Buchanan's argument for redirecting attention from paternalism to justice is relevant here. At a societal level, people with more autonomy enjoy better health than those with limited autonomy. Thus, "public health should focus on finding ways to expand individual autonomy, not restrict it." This focus should "foster responsible individuals who choose to take care of themselves and those around them." By paying attention to justice, or fair opportunity, we can correct institutional practices that unnecessarily put individuals at a disadvantage.

There are at least three immediate implications for surveillance. First, the principle of justice implies that surveillance systems should measure or otherwise account for impediments to fair opportunity—the actual levels of disparity across populations as well as the social structures that lead to inequity. Thus, surveillance systems should capture data equally across populations; equitable data capture relies on equal reporting across treatment providers, whether in private practice or at public clinics. Second, the administration of surveillance systems and dissemination of findings should ensure public participation, which in turn might both improve the practice of public health within communities and yield ongoing refinement in surveillance systems themselves. Third, transparent management of surveillance systems might foster credibility and community trust in public health efforts.

Resolving Competing Moral Considerations

When moral considerations lead to conflicting claims, how does a public health practitioner resolve the conflict? We have discussed two examples where reframing a problem helps to resolve the conflict: Burris's example in name-based reporting (*21*) shows how respect for persons can mitigate threats to beneficence, and Buchanan's example (*23*) demonstrates how the principle of justice (fair opportunity) can redirect a paternalistic intent toward respect for persons.

Childress et al. (*6*) describe a more general approach. Step 1 is to specify the ethical issues at play. Consider two issues in name-based HIV surveillance. Respect for persons might imply that patients should be informed that a positive test would be reported to state officials. Beneficence might require that no more risk is imposed (i.e., no more information is collected) than is needed to achieve the specific public health goals of surveillance. Step 2 is to weigh competing claims against each other. In the *Belmont Report*, the three principles start out with equal moral force. In public health ethics, it is conceivable that some considerations generally outweigh others because no general consensus yet exists regarding the relative weight of competing moral considerations. In the absence of consensus, Childress and coauthors enumerate five "justificatory conditions" intended to help determine whether promoting public health warrants overriding such values as individual liberty or justice in particular cases:

> Effectiveness: Show that infringing one or more general moral considerations will probably protect public health.
>
> Proportionality: Show that the probable public health benefits outweigh the infringed general moral considerations. All of the positive features and benefits must be balanced against the negative features and effects.
>
> Necessity: Show that an infringing policy must be necessary to realize the public health goal that is sought, such that a less infringing alternative is not suitable.
>
> Least infringement: Seek to minimize the infringement of general moral considerations.
>
> Public justification: Explain and justify infringements, whenever possible, to the relevant parties, including those affected by the infringement.

The second half of this chapter outlines concrete application of these conditions and presents specific rules and guidelines for ethical conduct of public health surveillance.

PRAGMATIC RULES AND GUIDELINES

Professional Codes of Conduct

Professional organizations have adopted codes of conduct that translate ethical standards into standards for professional practice (*29*). The American Public Health Association has endorsed 12 principles of the ethical practice of public health (*30–33*). The principles in the code guide, but do not prescribe, specific actions. Thomas (*34*) provides a genomics example, comparing and contrasting issues commonly raised in medical ethics. The code highlights issues that would not have come up directly in medically oriented discussions. The population orientation of the code supports considerations of how resource allocation benefits communities, where costs have to be balanced with other public health activities. The code's use of democratic processes points to the need to inform the public about the strengths, limitations, and costs of genomic tools and allow for the public to provide input on the use of genomic information such as in DNA databases. Further, the code highlights concerns about releasing genomic information that might potentially harm disenfranchised communities.

The American College of Epidemiology has endorsed ethics guidelines that outline core values, duties, and virtues in epidemiology and obligations of epidemiologists (*35,36*). The guidelines serve as the "basis for thoughtful reflection and sound judgment" rather than a step-by-step method for reaching decisions about ethical issues in epidemiologic research and practice. Guidelines relevant to public health surveillance include minimizing risks and providing benefits, ensuring equitable distribution of risks and benefits, protecting security and confidentiality, maintaining public trust, adhering to scientific standards, and involving community representatives.

Ethical Guidance Implicit in Model Legislation

In addition to professional codes, legal concepts can guide ethics in public health surveillance practice, as found in the Model State Public Health Privacy Act (37) and the subsequent Turning Point Model State Public Health Act (4, henceforth, Model Acts). The Model Acts were developed through consensus-building among national, tribal, state, and local public health representatives to remedy the fragmentation, inconsistency, and inadequacy of state laws on public health information privacy (38–41). These documents provide a model for protecting surveillance data without limiting the ability of public health agencies to act for legitimate public health purposes. Recent proposals for reform of national privacy protections have incorporated similar principles for ethical collection, storage, and use of public health data (42). Despite their limited success in actual legislative reform, they furnish a robust schema for the ethics of public health surveillance.

The guiding principles of the Model Acts (4: §5-101[b]) are grounded in the principles of beneficence, respect for persons, and justice and are consistent with the justificatory conditions:

> Public health authorities' actions should aim to achieve a public health purpose that sustains or furthers the public health (consistent with the principle of beneficence).
>
> Public health activities should be based in scientifically sound, evidence-based practices (beneficence).
>
> Interventions should be targeted to accomplish the public health activities and not apply to more individuals than necessary to achieve health. This is consistent with the condition of proportionality and fair distribution of burdens and benefits (justice). Similarly, when it is necessary to exercise public health powers that might restrict individual activity, public health should employ the least restrictive alternative that remains effective in protecting health and safety of the community (least infringement).
>
> Public health actions should not discriminate against individuals on the basis of their race, ethnicity, nationality, religious beliefs, sex, sexual orientation, or disability (respect for persons); should respect the dignity of individuals regardless of nationality or residency status (respect for persons); and should support community involvement and participation in achieving public health goals (public justification).

Box 9–1 itemizes guidelines distilled primarily from the Model Acts, under the rubrics of acquiring, using, disclosing, and storing surveillance data. We discuss and apply these guidelines in the next section.

Practical Application of Ethics in Surveillance

Public health surveillance typically includes data collection, data management and storage, and sharing and disseminating results. At each stage, surveillance

Box 9–1 Practical Application of Ethics in Public Health Surveillance

These guidelines are adapted primarily from the Model State Public Health Privacy Act (*37*) and Turning Point Model State Public Health Act (*4*). The Model Acts were developed over several years through partnerships of public health practitioners, national public health organizations, and representatives from the public and private sectors at the federal, tribal, state, and local levels (*41*). The Model Acts set a reference standard for the responsible acquisition, use, disclosure, and storage of identifiable health information and are applied here to public health surveillance.

Public health surveillance data should be acquired, used, disclosed, and stored for legitimate public health purposes.

> **Legitimate public health purpose** means a population-based activity or individual effort primarily aimed at the prevention of injury, disease, or premature mortality or the promotion of health in the community, including (*a*) assessing the health needs and status of the community through public health surveillance and epidemiologic research, (*b*) developing public health policy, and (*c*) responding to public health needs and emergencies.
>
> **Acquire** means to collect or gain control of identifiable surveillance data for legitimate public health purposes.
>
> **Use** means to employ identifiable surveillance data for a legitimate public health purpose.
>
> **Disclose** means to communicate identifiable surveillance data to any person or entity, other than a public health agency or authorized public health official.
>
> **Store** means to hold, maintain, keep, or retain identifiable surveillance data.

Public health surveillance data should be acquired for legitimate purposes and limited to that reasonably necessary to achieve the public health purpose.

> **Purpose**: Acquire only those surveillance data that relate directly to a legitimate public health purpose and are reasonably likely to achieve such purpose, consistent with governing law and available resources.
>
> **Identifiability**: Acquire nonidentifiable data whenever possible. Acquire identifiable data only if they are required to accomplish the legitimate public health purpose.
>
> **Limited scope**: Limit acquisition of surveillance data to the minimum amount of information needed.
>
> **Engagement**: Engage and notify affected communities and stakeholders prior to acquiring surveillance data.

Public health surveillance data may be used only for legitimate public health purposes.

> **Purpose**: After surveillance data are acquired for specific legitimate public health purposes, use them for those purposes. Use surveillance data for other legitimate public health purposes, including research, only with sufficient justification. The failure to use data for public health purposes must be justified.

(*continued*)

Identifiability: Use nonidentifiable data whenever possible.

Limited extent: Limit use of surveillance data to the minimum amount of information needed.

Dissemination: Release nonidentifiable, aggregate data in a manner that minimizes and fairly distributes possible burdens resulting from them. Disseminate nonconfidential results for public benefit.

Engagement: Engage and notify affected communities and stakeholders prior to disseminating surveillance data that might significantly impact an individual or community.

Identifiable public health surveillance data may be disclosed only when justified, for public health purposes, and subject to strict privacy and confidentiality standards.

Privacy and confidentiality: Strict norms of privacy and confidentiality must govern the disclosure of data. Whenever possible, disclose only nonidentifiable surveillance data.

Informed consent: Identifiable surveillance data should not be disclosed to any person or entity, other than a public health agency or authorized public health official, without the informed consent of the subject of the information.

Discretionary disclosure: Alternatives must be exhausted before it is justifiable to release individually identifiable data. Secondary recipients of identifiable surveillance data should not further disclose the data without authorization.

Compelled disclosure: Identifiable data may be disclosed without informed consent to appropriate authorities as required by law and to healthcare personnel in a medical emergency.

Public health surveillance data should be stored and managed in a physically and technologically secure environment.

Secure systems: Take appropriate measures to protect the physical and technological security of surveillance data. Limit and protect the places data are stored, the duration they are stored, and the means to access them.

Personal responsibility: Limit the persons who may access surveillance data. Each person who has authority to acquire, use, disclose, or store surveillance data assumes personal responsibility for preserving the security of the data.

Limited duration: Expunge surveillance data in a confidential manner when use of those data no longer furthers the legitimate public health purpose for which they were acquired.

practitioners might encounter issues that require thoughtful review of and reflection on ethical principles to decide on a course of action. We draw out some approaches to weigh various actions and consequences based on the ethical principles of beneficence, respect for persons, and justice and the justificatory conditions.

Accountability

As public servants, public health practitioners must be accountable for maintaining ethical practices in public health. This enhances public trust in the activities of public health institutions.

Establishing written policies and procedures is an important first step (*43*). Written procedures help to document and ensure standard approaches are used in various situations. These policies and procedures should be based on effective practices, current technology, empirical evidence, and sound ethics. Policies should be developed with the collaboration of persons involved in different aspects of surveillance, taking appropriate care to manage competing interests from those providing input. Policies and standards should cover data quality and require that data used to inform policies are sufficiently accurate and valid. Evaluations of data quality should take place at every stage of the surveillance process: during collection, management and storage, and analysis and use. These mechanisms are critical for justifying science-based public health policies and actions (*44*).

Surveillance practitioners can further ensure accountability by seeking review outside of their organization, whether through invited peer review, vetting by public health organizations, or publication. An autonomous body composed of persons familiar with ethics of public health surveillance might provide useful insight and feedback on proposed surveillance activities (*45*). It has been suggested that this be required (*46*).

Finally, procedures should allow for public notice to announce and justify surveillance activities at a broad level; additional engagement may be warranted for specific conditions or groups of conditions, depending in part on the public response itself. The public can be engaged through newsletters, websites, or public meetings with affected individuals and communities. The public should be told how community input will be obtained and used.

Ethical Considerations for Acquiring Data

When implementing new surveillance data collections, it is important for surveillance practitioners to articulate clearly the goal of the proposed data collection and the intended public health purpose—how the surveillance data collection activity will ultimately promote health or prevent disease. As Childress et al. (*6*) suggests, show that although data collection might infringe on liberty or privacy, it is worthwhile and likely to accomplish its purposes. Further, show whether the probable benefits outweigh the possible negative features or consequences of the data collections. If risks or harms are identified, consider how these risks or harms might be minimized while still achieving the identified goals.

Per the Model Acts, one should acquire the minimum amount of information necessary to achieve a public health purpose. Is the collection of personally identifiable data necessary, or can equally useful information be obtained using nonidentifiable data? If identifiable information must be used, the potential risks to individual privacy must be weighed against the potential benefits to the community of monitoring, preventing, or controlling a disease. The proposed data collection methods should be reasonable, scientifically reliable and valid, and likely to result in the data necessary to achieve the goal. The proposed data collection should be conducted with appropriate authority and consistent with existing laws and regulations. Planning includes other practical considerations, such as whether adequate staff and other resources are available to carry out the data collection, evaluation, and analysis.

Name-based HIV surveillance provides a useful example of ethical considerations when planning surveillance data collections (20,21). In the 1980s and 1990s in the United States, the value of and need for name-based surveillance systems were widely debated. Proponents thought that name-based systems provided the most standardized, high-quality data and would be more useful than anonymous or coded systems for interventions and referrals (condition of effectiveness). Opponents argued the risk to privacy was too great if data were inadvertently released or shared for purposes other than public health and that adequate quality data could be obtained without using names and that there was a suitable, less infringing alternative (condition of necessity). Programs had to demonstrate that the potential effectiveness at promoting public health goals outweighed potential or perceived risks (condition of proportionality). Some states implemented name-based HIV surveillance systems whereas others implemented systems that did not use names. HIV programs had to consider whether collection of sensitive information on sexual risk behaviors was critical for public health activities and whether the information could be adequately protected and used in a way that would not cause undue burden or further stigma in some communities. Some programs sought to address these issues through reaching out to affected communities and jointly assessing values, benefits, and harms (condition of public justification; *see also* ref. *47* regarding stakeholder theory). These consultations led to educating communities on the usefulness of the data and providing examples of how the data might be used or limited in release, as well as implementing policies and procedures that ensured security and confidentiality of the data. These efforts worked to build public trust in public health authorities and surveillance efforts and enhance transparency.

Lab-based reporting of diabetes indicators to New York City health officials provides another example (48–50). In addition to expanding diabetes surveillance, this name-based registry would be used to provide information on patients thought to evidence poor glycemic control to the individuals and their physicians. Despite strong confidentiality protections, this initiative was perceived as violating privacy and choice, liable to drive patients from care or physicians to shun difficult cases, and lacking increased resources for services. Proponents argued for the prospect of improved access to appropriate care (principle of justice) with potential for little discernible harm.

Ethical Considerations for Using and Disclosing Data

It is ethical to acquire surveillance data only if those data are put into use. The risks to privacy and liberty are justified only if the data are analyzed and disseminated for a public health purpose aimed at monitoring, preventing, or controlling disease or improving or protecting health (51). Even considering these potential benefits, the ethics of surveillance should include a code of restraint "to preserve fairly and appropriately the negative rights of citizens to noninterference" (7).

Fairchild et al. (52) propose a detailed code for using and disclosing identifiable data to achieve legitimate public health purposes. Under this code, data use and disclosure activities are associated with incremental rules of restraint, starting with the obligation to use data once collected, and ranging over disclosures within public health agencies; aggregate releases; releasing anonymous, individual-level data; disclosure to the public; and exceptional disclosure for nonhealth ends.

Disclosure within or among public health agencies:
The burden or risk of sharing identifiable data with other programs within a public health agency for related public health purposes is considered minimal if it is being shared for a legitimate public health purpose and the data have equivalent security protections. The ease of access to data within an agency does not negate the need to justify the use of the data. Thus it is necessary to review how the data will be used. It is possible to justify sharing identifiable surveillance data with another public health program to initiate a public health intervention, such as partner notification for an infectious disease. Sharing of data from a surveillance program might be the most efficient, cost-effective, and timely way of providing data to initiate a public health intervention (53). However, the proposed intervention must be proven to be a necessary, valid, and acceptable public health approach to justify the sharing of data.

Release to the public:
For most purposes, such as monitoring of disease trends, it is sufficient to release de-identified or aggregate data consistent with confidentiality standards that protect individual privacy. Policies should restrict any portion of a release that might lead to indirect identification of individuals. For example, when releasing data about a community with few members of an ethnic group or age group in a specified geographic area, a person might be identified by the combination of these characteristics. It might not be possible, however, to eliminate all risk to vulnerable populations and the obligation to use the data to help these groups could outweigh limited or short-term harms (54). For example, the potential burden or stigma brought on by reporting aggregate data suggesting high rates of alcohol and drug use in a small community must be weighed against the potential benefits to this community through potential additional resources for drug and alcohol treatment services afforded by releasing the data. Such data release might be justified and additional steps taken to help minimize the burden to these groups through a process of public justification in the affected community, where the data are explained and potential consequences of further dissemination or publication of the data discussed.

Disclosure to the public:
Disclosing identifiable public health data outside public health institutions requires a more stringent standard, even when data are shared for public health purposes. Health authorities might need to disclose a person's identity in an effort to avert a threat to the community. Community norms for the health departments' disclosing personal health information have evolved as norms for preserving confidentiality have emerged over time (55). Such public disclosures can only be ethically

justified if all alternative approaches have been exhausted and no other means are available to protect the public's health. In those rare instances, the principle of respect for persons dictates using the least intrusive measures available to achieve the public health goal and avert the threat (52).

Disclosure for nonhealth purposes:
Public health authorities might be compelled, after exhausting all other means to address or eliminate a public health threat, to seek the assistance of law enforcement or other officials to enforce public health measures. In these cases, it might be necessary to share identifiable data obtained through public health surveillance with law enforcement to achieve a public health goal. Fairchild et al. (52) note that "public health data acquired without consent pursuant to public health goals represent information that in other social domains might be provided under far more restrictive circumstances, e.g., where there exists a right to remain silent or an obligation to obtain a court order." In some cases, additional legal protections, such as an assurance of confidentiality under §308(d) of the Public Health Service Act (56), might be available to secure surveillance data against compelled disclosure. Surveillance data may be shared ethically only for non-public health purposes under extreme and compelling circumstances where the consequence of not doing so would result in significant harm to an individual or the public's health.

Surveillance programs should establish data-release policies to ensure that the data are released in a way that is consistent with the public health purpose but that cannot identify individuals or cause undue burden to groups of individuals or communities (57,58). Policies should delineate the exceptional circumstances in which release of identifiable data is warranted and how confidentiality will be protected (57,58). Published standards and recommended practices for de-identification of data can be used to guide policy development (59–63).

Population-based cancer registries illustrate issues in data sharing. Cancer cases are registered without patient consent, raising privacy concerns when using registry data to recruit for research (64) weighed against the need for valid and generalizable results from cancer research. Across different registries, physicians play different gate-keeping roles for patient access and privacy. In pursuit of improved cancer surveillance, prevention, and care, national leaders advocate for making "all cancer data systems linkable to each other … [with] privacy, confidentiality, and discrimination protections in place" (65).

Ethical Considerations for Managing and Storing Data

Public health agencies and staff that conduct public health surveillance must ensure that data are collected and held in a confidential manner and that adequate security measures are taken to protect surveillance data (42). Recommended security provisions include a variety of procedural and technical approaches (57,59) that cover how data are obtained, transferred, accessed, stored, and subsequently used or shared. Appropriate security protections include maintaining data in physically and technologically secure environments. Paper copies should be limited in number and stored in locked cabinets;

office space should be locked and provide limited access; and offices should be located in secured buildings that require authorization for entry. Paper copies may be transported by secure mail or locked brief cases. The minimum information should be included when paper copies are transported. The number and content of databases should be kept to the minimum possible; for example, analysis datasets should be anonymized. All computers and digital devices to store or access data should limit and authenticate a controlled number of users. Electronic data files can be stored in encrypted format. Data stored on computer networks should use firewalls, routers, and other mechanisms to limit access. Data should be encrypted for digital transmission to prevent reading by unauthorized individuals.

Written procedures should be available to all persons with access to the data and should clearly state roles, responsibilities, and consequences for violating policies. Access to surveillance data should be kept to a minimum and authorized access limited to those that have a justifiable need based on their role and job duties. It is good practice to incorporate a confidentiality statement of agreement for individuals working with surveillance data, which indicates they have read and understood the policies and their responsibilities and agree to abide by rules. Some agencies have incorporated specific sanctions into these agreements, including fines or loss of employment. Procedures for investigating breaches in policies should be incorporated and clearly stated. These procedures and agreements should be reviewed in routine, periodic staff training that adjusts to important changes in activities and evolving technologies.

CONCLUSIONS

Public health surveillance is essential for population well-being. This core obligation of government must be carried out with full sensitivity to relevant ethical considerations. We have outlined a set of concepts for analyzing the ethical dimensions of surveillance activities and shown pragmatic applications of these principles and conditions to routine collection, management, and sharing of data collected for public health surveillance.

Despite a substantial, intimate relationship between ethics and law, ethical dimensions are separate and distinguishable from legal and regulatory concerns. (Chapter 10 elucidates specific legal issues in surveillance.) Biomedical research ethics is the touchstone but ethical conduct of public health surveillance requires us to move past the formal demarcation between research and practice to focus first on intended benefits. Principles of human rights, justice, paternalism, and promotion of autonomy contribute to the construction of an ethic for public health surveillance. These ethical principles form the foundation on which leading model legislation has been erected.

As the field of public health ethics matures, it will further differentiate itself from biomedical ethics. The discourse on ethics of public health surveillance will become more refined, as well.

REFERENCES

1. Committee for the Study of the Future of Public Health, Institute of Medicine (U.S.). *The Future of Public Health*. Washington: National Academies Press; 1988.
2. Committee on Assuring the Health of the Public in the 21st Century, Institute of Medicine (U.S.). *The Future of the Public's Health in the 21st Century*. Washington: National Academies Press; 2002.
3. Gostin LO. Health of the people: the highest law? *J Law Med Ethics* 2004;32(3):509–515.
4. The Turning Point Public Health Statute Modernization Collaborative. *The Turning Point Model State Public Health Act: A Tool for Assessing Public Health Laws*. September 2003. http://www.turningpointprogram.org/Pages/pdfs/statute_mod/MSPHAfinal.pdf. Accessed February 2, 2009.
5. Callahan D, Jennings B. Ethics and public health: forging a strong relationship. *Am J Public Health* 2002;92(2):169–176.
6. Childress JF, Faden RR, Gaare RD, *et al*. Public health ethics: mapping the terrain. *J Law Med Ethics* 2002;30:170–178.
7. Kass NE. An ethics framework for public health. *Am J Public Health* 2001;91(11):1776–1782.
8. Levin BW, Fleischman AR. Public health and bioethics: the benefits of collaboration. *Am J Public Health* 2002;92(2):165–167.
9. Roberts MJ, Reich MR. Ethical analysis in public health. *Lancet* 2002;359:1055–1059.
10. The National Commission for the Protection of Human Subjects of Biomedical and Behavioral Research. *The Belmont Report: Ethical Principles and Guidelines for the Protection of Human Subjects of Research*. Department of Health, Education, and Welfare; April 18, 1979.
11. Beauchamp TL, Childress JF. *Principles of Biomedical Ethics*, 1st ed. New York: Oxford University Press; 1979.
12. Beauchamp TL, Childress JF. *Principles of Biomedical Ethics*, 5th ed. New York: Oxford University Press; 2001.
13. Mann JM. Medicine and public health, ethics and human rights. *Hastings Cent Rep* 1997;27(3):6–13.
14. National Bioethics Advisory Commission. *Ethical and Policy Issues in Research Involving Human Participants*. Bethesda, Maryland; August 2001. *Report and Recommendations of the National Bioethics Advisory Commission*; Volume I.
15. Federal Policy for the Protection of Human Subjects (45 CFR part 46).
16. Centers for Disease Control and Prevention. *Guidelines for Defining Public Health Research and Public Health Non-Research*. http://www.cdc.gov/od/science/regs/hrpp/researchDefinition.htm. Revised October 4, 1999. Accessed February 2, 2009.
17. Hodge JG, Gostin LO. Public health practice vs. research: a report for public health practitioners including cases and guidance for making distinctions. Council of State and Territorial Epidemiologists; May 24, 2004. http://www.cste.org/pdffiles/newpdf-files/CSTEPHResRptHodgeFinal.5.24.04.pdf. Accessed February 2, 2009.
18. Hodge JG. An enhanced approach to distinguishing public health practice and human subjects research. *J Law Med Ethics* 2005;33(1):125–141.
19. Gostin LO, Hodge JG. Personal privacy and common goods: a framework for balancing under the national health information privacy rule. *Minn Law Rev* 2002;86:1430–1479.

20. Bayer R, Fairchild AL. The genesis of public health ethics. *Bioethics* 2004;18(6):473–492.

21. Burris S. Surveillance, social risk, and symbolism: framing the analysis for research and policy. *J Acquir Immune Defic Syndr* 2000;25:S120–S127.

22. Jones MM, Bayer R. Paternalism & its discontents: motorcycle helmet laws, libertarian values, and public health. *Am J Public Health* 2007;97(2):208–217.

23. Buchanan DR. Autonomy, paternalism, and justice: ethical priorities in public health. *Am J Public Health* 2008;98(1):15–21.

24. *Healthy People 2010*. Washington: US Department of Health and Human Services; 2000.

25. Kass NE. Public health ethics: from foundations and frameworks to justice and global public health. *J Law Med Ethics* 2004;32:232–242.

26. Gostin LO, Lazzarini Z. *Human Rights and Public Health in the AIDS Pandemic*. New York: Oxford University Press; 1997.

27. Gostin LO. Public health, ethics, and human rights: a tribute to the late Jonathan Mann. *J Law Med Ethics* 2001;29:121–130.

28. Gruskin S. Ethics, human rights, and public health. *Am J Public Health* 2002;92(5):698.

29. Weed DL, McKeown RE. Science, ethics, and professional public health practice. *J Epidemiol Community Health* 2003;57:4–5.

30. American Public Health Association. Ethical Guidelines. http://www.apha.org/programs/education/progeduethicalguidelines.htm. Accessed February 2, 2009.

31. Public Health Leadership Society. Principles of the Ethical Practice of Public Health, Version 2.2, 2002. http://209.9.235.208/CMSuploads/PHLSethicsbrochure-40103.pdf. Accessed February 2, 2009.

32. Thomas JC, Sage M, Dillenberg J, Guillory VJ. A code of ethics for public health. *Am J Public Health* 2002;92(7):1057–1059.

33. Stefanak M, Frisch L, Palmer-Fernandez G. An organizational code of public health ethics: practical applications and benefits. *Public Health Rep* 2007;122:548–551.

34. Thomas JC, Irwin DE, Zuiker ES, Millikan RC. Genomics and the Public Health Code of Ethics. *Am J Public Health* 2005;95(12):2139–2143.

35. Weed DL, Coughlin SS. New ethics guidelines for epidemiology: background and rationale. *Ann Epidemiol* 1999;9:277–280.

36. American College of Epidemiology. American College of Epidemiology ethics guidelines. *Ann Epidemiol* 2000;10:487–497.

37. Gostin LO, Hodge JG. *The Model State Public Health Privacy Act*. 1999. http://www.publichealthlaw.net/ModelLaws/MSPHPA.php. Accessed February 2, 2009.

38. Gostin LO, Lazzarini Z, Neslund VS, Osterholm MT. The public health information infrastructure: a national review of the law on health information privacy. *JAMA* 1996;275(24):1921–1927.

39. Gostin LO. Public health law reform. *Am J Public Health* 2001;91(9):1365–1368.

40. Gostin LO, Hodge JG, Valdiserri RO. Informational privacy and the public's health: the Model State Public Health Privacy Act. *Am J Public Health* 2001;91(9):1388–1392.

41. Hodge JG, Gostin LO, Gebbie K, Erickson DL. Transforming public health law: the Turning Point Model State Public Health Act. *J Law Med Ethics* 2006;34(1):77–84.

42. Lee LM, Gostin LO. Ethical collection, storage, and use of public health data—a proposal for a national privacy protection. *JAMA* 2009;302(1)82–84.

43. National Public Health Performance Standards Program. *10 Essential Public Health Services*. Centers for Disease Control and Prevention. http://www.cdc.gov/od/ocphp/

nphpsp/EssentialPublicHealthServices.htm. Updated October 15, 2008. Accessed February 4, 2009.

44. Centers for Disease Control and Prevention. Guidelines for Ensuring the Quality of Information Disseminated to the Public. http://www.cdc.gov/maso/qualitycontrol/Guidelines.htm. Last revised, December 13, 2006. Accessed February 2, 2009.

45. Baily MA, Bottrell M, Lynn J, Jennings B. The ethics of using QI methods to improve health care quality and safety. *Hastings Cent Rep* 2006;36(4):S1–S40.

46. Fairchild AL, Jones MM. Ethics and the conduct of public health surveillance. In: M'ikanatha NM, Ruth Lynfield R, Van Beneden CA, de Valk H, eds. *Infectious Disease Surveillance*. Oxford, England: Blackwell Publishing; 2007.

47. Bernheim RG, Nieburg P, Bonnie RJ. Ethics and the practice of public health. In: Goodman RA, ed. *Law in Public Health Practice*, 2nd ed. New York: Oxford University Press; 2007.

48. Fairchild AL. Diabetes and disease surveillance. *Science* 2006;313(5784):175–176.

49. Gostin LO. "Police" powers and public health paternalism: HIV and diabetes surveillance. *Hastings Cent Rep* 2007;37:9–10.

50. Goldman J, Kinnear S, Chung J, Rothman DJ. New York City's initiatives on diabetes and HIV/AIDS: implications for patient care, public health, and medical professionalism. *Am J Public Health* 2009;98(5):807–813.

51. CDC/ATSDR Policy on Releasing and Sharing Data. Centers for Disease Control and Prevention. http://www.cdc.gov/od/foia/policies/sharing.htm. Updated September 7, 2005. Accessed February 4, 2009.

52. Fairchild AL, Gable L, Gostin LO, Bayer R, Sweeney P, Janssen RS. Public goods, private data: HIV and the history, ethics, and uses of identifiable public health information. *Pub Health Rep* 2007;122(Suppl 1):7–15.

53. Centers for Disease Control and Prevention. Recommendations for partner services programs for HIV infection, syphilis, gonorrhea, and chlamydial infection. *MMWR Recomm Rep* 2008;57(RR-9):1–83.

54. Bernheim RG. Public health ethics: the voices of practitioners. *J Law Med Ethics* 2003;31(4 Suppl):104–111.

55. Fairchild AL, Bayer R, Colgrove J. *Searching Eyes: Privacy, the State, and Disease Surveillance in America*. Berkeley, CA: University of California Press; 2007.

56. Privacy Legislation and Regulations. Centers for Disease Control and Prevention. http://www.cdc.gov/od/science/regs/privacy/#assurances. Updated October 14, 2008. Accessed February 4, 2009.

57. Centers for Disease Control and Prevention and Council of State and Territorial Epidemiologists. *Technical Guidance for HIV/AIDS Surveillance Programs, Volume III: Security and Confidentiality Guidelines*. Atlanta, Georgia: Centers for Disease Control and Prevention; 2006. http://www.cdc.gov/hiv/topics/surveillance/resources/guidelines/guidance/index.htm. Accessed February 4, 2009.

58. CDC-CSTE Intergovernmental Data Release Guidelines Working Group Report. *CDC/ATSDR Data Release Guidelines and Procedures for Re-release of State-Provided Data*. January, 2005. http://www.cdc.gov/od/foia/policies/drgwg.pdf. Accessed February 4, 2009.

59. Committee on the Role of Institutional Review Boards in Health Services Research Data Privacy Protection, Division of Health Care Services, Institute of Medicine (U.S.). *Protecting Data Privacy in Health Services Research*. Washington, DC: National Academies Press, Washington, 2000.

60. Doyle P, Lane J, Theeuwes J, Zayatz L, eds. *Confidentiality, Disclosure and Data Access: Theory and Practical Applications for Statistical Agencies*. New York: North Holland; 2001.

61. *Record Linkage and Privacy: Issues in Creating New Federal Research and Statistical Information.* No. GAO-01-126SP. Government Accountability Office; April 2001.

62. Confidentiality and Data Access Committee. *Identifiability in Microdata Files.* Office of Management and Budget; 2002.

63. Federal Committee on Statistical Methodology. *Statistical Policy Working Paper 22: Report on Statistical Disclosure Limitation Methodology.* Office of Management and Budget; 2005.

64. Beskow LM, Sandler RS, Weinberger M. Research recruitment through US central cancer registries: balancing privacy and scientific issues. *Am J Public Health* 2006;96(11):1920–1926.

65. Hiatt RA. The future of cancer surveillance. *Cancer Causes Control* 2006;17:639–646.

10

Legal Considerations in Public Health Surveillance in the United States

VERLA S. NESLUND, RICHARD A. GOODMAN,
JAMES G. HODGE, Jr., AND JOHN P. MIDDAUGH

INTRODUCTION

Public health surveillance is a critical, basic function carried out by public health agencies at local, state, and federal levels. Each of the 50 states operates and maintains public health surveillance systems, not only to monitor notifiable disease conditions caused primarily by infectious pathogens but also to monitor noninfectious conditions (e.g., injuries, cancer, lead exposure, and birth defects) and public health indicators, such as behavioral risk factors for injuries and chronic conditions (*1,2*). Along with the traditional collection and analysis of vital records, state-level surveillance forms the foundation for national-level surveillance systems, which might be coordinated by federal agencies such as the Centers for Disease Control and Prevention (CDC), the National Cancer Institute (NCI), and the National Institutes of Health (NIH) (*1–3*).

Public health surveillance is the first step in a series of activities to protect the public's health. These activities range from outbreak response, to conduct of analytic studies, to implementation and enforcement of control measures such as vaccination, chemoprophylaxis, isolation and quarantine, or even seizure or destruction of property.

This chapter provides an overview of the legal issues relating to public health surveillance. It discusses the general legal authorities for public health surveillance set forth in constitutional, statutory, and regulatory laws; legal milestones in the evolution of public health surveillance and disease control in the United States (see Box 10–1); and legal issues related to the collection, analysis, and dissemination of surveillance data for public health practice and research activities. In addition, the chapter presents information about new surveillance challenges beyond traditional infectious disease models, including the influence of bioterrorism preparedness on surveillance activities.

Box 10–1 Legal Milestones in the Evolution of Public Health Surveillance, Outbreak Investigations, and Disease Control

A form of surveillance was employed in colonial America as early as 1741, when the colony of Rhode Island passed an act requiring tavern keepers to report contagious diseases among their patrons (4). Two years later, the colony enacted a law requiring the reporting of smallpox, yellow fever, and cholera. In 1874, systematic reporting of disease in the United States began when the Massachusetts State Board of Health initiated voluntary weekly reporting of common diseases by physicians who used a postcard reporting format (5). The collection of morbidity data to be used by the U.S. Marine Hospital Service, the forerunner to PHS, for quarantine measures against selected diseases (e.g., cholera and yellow fever) was authorized by Congress in the Quarantine Act of 1878 (6). Fifteen years later, Michigan became the first jurisdiction in the United States to require reporting of specific infectious diseases (4).

The federal Quarantine Act of 1893 authorized the weekly collection of data from all states (7). By 1901, all states required that selected infectious diseases be reported to local health authorities. As the result of the intervening epidemic of polio in 1916 and pandemic of influenza in 1918, all states were participating in national morbidity reporting by 1925 (5). In 1961, CDC—at that time bearing the name "Communicable Disease Center"—became responsible for receipt of reports of notifiable conditions and for weekly dissemination of such data through the *Morbidity and Mortality Weekly Report*, a publication that by 1994 had begun to make these data available online. The Public Health Service Act authorized CDC to collect, collate, and analyze notifiable disease data at the national level; but in fact, state health agencies provide these data to the federal government on a voluntary, cooperative basis. Moreover, each state promulgates its own set of conditions by legislative enactment or regulation (5,8).

Influence of Smallpox on Public Health Laws

Smallpox, the only disease to have been eradicated from the world, played an especially profound role in influencing the evolution of the legal basis for the control of infectious diseases in the United States; many of the key developments have been reported by Dr. Donald R. Hopkins (9). An early example of the use of the functional strategies of local quarantine and isolation to prevent the spread of smallpox during the colonial era was an order issued in East Hampton, Long Island, in 1662. In 1676, the colony of Virginia legislated mandatory home isolation of persons with smallpox. During a protracted outbreak in 1702, the Massachusetts Bay Colony enacted a law authorizing selectmen of local towns to carry out isolation and quarantine; this act superseded vaguer authority previously delegated by the governor to selectmen. The Massachusetts Bay Colony authorized additional measures in 1731 with enactment of "An Act to Prevent Persons from Concealing the Small Pox," which required household heads to report cases to selectmen and to display a red flag on the home to warn others (9).

As part of a more concerted effort to control smallpox, in 1813, the U.S. Congress established a National Vaccine Agency as part of the "An Act to Encourage Vaccination"; however, the Agency was closed and the act repealed in 1822 at the recommendation of a Congressional committee investigating a cluster of deaths in persons who inadvertently had been vaccinated with real smallpox scabs (9–11). As

(continued)

the 19th century progressed, legislators were faced with the challenge of balancing the need for control measures, such as vaccination to protect communities, against evolving beliefs regarding personal freedom of choice. However, in the setting of an epidemic in Boston during 1855, the state legislature enacted "the first mandatory school vaccination law in the United States," although this law was not enforced until an epidemic wave in the early 1880s (9). Similarly, in Atlanta, regulations mandating vaccination of schoolchildren were enforced only months before an outbreak in that city in 1882. Improvement in the smallpox situation led to public resistance to vaccination and vaccination laws in the early 1900s, and California went so far as to repeal its law mandating vaccination for schoolchildren. However, in 1922, after a resurgence of smallpox beginning in 1920, the U.S. Supreme Court held that school authorities could mandate vaccination for school entry, regardless of whether an immediate local smallpox threat existed (9,12).

Smallpox precipitated one of the most important—if not *the* most important—appellate decisions involving U.S. public health practice: the 1905 U.S. Supreme Court case of *Jacobson v. Massachusetts* (13). In that case, the facts of which emerged during a smallpox epidemic in 1902, the defendant, Henning Jacobson, refused smallpox vaccination as ordered by the Cambridge Board of Health pursuant to its authorities under Massachusetts law. Jacobson was found guilty of violating the law and appealed the verdict first to the state's Supreme Judicial Court, and then to the U.S. Supreme Court. In its opinion, the Supreme Court upheld the validity of the Massachusetts statute and stated that "[u]pon the principle of self-defense, of paramount necessity, a community has the right to protect itself against an epidemic of disease which threatens the safety of its members." The impact of this case on public health practice has endured for over a full century, and the holding has provided constitutional support not only for vaccination laws but also for many other public health laws (14).

As a historical footnote, in addition to prompting laws and other control measures, smallpox affected the legislative and judicial processes in colonial America in other ways. For example, in 1636 and 1659, the General Court of the Massachusetts Bay Colony was forced to convene in locations outside of Boston, where it usually met, to escape smallpox outbreaks in the city. Similarly, in 1696, an outbreak in Jamestown, Virginia, caused the colony's assembly to recess; and in 1702, smallpox in Manhattan caused both the assembly and Supreme Court to adjourn to Long Island (9).

Impact of Other Infectious Disease Influences on Present-Day Laws

Although smallpox represents one of the earliest of the infectious disease problems prompting legislative responses in the United States, many other infectious diseases fundamentally influenced present-day laws related to infectious diseases (15). For example, epidemics of yellow fever and cholera during the 1800s also led to enactment of state and local disease-control laws providing for sanitation, quarantine, and isolation. Recognition of the impact of tuberculosis led to changes in disease reporting and surveillance, including establishment of case reporting in New York in the 1890s, and syphilis-control initiatives in the early 1900s prompted enactment of laws for premarital screening, reporting, contact tracing, and involuntary treatment (15). The federal government had only limited early involvement in public health, including the control and prevention of infectious diseases; examples of such involvement included "An Act relative to Quarantine," passed in 1796 and authorizing the President to direct federal officials "to aid in the execution of quarantine, and also in the execution of

(continued)

the health laws of the states," and the 1813 act to encourage smallpox vaccination, as noted above (*10,16*).

Some of the earliest sanitary legislation in the American colonies was enactment in 1647 or 1648 by the General Court of the Massachusetts Bay Colony that provided for maritime quarantine against ships from the yellow fever-affected West Indies (*17*). In 1678, local regulations against smallpox were adopted in Boston, Salem, and Plymouth, and in 1742, the Massachusetts Bay Colony passed a law to prevent smallpox and other infectious sickness. The first local boards of health in the United States were created during 1793 to 1794 in Baltimore and Philadelphia as a consequence of a yellow fever epidemic (*17*).

GENERAL LEGAL AUTHORITIES FOR PUBLIC HEALTH SURVEILLANCE

U.S. Constitution

Both federal and state governments have inherent powers to protect the public's health. Article 1, Section 8, of the U.S. Constitution authorizes Congress to impose taxes to "provide for the general [w]elfare of the United States" and to regulate interstate and foreign commerce. The Public Health Service (PHS) and CDC are examples of federal agencies that might be supported generally by the authority of the welfare clause. Through its constitutional powers to regulate interstate commerce and tax and spending, the federal government oversees health-related activities such as the licensing and regulation of drugs, biological products, and medical devices. Although the provisions in the federal Constitution are broad, the activities of the federal government relating to health and welfare nonetheless must fit within the enumerated powers.

By contrast, the public health powers of a state are extensive, rooted in its inherent sovereign powers to protect the peace, safety, health, and general welfare of its citizens. The Tenth Amendment to the U.S. Constitution specifically reserves all powers not expressly granted to the federal government nor otherwise prohibited by the Constitution to the states. Unlike the federal government, the states have vast, sovereign authority, pursuant to their "political powers," which include the intrinsic right to pass laws and to take other measures necessary to protect the public's health and safety. In many instances, states have delegated their public health responsibilities to county or municipal governments, which likewise exercise the state's broad authority to examine, treat, and quarantine or isolate citizens in the case of certain contagious diseases to protect the public health. The state's public health laws include not only the established statutes of the state but also regulations, executive orders, and other directives from health authorities that might have the force of law.

State Police Powers and Public Health

The exercise of the states' police powers with respect to public health matters has limitations. The U.S. Constitution provides procedural safeguards to ensure the exercise of these powers is not excessive or unrestrained. The Fourth Amendment protects citizens from unlawful searches and seizures, and the Fifth Amendment prohibits the federal government from depriving any persons of life, liberty, or property without due process of law. The Fourteenth Amendment imposes similar due process obligations on states, and specifically incorporates other federal constitutional protections to state and local governments. Substantive due process requires that government act in a manner that is not arbitrary or capricious when such actions might deprive persons of their right to life, liberty, or property. This form of due process might, for example, require that government use the least restrictive alternative to achieve the state's interest when the exercise involves limitations of the individual's personal liberty. Procedural due process demands the government use even-handed and impartial procedures in exercising its police power. The basic elements of due process include notice to the person involved, opportunity for a hearing or similar proceeding, and the right to representation by counsel (in certain instances).

MANDATORY REPORTING OF DISEASES AND CONDITIONS

Public health surveillance systems in the United States are legally supported by states' police powers. These state-based systems require reporting with patient identifiers of diseases and conditions of pubic health interest by health-care professionals, pharmacists, diagnostic laboratories, clinical facilities, schools, daycare centers, and others (18–20). All states have laws and regulations that mandate the reporting of a list of diseases and conditions, as well as prescribe the timing and nature of information to be reported, including patient identifying information, and penalties for noncompliance (18). Most states also offer specific legal protections for the privacy of the identifiable data they collect through public health surveillance systems (19). The specific legal mechanisms that authorize required disease reporting vary greatly among states and territories. In some states, disease reporting is mandated by antiquated statutes that have not been revised in decades. Other states have general statutes that empower the health commissioner or state boards of health to create, monitor, and revise the list of reportable diseases and conditions (21). Some states require reports via statutes and health department regulations (22). All states, however, periodically update their disease reporting lists through public processes of administrative and legal rule making. Although state disease reporting generally is mandated by law or regulation, reporting of disease and death information by the state or territorial health department to CDC is voluntary and does not typically include providing patient-identifying information, which is held confidentially by the states.

The scope and nature of reporting requirements vary considerably by state, differing, for example, by the number of conditions required for reporting, period within which conditions must be reported, agencies to which reports must be submitted, and persons or sources required to report. Despite legal requirements for reporting, adherence to and completeness of reporting also vary substantially by infectious disease agent, ranging from 6% to 90% for different common infectious conditions (23). Disease reporting is an efficient and effective, proven mechanism to monitor diseases of public health importance. The completeness of disease reporting is highly correlated with the severity and importance of immediate public health actions that ensure upon identification of the disease. For example, diseases such as human rabies, botulism, ciguatera poisoning, or meningococcal meningitis tend to have close to 100% reporting, whereas diseases such as Chlamydia, gonorrhea, and hepatitis might capture as few as 10% of actual cases. Epidemiologists monitor each of the diseases and periodically conduct special case ascertainment studies to validate the estimates of the completeness of reporting and the true disease burdens of the populations. Deficiencies in reporting by physicians are accounted for, in part, by limitations in physicians' knowledge of reporting requirements and procedures, as well as the assumption that laboratories have reported cases of infectious diseases (18,24). A dramatic exception was engendered by linking Ryan White Care Act (25) funding to AIDS case counts. Because the number of reported cases determined the fate of millions of dollars of federal funding, the disease reporting system attempts to ascertain all cases of disease.

The Role of Council of the State and Territorial Epidemiologists in Standardizing Reportable Diseases and Conditions

Beginning in 1951, the Council of State and Territorial Epidemiologists (CSTE) was authorized by its parent body, the Association of State and Territorial Health Officials (ASTHO), to decide what diseases states should report to the Public Health Service (PHS). In consultation with CDC, CSTE annually recommends additions and deletions to the list of diseases and conditions.

An assessment of state laws and regulations in 1989 highlighted an important impediment to the surveillance and control of infectious diseases—namely, variations in case definitions the states used for identifying and acting on reports of cases and the effect of lack of uniformity on limiting the ability to compare patterns of infectious disease occurrence among states. For example, some states required reporting of any person with a positive culture for *Salmonella*, whereas others required reporting of only culture-positive persons who were symptomatic (4). To address these differences and to facilitate comparison of surveillance among states, CSTE and CDC developed and updated standardized case definitions for the nationally notifiable infectious diseases (26). Implementation of uniform case definitions and related procedures were expected to provide for interstate reciprocal notification for cases of infectious disease when onset was in one state but the patient was hospitalized in or transferred to another state and cases for which public health action (e.g., contact tracing) might be involved in different states. However, reporting requirements by state continue to differ: as of January 1999, of the 52 infectious conditions agreed on for national surveillance, only 19 were reportable in all states (19).

In 1995 and 1996, CDC and CSTE expanded the list beyond the traditional collection of infectious diseases, recommending that elevated blood lead levels, silicosis, and acute pesticide poisoning be added (19). The number of diseases and conditions on the list varies from year to year but is usually 65 to 75. The list of diseases and conditions under national surveillance is published each year in the annual summary of notifiable diseases in the *Morbidity and Mortality Weekly Report* (*MMWR*). CSTE also keeps information about state disease and condition reporting requirements on its website (*27*).

Enforcement of Reporting Laws

Few states choose to penalize health-care providers for not reporting notifiable conditions, although disciplinary measures may be invoked in instances when failure to report has serious untoward effects. For example, the California Board of Medical Quality Assurance took action against a physician in that state for "gross negligence and incompetence, failure to report to local health authorities a suspected case of an infectious disease in a known food handler" (*28*). At that time, California law set forth legal responsibility of physicians, dentists, nurses, and others to notify local health authorities of persons ill with specified infectious diseases. In this instance, the physician had examined a patient he knew to be a food handler. Although the physician recognized the patient was jaundiced and possibly had hepatitis, he failed to report the patient's condition to local public health authorities. An outbreak of foodborne hepatitis followed in which at least 62 cases of hepatitis were associated with the food handler; one person died. In suspending the physician's license for 1 year (the suspension was stayed and the physician was placed on 5 years of probation), the California Board of Medical Quality Assurance declared that the "failure to report a suspected if not a known case of an infectious disease in a food handler was an extreme departure from the standard practice of medicine" (*28*).

EMERGING DEVELOPMENTS IN PUBLIC HEALTH SURVEILLANCE

Historically, public health surveillance was largely for infectious diseases and based on mandatory reporting of individual cases of disease. Increasingly in the past 20 years, use of mandatory reporting as a surveillance method has been expanded through changes in state public health reporting statutes, regulations, or executive orders to include conditions and syndromes beyond infectious diseases (*29*). These especially include cancer, birth defects, injuries, fatalities, and chemical exposures. During the past 5 years, there has been expanded attention to emerging infectious diseases, diseases that might result from bioterrorism, and other urgent threats.

Through collaboration between CSTE and CDC, newer methods have been developed as a basis for state and national public health surveillance. These include use of the Behavioral Risk Factor Surveillance System to monitor prevalence of health risk behaviors such as tobacco use (*30*) and a variety of methods to monitor occupational disease, chronic conditions, and injuries. Methods range from telephone surveys (Youth Risk Behavior Surveillance) system to the development and maintenance of cancer registries, trauma registries, and birth defect registries to use of hospital discharge databases, Medicare and Medicaid databases, and worker compensation databases. Similarly to updating the national list of notifiable infectious diseases and case definitions, a collaborative process exists to develop, define, and update a national list of chronic disease indicators (*31*). CSTE maintains information on its website to identify indicators for chronic disease surveillance, including access to current data to assist public health practitioners assess indicators for their locales. In addition, publication of data on matters such as firearm-related injuries has significantly increased awareness of these public health issues, as well as the importance of surveillance to the consideration of law and policy interventions.

These newer surveillance methods use mandatory reporting dependent upon state public health police powers. They also use voluntary processes, such as willingness of the public to respond to a telephone survey, or employ existing databases from which individual identifier information usually is removed. However, their public health use is facilitated by the broad authority of state public health officials to obtain public health surveillance data.

LEGAL ISSUES RELATED TO DATA COLLECTION, ANALYSIS, AND DISSEMINATION

The processes of collecting data for public health surveillance, as part of an outbreak investigation for other epidemiology activities, might invoke numerous legal considerations, including: *(1)* protection available under state or federal law during and after the investigation for the confidentiality of records collected and generated in relation to the investigation; *(2)* privacy provisions for medical and other information; *(3)* required reporting of particular diseases or conditions; *(4)* status of information in investigative files under the federal Freedom of Information Act (FOIA) (5 U.S.C. §552) or state FOIA counterparts (and their usual exemption from FOIA requirements); and *(5)* the possible applicability of federal or state human subjects research regulations, including the need for review of study protocols by institutional review boards and the need for informed consent for participation in the investigation or for procedures related to the investigation, if activities being conducted involve research and not public health practice.

To determine what records will be kept or generated and where and how such records will be stored, federal, state, and local public health officials need to be familiar with legal protections applicable to documents and other records that will be examined, extracted, and compiled in association with the surveillance activity. Most states provide specific statutory and regulatory privacy protection over medical and public health records. In general, the privacy protection prevents the disclosure of a personally identified record without the consent of the person on whom the record is maintained. Accordingly, state law generally protects such medical records. Furthermore, such state laws frequently require that only certain authorized personnel have access to such private records and that such records be maintained in a secure manner. Public health investigators usually would be authorized access to such records for surveillance and related public health activities but would be bound to maintain the records in a manner that would protect the privacy of the identifiable information from unauthorized or inadvertent disclosure.

In the course of surveillance activities, public health personnel might create or compile a variety of documents, including questionnaires, forms, notes, copies, or extractions of patient or other records, letters, reports, memoranda, drafts, manuscripts, and final reports. Depending on the nature of the records, these documents might not be protected from disclosure to the public by state or federal laws (such as state laws protecting public health and medical records), public health investigators should assume that all records collected might at some point be open to public scrutiny. This may include personal notes by the public health investigator, drafts of documents retained in the files, and other related information within the scope of the request.

HEALTH INFORMATION PRIVACY IN EPIDEMIOLOGIC PRACTICE

An effective surveillance system includes the capacity for data collection and the ability to disseminate the data to persons who can undertake prevention and control activities. The collection of vital records and other data for public health practice, surveillance, and during epidemic investigations implicates a variety of legal issues and considerations, which also are relevant to information gathering necessary for other basic disease-control activities (e.g., surveys, special studies, categorical disease-control programs, and program evaluation). Increasingly, surveillance is used for investigating the range of conditions affecting health, including, for example, injuries, chronic diseases, environmental exposures, and maternal and child health activities (*32*). The underlying issues attendant to data collection in these situations are balancing the need for access to medical and other records against individuals' interests in privacy through the imposition of strict limits on access. These legal considerations, most of which are addressed by statutes or regulations, include protections available during and after records are developed for a public health surveillance activity; special privacy provisions for medical and other information; and mandated reporting of specific infectious conditions, as noted above.

Protecting the privacy, confidentiality, and security of health data, whether in a research or public health activity, is fundamental to responsible data collection and sharing practices. Although often used interchangeably, the terms *privacy*, *confidentiality*, and *security* have distinct legal and ethical meanings with respect to identifiable health information (*33*). Health information privacy broadly refers to the rights of individuals to control acquisition, uses, or disclosures of their identifiable health data. The closely related concept of confidentiality refers to the obligations of those who receive information to respect the privacy interests of individuals who are the subjects of the data.

Security is different from confidentiality in that it refers to technological or administrative safeguards or tools to protect identifiable health data from unwarranted access or disclosure. Maintaining information security has become increasingly more difficult in the modern era of digitized exchanges and large electronic health databases that can be hacked or infiltrated through unlawful invasions. However, electronic health systems also hold great promise for improving health care and public health efficiency as well as for protecting privacy and security (34).

Varied privacy and security laws and policies for sharing health data reflect the fragmented nature of legal protections of health information privacy. Neither constitutional principles nor judicial decisions focused on common law concepts of duties of confidentiality support an individual's broad expectation of health information privacy. Rather, federal and state statutes and regulations are the dominant basis for health information privacy protections in the United States (33). Arrays of significant federal and state laws, discussed below, are intended to safeguard health information privacy.

FEDERAL PUBLIC HEALTH INFORMATION PRIVACY LAWS

The federal Privacy Act of 1974 applies whenever information is collected and maintained by a federal agency in a system of records in which the information is retrieved by an individual's name, identification number, or other identifier (35). The Privacy Act was the first national law to introduce fair information practices that allow individuals to access their own government-held information. A person also may seek amendments to information that is not accurate, relevant, or complete. Among other things, the Privacy Act protects individual privacy by (1) specifying the situations in which a person's health information could be disclosed without individual consent and which situations require consent; (2) proscribing government maintenance of identifiable health information that is irrelevant and unnecessary to accomplish the agency's purpose; (3) requiring agencies to publish a notice about each record system describing its purpose and identifying disclosures outside the agency (e.g., "routine uses") that the agency has made administratively; and (4) requiring agencies to inform individuals of the statutory basis for collecting health information, purposes for which it is used, and consequences for not supplying the information.

The Freedom of Information Act (FOIA) of 1988 provides that agency records created or maintained by an agency and under its control are available to the public unless specifically exempted from disclosure (36). The Act contains nine exemptions, several of which help protect the privacy of some public health data, including the following:

> *Interagency and intra-agency communications.* Exemption (b) (5) permits the federal government to withhold from disclosure interagency and

intra-agency memoranda or letters that would not available "to a party other than an agency in litigation with the agency." This exemption may be used by the agency data holder, for example, to protect from disclosure a draft memorandum written by the investigator to his or her supervisor describing the early findings of an epidemiologic investigation.

Personnel and medical records. Exemption (b) (6) permits an agency data holder to withhold from mandatory disclosure "personnel and medical files and similar files the disclosure of which would constitute a clearly unwarranted invasion of personal privacy." This exemption may be invoked to protect confidential medical information about a person contained in an agency record.

Information otherwise exempt from disclosure by statute. Exemption (b) (3) provides that a federal agency may withhold from disclosure information "specifically exempted from disclosure by statute." For example, if a federal epidemiologic investigation is conducted under an assurance of confidentiality authorized by a federal statute (discussed below), the information collected pursuant to the confidentiality assurance may be exempted from disclosure under FOIA.

Additional privacy protections for research and other health data are found in the Public Health Service Act (PHSA) (*37*). Sections 308(d) and 924(c) of the PHSA provide strong protection for identifiable information collected respectively by CDC's National Center for Health Statistics and the U.S. Department of Health and Human Services (DHHS) Agency for Healthcare Research and Quality (*38*). Assurances of confidentiality under Section 308(d) can be used to protect individuals and institutions providing information. Section 308(d) provides that: "No [identifiable] information...may be used for any purpose other than the purpose for which it was supplied unless such establishment or person has consented..."

Certificates of confidentiality, available to researchers within or outside government, are authorized under PHSA Section 301(d) (*39*). DHHS can grant these certificates to protect research participants from legally compelled disclosures of identifiable health information. Section 301(d) provides that health researchers can "protect the privacy of [research participants] by withholding from all persons not connected with the conduct of such research the names or other identifying characteristics of such [participants]." Researchers generally seek this confidentiality protection only when the health information collected is so sensitive (e.g., related to sexual practices or illegal conduct) that research subjects probably either would not participate or would provide inaccurate or incomplete responses without such protections.

Before DHHS introduced the Privacy Rule promulgated pursuant to the Health Insurance Portability and Accountability Act (HIPAA) of 2000 (*40*), no comprehensive federal information privacy law existed. Rather, federal privacy laws generally applied to certain types of health information collected, maintained, or funded by the federal government through its specific agencies (e.g., Centers for Medicare and Medicaid Services, NIH, CDC). The HIPAA Privacy Rule, which became fully effective on April 14, 2004 (*41*), gives patients more control over their health information, sets boundaries on use and release of health records, and establishes safeguards that health-care providers and others must achieve to protect the privacy of health information. It provides the first national standards for the protections of identifiable health information as applied to three types of covered entities: health, health-care clearinghouses, and health-care providers who conduct certain health-care transactions electronically (*42,43*), and others performing "covered functions." Although the Privacy Rule sets a national floor of privacy protections for many exchanges of identifiable health data, it does not pre-empt more stringent state and local privacy laws (*44*).

In general, the Privacy Rule established standards for covered entities to use and disclose protected health information (PHI), which includes individually identifiable health information (*42,45*). A covered entity must use or disclose PHI only as required or permitted by the Privacy Rule. It requires disclosures (without written authorization) in only two instances: first, to the individual and second, to DHHS for compliance investigations, reviews, or enforcement actions. The Privacy Rule expressly permits PHI to be shared for specified public health purposes with specific, individual written authorization. A covered entity may disclose PHI to a public health authority (or to an entity working under a grant of authority from a public health authority) that is legally authorized to collect or receive the information for the purposes of preventing or controlling disease, injury, or disability or conduct public health surveillance, investigations, and interventions.

The HIPAA Privacy Rule also permits entities to make nonconsensual disclosures to public health authorities that are required by other laws [45 CFR 160.203 (c), 45 CFR 164.512 (b)], including laws that require disclosures for public health purposes. For example, to protect the health of the public, public health officials might need to obtain information related to persons affected by a disease. In certain cases, they might need to contact those affected to determine the cause of the disease to allow for actions to prevent further illness. The Privacy Rule allows for the sharing of PHI with public health authorities who are authorized by law to collect or receive such information to aid them in their mission of protecting the health of the public. Examples of such activities include those directed at the reporting of a disease or injury, reporting adverse events, reporting births and deaths, and investigating the occurrence and cause of injury and disease.

MINIMUM NECESSARY STANDARD

The Privacy Rule usually directs covered entities to limit the amount of information disclosed to the minimum necessary to achieve the specified goal [45 CFR §164.514(d) (1)]. This requirement usually applies to disclosures for a public health agency. It would not apply, however, if the disclosure were required by law, authorized by the individual, or for treatment purposes. A covered entity can also reasonably rely on a public official's determination that the information requested is the minimum necessary for the public health purpose.

The Family Educational Rights and Privacy Act (FERPA) (*46*) was designed to protect the privacy of student educational records and applies to all schools that receive funds under applicable U.S. Department of Education programs. It prohibits release to third parties of identifiable, nondirectory information gathered in a school setting by school employees or institutions and cannot be released without explicit parental consent or the consent of an eligible student over the age of 18 years. FERPA has no specific exception for public health purposes other than a narrowly construed exception for emergencies to protect the health or safety of the student or other persons, but the Act does not define "emergency."

After the passage of HIPAA, schools began to re-examine their privacy protections. Subsequently, the U.S. Department of Education began issuing administrative guidance that broadened the scope of FERPA to include student health records and restricted provision of health information to public health authorities. This guidance has been viewed by many as a serious barrier to good public health practice and has also had the effect of instructing state-licensed medical doctors not to comply with state laws that require medical doctors to report diseases of public health significance, potentially exposing those doctors to the risk of discipline by state boards of medicine and to civil liability for failing to report.

As a result of increasing recognition of the serious threats to public health caused by these recent administrative interpretations, several major health and public health organizations have passed resolutions calling for a remedy to the current situation by authorizing disclosure of health information to public health authorities in a fashion similar to the public health exception in HIPAA.

Specific provisions of the E-Government Act of 2002 protect the confidentiality of federal government statistical collections of identifiable information, including health information (*47*). The act restricts the use of information gathered for statistical uses to the purposes for which it is gathered and penalizes unauthorized disclosures. It also requires federal agencies to conduct privacy assessments before developing or procuring information technology that collects, maintains, or disseminates identifiable information.

Whereas the Privacy Act, FOIA, and E-Government Act apply to all federal agencies, other federal privacy laws and regulations relate to particular government programs or agencies. For example, a federal statute protects the privacy of health information generated in federally assisted specialized substance abuse facilities.

STATE AND LOCAL PUBLIC HEALTH INFORMATION PRIVACY LAWS

Although many states have statutory laws similar to the federal Privacy Act and FOIA, and a few (e.g., California, Rhode Island, Maryland, Montana, and Washington) have passed additional privacy protections, most do not have comprehensive statutes regulating the acquisition, use, and disclosure of individual health data (*33*). Rather, state privacy laws tend to regulate specific data recipients (e.g., public health agencies, health insurers); certain medical tests, diseases, or conditions (e.g., genetic tests, HIV status, mental disorders); or particular data sources (e.g., nursing or health-care facilities).

Significant additional privacy protections of public health data are featured in the Model State Public Health Information Privacy Act of 1999 (*48*) and, more recently, the Turning Point Model State Public Health Act of 2003 (*49*). Both model acts introduce modern privacy language to protect the privacy and security of identifiable health data acquired, used, disclosed, or stored by state public health agencies while preserving the ability of state and local health departments to use health data responsibly for the common good.

TERRORISM-RELATED PUBLIC HEALTH SURVEILLANCE

Terrorism-related concerns have led to efforts to examine the adequacy of disease reporting laws and disease-specific surveillance to meet the challenge of detecting acts of bioterrorism as rapidly as possible to minimize their health, social, and psychological consequences. In 2002, CDC reported on an examination of disease reporting laws of 54 jurisdictions, including all 50 states, to determine how many had laws mandating the reporting of diseases caused by "critical biological agents" (*50*)—agents designated by CDC with the potential for use in a bioterrorist weapon. The study showed that particular deficiencies existed for the immediate reporting of diseases associated with Category A agents (i.e., anthrax, botulism, viral hemorrhagic fevers, plague, smallpox, and tularemia). Although anthrax, botulism, and plague were immediately reportable in most jurisdictions, tularemia was immediately reportable in less than half of the jurisdictions. The findings underscored the need for states and other jurisdictions to review existing disease reporting laws to determine whether they include the most critical biologic agents associated with bioterrorism (*50*), an activity that has become a requirement of federal public health preparedness funding (*51*).

To speed up reporting of some diseases and laboratory findings, use of electronic data captured from laboratories (electronic laboratory reporting) and Web-based clinical facility and provider reporting increasingly are replacing paper and mail-based reporting (*52–54*). In some states, disease reporting regulations have been modified to provide a legal basis for such electronic reporting (*55*).

In addition, syndromic surveillance—use of real-time data from existing systems that record events such as emergency department visits, emergency system (911) calls, and pharmacy purchases— is being explored at both the state and national levels to detect unusual disease activity up to several days before reporting of any specific diagnostic information by providers and to help monitor the scope and duration of outbreaks, including those detected by other means (*56–58*). An analysis of statutes and regulations in New York City and New York State led to the conclusion that New York City had ample authority for its syndromic surveillance activities (*59*), and at least three states (Iowa, Nevada, and Arizona) have passed explicit statutory language authorizing syndromic surveillance (*60–63*).

The anthrax attacks of 2001 and increased recognition of the potential for criminal behavior and other deliberate actions to cause disease outbreaks have crystallized the concept of "forensic epidemiology." Forensic epidemiology has been characterized as "the use of epidemiologic methods as part of an ongoing investigation of a health problem for which there is suspicion or evidence regarding possible intentional acts or criminal behavior as factors contributing to the health problem" (*64*). The operational challenges during joint public health and law enforcement investigations of such problems implicate several relatively new legal issues that, in turn, have stimulated development of new legal frameworks for interdisciplinary collaboration, such as the "agreement regarding joint field investigations following a suspected bioterrorist incident" entered into by the City of New York Department of Mental Health and Hygiene, the City of New York Police Department, and the Federal Bureau of Investigation field office in New York City (*65*).

STATE AND FEDERAL COOPERATION IN EMERGENCY RESPONSES

Beginning in 1999, federal government initiatives designed to improve national public health capabilities to respond to acts of terrorism raised questions about the adequacy of state quarantine, isolation, and other compulsory public health powers. Preliminary review of state quarantine, isolation, and other critical agent laws conducted informally by CDC in 2000 showed that most of these laws had not been revised since the 1940s—probably because voluntary cooperation of the public and advances in medical interventions used compulsory actions less frequently. However, in the context of public health threats related to potential bioterrorism events, the infrequent use of such actions also presented the possibility that public health officials were inexperienced or unfamiliar with the proper procedures for invoking the compulsory powers. Accordingly, CDC and other federal officials involved in terrorism preparedness have suggested that states examine public health laws, including quarantine and isolation powers, that affect their abilities to effectively respond to potential chemical and biological threats. Such assessments can help ensure that the laws enable public health officials to act promptly while providing adequate due process protections for individuals who may be detained as part of a terrorism response. In addition, terrorism initiatives increasingly focus on the need for advance coordination, planning, pharmaceutical stockpiling, and training that involves public health officials and officials from various law enforcement, emergency response, and other civilian agencies, as well as military intelligence experts.

The events following the September 11, 2001 attacks in New York City and Northern Virginia illustrate the strengths of and challenges to traditional concepts of primary state and local responsibility for public health investigations. The catastrophic nature of the events rapidly taxed the ability of local and state public health officials to respond to the needs for surveillance of hospital and emergency department admissions, injuries, hospital-based syndromic surveillance (*56*), and various environmental monitoring activities. Resources from

CDC and other public health agencies had to be deployed to help gather this important surveillance information. Yet, the legal authority and oversight for most of these public health activities remained with local and state public health officials. The consistency in training, advance planning, and prior collaborative relationships between state, municipal, and local public health practitioners made possible an effective response during this emergency situation. In the aftermath of the events of September 11, 2001 and the anthrax attack in the United States, a draft model law, The Model State Emergency Health Powers Act, was created and made available for public review and use to strengthen preparedness (66).

CONCLUSIONS

The epidemiologist should understand that the basic authority of public health officials to conduct public health surveillance is the state's inherent police powers. Federal and state laws that govern the health and safety of the public are enacted pursuant to this broad authority. These laws provide not only for the state to have access to medical and other records for the purposes of public health surveillance but also for protection of the individual's interest in privacy by placing strict limits on access to medical, hospital, and public health records. Although public health surveillance and interventions usually rely on the voluntary cooperation of individuals and institutions, federal and state laws provide authority for the use of compulsory measures when necessary for the protection of the public health and safety.

Public health surveillance personnel are certainly not expected to know every facet of public health law. Yet they should have an appreciation of the legal issues that pertain to surveillance, privacy of medical records, and the legal responsibilities of both federal and state governments. The quality, quantity, and ease of collecting epidemiologic data can be enhanced materially by an awareness of these issues and, if necessary, consultation with the legal profession.

Acknowledgments   We acknowledge David W. Fleming, whose work on a corollary chapter, "Frontline Public Health: Surveillance and Outbreak Investigations," Law in Public Health Practice, New York:Oxford University Press, 2003:143–159, contributed in part to this chapter.

REFERENCES

1. Centers for Disease Control and Prevention. Summary of notifiable diseases, United States, 2003. *MMWR* 2005;52:2–3.
2. Centers for Disease Control and Prevention. Surveillance for certain health behaviors among selected local areas—United States, Behavioral Risk Factor Surveillance System, 2002. *MMWR* 2004;53(SS-5):2–3.
3. Ries LAG, Eisner MP, Kosary CL, *et al.*, eds. *SEER Cancer Statistics Review, 1975–2001.* Bethesda, MD: National Cancer Institute, 2004. http://seer.cancer.gov/csr/1975_2001. Accessed November 16, 2005.

4. Thacker SB. Historical development. In: Lee LM, Teutsch SM, Thacker SB, St Louis ME, eds. *Principles and Practice of Public Health Surveillance*, 3rd ed. New York: Oxford University Press, 2010: 1–17.
5. Chorba TL, Berkelman RL, Safford SK, Gibbs NP, Hull HF. The reportable diseases: I. Mandatory reporting of infectious diseases by clinicians. *JAMA* 1989;262:3018–3026.
6. Act of Apr 29, 1878, Ch 66, 20 Stat 37.
7. Act of Feb 15, 1893, Ch 114, 27 Stat 449, *amended* by Act of June 19, 1906, Ch 3433, 34 Stat 299.
8. Koo D, Wetterhall SF. History and current status of the National Notifiable Diseases Surveillance System. *J Public Health Manag Pract* 1996;2:4–10.
9. Hopkins DR. *Princes and Peasants: Smallpox in History*. Chicago: University of Chicago Press; 1983.
10. Act of Feb 27, 1813, Ch 37, 2 Stat 806, *repealed* by Act of May 4, 1822, Ch 50, 3 Stat 677.
11. Furman B. *A Profile of the United States Public Health Service*, 1798–1948. Washington, DC: US Department of Health, Education, and Welfare, 1973 (DHEW publication no [NIH] 73-369).
12. *Zucht v King*, 260 US 174 (1922).
13. *Jacobson v Massachusetts*, 197 US 11 (1905).
14. Parmet WE, Goodman RA, Farber A. Individual rights versus the public's health—100 years after *Jacobson v Massachusetts*. *N Engl J Med* 2005;352:652–654.
15. Gostin LO, Burris S, Lazzarini Z. The law and the public's health: a study of infectious disease law in the United States. *Columbia Law Rev* 1999;99:59–128.
16. Act of May 27, 1796, Ch 31, 1 Stat 474, repealed by Act of Feb 25, 1799, Ch 12, 1 Stat 619.
17. Tobey JA. *Public Health Law*, 3rd ed. New York: Commonwealth Fund; 1947.
18. Chorba TL, Berkelman RL, Safford SK, Gibbs NP, Hull HF. The reportable diseases: I. Mandatory reporting of infectious diseases by clinicians. *JAMA* 1989;262:3018–3026.
19. Roush S, Birkhead GS, Koo D, Cobb A, Fleming D. Mandatory reporting of diseases and conditions by health care professionals and laboratorians. *JAMA* 1999;282:164–170.
20. Thacker SB. Surveillance. In: Gregg MB, Dicker RC, Goodman RA, eds. *Field Epidemiology*. New York: Oxford University Press, 1996: pp. 16–32.
21. Gen Stat of Conn (revised to January 1, 2005), §19a-2a, Powers and duties, Volume 6, 787.
22. Public Health Code (revised through Sept. 21, 2004). Reportable Diseases and Laboratory Findings, §19a-36-A7, Diseases not enumerated, p. 529. http://www.dph.state.ct.us/phc/phc.doc. Accessed November 16, 2005.
23. Thacker SB, Berkelman RL. Public health surveillance in the United States. *Epidemiol Rev* 1988;10:164–190.
24. Konowitz PM, Petrossian GA, Rose DN. The underreporting of disease and physicians' knowledge of reporting requirements. *Public Health Rep* 1984;99:31–35.
25. Pub L. 101-381, 104 Stat.576 (Aug. 18, 1990).
26. Centers for Disease Control and Prevention. Case definitions for infectious conditions under public health surveillance. *MMWR* 1997;46(RR-10):1–64.
27. Council of State and Territorial Epidemiologists. State Reportable Conditions Websites. http://www.cste.org/dnn/ProgramsandActivities/PublicHealthInformatics/PHIStateReportableWebsites/tabid/136/Default.aspx. Accessed June 24, 2009.

28. California Department of Health Services. Disciplinary action by Board of Medical Quality Assurance for failure to report a reportable infectious disease. *California Morbidity* 1978 (August 11).

29. Fidler DP, Heymann DL, Ostroff SM, O'Brien T. Emerging and reemerging infectious diseases: challenges for international, national, and state law. *International Lawyer* 1997;31:773–799.

30. Centers for Disease Control and Prevention. Addition of prevalence of cigarette smoking as a nationally notifiable condition—June 1996. *MMWR* 1996;45:537.

31. Centers for Disease Control and Prevention. Indicators for chronic disease surveillance. *MMWR* 2004;53 (RR-11):1–8.

32. Birkhead GS, Maylahn CM. State and local public health surveillance in the United States. In: Lee LM, Teutsch SM, Thacker SB, St Louis ME, eds. *Principles and Practice of Public Health Surveillance*, 3rd ed. New York: Oxford University Press; 2010:381–398.

33. Hodge JG. Jr.Health information privacy and public health. *J Law Med Ethics* 2004; 31:4:663–671.

34. Hodge JG Jr, Gostin LO, Jacobson P. Legal issues concerning electronic health information. *JAMA* 1999; 282:1466–1471.

35. 5 USC 552(a) (1988).

36. 5 USC 552 (1988).

37. 42 USC 301, et seq.

38. 42 USCA 242m(d) and 299c-3 (2001).

39. 42 USCA 242m(d) (1997).

40. Pub L 104-191, 110 Stat 1936 (1996).

41. 45 CFR Parts 160 and 164 (2004); http://www.dhhs.gov/ocr/combinedregtext.pdf. Accessed December 7, 2008.

42. Centers for Disease Control and Prevention. HIPAA Privacy Rule and Public Health: Guidance from CDC and the U.S. Department of Health and Human Services. *MMWR* 2003; 52(S-1):1–12.

43. Gostin LO, Hodge JG Jr. Personal privacy and common goods: a framework for balancing under the National Health Information Privacy Rule. *Minn Law Rev* 2002;86:1439–1480.

44. 45 CFR 164.502(a)(2) (2003).

45. Department of Health and Human Services, OCR Privacy Brief. *Summary of the HIPAA Privacy Rule: HIPAA Compliance Assistance*, 2003. HHS.gov/ocr/privacy summary. Accessed September 12, 2005.

46. 20 USC 1232g; 34 CFR Part 99.

47. Pub L 107-347 (2002).

48. Gostin LO, Hodge JG Jr, Valdiserri RO. Informational privacy and the public's health: the model state public health privacy Act. *Am J Public Health* 2001;91(9):1388–1392.

49. Turning Point Model State Public Health Act (Sept. 19, 2003). www.turningpointprogram.org. Accessed December 7, 2008.

50. Horton H, Misrahi JJ, Matthews GW, Kocher PL. Critical biological agents: disease reporting as a tool for bioterrorism preparedness. *J Law Med Ethics* 2002;30:262–266.

51. Centers for Disease Control and Prevention. *Continuation Guidance—Budget Year 5. Attachment B. Focus B: Surveillance and Epidemiology Capacity.* June 14, 2004:1–8. http://www.bt.cdc.gov/planning/continuationguidance/pdf/epidemiology_capacity_attachb.pdf. Accessed September 4, 2005.

52. Effler P, Ching-Lee M, Bogard A, Ieong M, Nekomoto T, Jernigan D. Statewide system of electronic notifiable disease reporting from clinical laboratories. *JAMA* 1999;282:1845–1850.

53. Backer HD, Bissel SR, Vugia DJ. Disease reporting from automated laboratory-based reporting system to a state health department via local health departments. *Public Health Rep* 2001;116:257–265.

54. Jernigan DB. Electronic laboratory-based reporting: opportunities and challenges for surveillance. *Emerg Infect Dis* 2001;7(3 Suppl):538.

55. See, for example, 33 Pennsylvania Bulletin (Pa.B) 2439 (effective Nov. 16, 2003) (under authority of 28 Pa.Code Section 27.4); 6 Code of Colorado Regulations (CCR) 1009-1, Reporting of Selected Cases of Morbidity and Mortality (effective September 30, 2004); Administrative Rules of South Dakota (ARDS) 44:20:02:06 (under authority of SDCL 34-22-9) (effective Dec. 7, 2003); Washington Administrative Code (WAC) 246-101-110(2) (effective Dec. 2004).

56. Henning K. What is syndromic surveillance? *MMWR* 2004;53(Suppl):7–11.

57. Centers for Disease Control and Prevention. Framework for evaluating public health surveillance systems for early detection of outbreaks: recommendations from the CDC working group. *MMWR* 2004;53(RR-5):2–3.

58. Loonsk J. Biosense—a national initiative for early detection and quantification of public health emergencies. *MMWR* 2004;53(Suppl):53–55.

59. Lopez W. New York City and state legal authorities related to syndromic surveillance. *J Urban Health* 2003;80(2 Suppl 1):i23–i24.

60. Drociuk D, Gibson J, Hodge JG Jr. Health information privacy and syndromic surveillance systems. *MMWR 2004*;53(Suppl):221–225.

61. Iowa Code, Title 4, Subtitle 2, Ch 139, §139A.3A (2005).

62. Nev Rev Stat, Ch 441A, §441 A.125 (2003).

63. Ariz Rev Stat, Title 36, §36-782 (2005).

64. Goodman RA, Munson JW, Dammers K, Lazzarini Z, Barkley JP. Forensic epidemiology: law at the intersection of public health and criminal investigations. *J Law Med Ethics* 2003;31:684–700.

65. Centers for Disease Control and Prevention, Public Health Law Program. Agreement regarding joint field investigations following a suspected bioterrorist incident. http://www2a.cdc.gov/phlp/docs/Investigations.pdf. Accessed November 16, 2005.

66. Gostin LO, Sapsin JW, Teret SP, *et al.* The Model State Emergency Health Powers Act: planning for and response to bioterrorism and naturally occurring infectious diseases. *JAMA* 2002;288:622–628.

11

Public Health Surveillance for Infectious Diseases

CHRIS A. VAN BENEDEN AND RUTH LYNFIELD

INTRODUCTION

Infectious diseases remain among the top causes of disease and death worldwide, despite advances in the prevention and treatment of infectious diseases, improved living conditions, and development of effective vaccines and antimicrobials. According to the World Health Organization (WHO), of the 10 leading causes of death globally, 4 are infectious and include lower respiratory infections, diarrheal diseases, HIV/AIDS, and tuberculosis (*1*). These infections accounted for an estimated 9.8 million deaths, 17% of all deaths in 2004. The majority of deaths resulting from these four infections (7.2 million) occurred in low-income countries, where the percentage of infections among the 10 leading causes of death is higher (34%), partially because of the additional impact of malaria and neonatal infections. Infections were estimated to account for 258 million disability adjusted life years (DALYs) worldwide in 2004 (*1*), representing both the years of life lost due to premature death and the years of healthy life lost due to poor health or disability.

Although infections have plagued humans for millennia, both well-established and novel aspects of these diseases make surveillance challenging and intriguing. Human pathogens constantly evolve, resulting in new agents and new mechanisms of transmission. Contact between humans and pathogens have changed over time as a result of human intrusion into previously uninhabited environments, increasing and more rapid global travel, and expansion of international food trade. Better integration of public health surveillance systems across the globe using standardized case definitions, careful data integration and well-established communication pathways are essential. Surveillance is needed not only for human diseases but for animal reservoirs and vectors of human infections. This is well-articulated in the concept of "one world, one health," which emphasizes the importance of an integrated approach toward understanding public health, veterinary health, microbes, and the environment (*2*). Public health agencies must now prepare for new, emerging, and potentially volatile global pathogens such as pandemic influenza or SARS. The rapidly changing world of information technology has both advanced surveillance methods and brought additional challenges. More detailed pathogen information, as found in molecular and genetic characterization, is now available for multiple organisms that increase our understanding of bacterial and viral epidemiology and pathology. This, in turn, helps researchers develop new or improved vaccines and therapies. The prolonged survival of people with immune compromising conditions (HIV, cancer) and growing antibiotic pressure have resulted in modifications of both hosts and pathogens.

There are multiple reasons to monitor infectious diseases. Detection of outbreaks enables rapid investigation, pathogen identification, and response. Surveillance data can garner government attention to a previously unrecognized or underappreciated illness, keeping local community and appropriate civic and political leaders aware of health burdens and costs to the population. Surveillance is used to establish baseline disease rates; identify new and emerging infections; monitor the impact and effectiveness of public health interventions such as vaccines, environmental remediation, vector control, and prophylactic use of antimicrobials; guide vaccine development and clinical management in the context of local antimicrobial resistance; and direct allocation of resources for disease prevention and treatment programs (3).

In this chapter, we apply five principles of public health surveillance to the area of infectious diseases, providing examples of various barriers and complexities of building surveillance systems that are specific to tracking infections. We also describe successes and provide examples of recent innovative approaches to surveillance of infectious diseases. We hope the reader will be better equipped to develop and maintain robust surveillance for infectious diseases and be prepared for the associated unique challenges and benefits of a strong infectious disease surveillance system.

SYSTEM DEVELOPMENT AND DATA COLLECTION

Setting up a Surveillance System

It is important to consider carefully the need for a new infectious disease surveillance system. Public health resources typically are limited, and any new system involves an investment of human and fiscal capital. In addition, it frequently takes several years before a surveillance system functions optimally. Before developing a new system, one must consider the following: Does the disease have a high morbidity or mortality (e.g., anthrax)? Can disease episodes be measured? Is the disease pathogen-specific (e.g., pneumococcus) or syndrome-specific (e.g., pneumonia)? Do effective prevention and control measures exist? Do these measures consume substantial resources? Are surveillance data needed to develop prevention and control measures and to monitor their impact? Can an existing system be modified to incorporate surveillance for the disease of interest? Will the system be ongoing or will it be time-limited to address a specific event (e.g., monitoring emergency room visits in a city hosting the Olympics during the period of the Olympic events)?

Components of an Infectious Disease Surveillance System

The first issue to address is what is under surveillance. Is it a human disease that is pathogen specific, so that the data can be acquired from a laboratory test (e.g., a positive blood culture for pneumococcus)? In other words, can it be measured by a laboratory-based system? Or, is it syndrome specific (cases of hospitalized pneumonia) and thus dependent on clinicians reporting? Or, is the surveillance for vectors of human disease such as monitoring mosquito pools for West Nile virus, or surveillance of animals that might be indicative of potential human disease, such as monitoring dead crows for West Nile virus? Alternatively, surveillance can be done using environmental samples, such as assessing *Cryptococcus gattii* in trees, soil, water, and air.

Next, it is important to determine whether the total population in a public health jurisdiction is under surveillance (population-based) or if surveillance will occur at a facility or group of facilities (sentinel site). Is the catchment area city or countywide, statewide, national, regional, industry-wide (e.g., poultry workers), or global?

Historically surveillance has been classified as active or passive. Active surveillance refers to active effort put in by the public health entity to collect case data. Passive surveillance usually refers to data supplied by reporters to the public health entity without active outreach by the public health entity. In an active system, surveillance officers employed by a public health entity typically contact laboratories or health-care providers for data and often will audit laboratories or query infection control professionals (ICPs) or medical records to ensure the completeness of data.

With the widespread use of electronic data systems and the development of data standards, more reporting is occurring through electronic information systems. These systems have the potential advantages of being more accurate, timely, and less resource intensive. Data can be captured digitally at the reporting site and transmitted electronically to the public health entity. Systems are being developed that allow data analysis at the local level, as well as upstream, at a more central site.

Prospective, active, laboratory-based, population-based surveillance is considered the "gold standard" because this method consistently captures the highest percentage of diagnosed cases in a well-defined population, often reaching nearly 100%. Unlike sentinel surveillance, population-based surveillance also captures all cases corresponding to an underlying surveillance population. These health data can be used to estimate the burden of disease and mortality, calculate specific incidence rates, monitor trends, and evaluate the impact of interventions over time. The results can be generalized to a larger area with similar population characteristics. However, this kind of surveillance is the most resource intensive and might not be needed to address a particular surveillance question.

Some examples of infectious disease surveillance systems include the following: global surveillance for circulating strains of influenza (4,5), regional surveillance for tuberculosis in the European Union (EuroTB supranational surveillance) (6), national surveillance for measles in the United States (7), state surveillance for Unexplained Death of Probable Infectious Etiology in Minnesota (8), sentinel site surveillance for community-associated methicillin-resistant *Staphylococcus aureus* (9), and fever surveillance at the Singapore airport during the severe acute respiratory syndrome (SARS) epidemic (10).

Diverse goals of infectious disease surveillance have been addressed by a variety of surveillance methods, including passive versus active systems, sentinel versus population-based systems, and specific pathogen or disease versus syndrome-based systems. A national passive system in the United States is the Vaccine Adverse Effect Reporting System (VAERS) (*11*). In VAERS, adverse events occurring after an immunization are reported to a central, national system by clinicians, public health professionals, or members of the public. An example of a national sentinel site system is the Gonococcal Isolate Surveillance Project (GISP), in which participating clinics in 25 to 30 U.S. cities submit a subset of bacterial isolates obtained from men with gonococcal urethritis to the Centers for Disease Control and Prevention (CDC) for antimicrobial susceptibility testing (*12*). A syndrome-based, passive system is the sentinel site reporting system for influenza-like illness that occurs in participating U.S. clinics (ILINet) (*13*). A sentinel site system in acute care facilities is the National Healthcare Safety Network (NHSN) (*14*), which collects data on hospital-associated infections in participating hospitals in the United States. This system is expanding rapidly and is described in Chapter 15. An active, laboratory- and population-based system is the Active Bacterial Core surveillance system (ABCs) of the U.S. CDC's Emerging Infections Program. This system tracks a number of invasive bacterial infections in 10 geographically disparate surveillance sites in the United States. ABCs is used to monitor disease trends and to calculate age- and race-specific rates of disease (*15*). Vaccine-effectiveness studies and risk factor studies can be built upon this population-based system. Although it is resource intensive, data are highly accurate because of audits and other checks built into the surveillance system, and because it is a population-based system, data can be generalized to other similar populations.

Table 11–1 outlines the steps involved in developing an infectious disease surveillance system. Table 11–2 outlines examples of innovative surveillance systems.

DATA MANAGEMENT AND INFORMATION INTEGRATION

The quality of information obtained from all surveillance systems depends on the availability and accuracy of the source data, the accuracy and completeness of data entry onto paper or into an electronic format, and appropriate integration of data from multiple sources. Accurate mapping of all data elements from electronic data sources is critical (for further detailed discussion, *see* Chapter 5). Matching algorithms for de-duplication, linking data to existing records, and importing new records must be defined, validated, and reassessed periodically (*see* Chapter 4). To ensure high-quality data on an ongoing basis, procedures must be established that include well-documented instructions on data collection and form completion, training on data entry, and training on definitions (e.g., data elements). Ongoing assessment of data quality is important, as is routine feedback about common errors.

Data management and information integration is a rapidly changing field. The availability and use of electronic resources have increased available data and

Table 11–1 Steps in Infectious Disease Surveillance System Development

Step	Detailed components of surveillance system development
1. Engage partners	• Engage various stakeholders (e.g., ICPs, clinicians, laboratorians, local public health staff, surveillance officers, government and academic partners) early in planning.
2. Develop clear case definition	• Incorporate person, place, and time. • Ensure that definition is standardized and measurable. • Incorporate readily available, sensitive, and specific diagnostic test(s) as appropriate. • In outbreak settings, include cases meeting predefined clinical criteria (but not laboratory criteria) if linked epidemiologically to a laboratory-confirmed case. • Exclude clinical judgment in clinical case definitions; make criteria objective.
3. Define the denominator	• Ensure appropriate pairing of cases (numerator) and surveillance population (denominator) in population-based surveillance. • Define population using appropriate, available sources (e.g., census data for residents of a specific geographic area, birth certificates for number of resident live births, and employee lists for workers in a particular industry). • Determine where the resident population seeks health care. • Determine how to count transient populations (e.g., college students or migrant workers).
4. Identify and report cases	• Determine rapidity of reporting: immediately or within 24 hours if quick action required (e.g., meningococcal case or a potential foodborne outbreak), or, less urgently but in a timely fashion if data are used to assess impact of intervention (e.g., pneumococcal disease in a vaccinated population). • Review data sources: *Primary*: Medical records, laboratory reports, and case interview return. *Secondary*: Reports from media or sentinel populations (e.g., hotline at a local health department). • For syndromic or aberration surveillance, use automated data extraction from emergency departments, emergency call centers, or poison control hotlines. • For active laboratory-based surveillance, review electronic summary reports and contact laboratories on a regular basis; report cases via phone, fax, mail or secure Internet site.
5. Collect data	• Use standardized data collection forms and standardized questions for interviews. • Include key data elements: person (e.g., demographic information encompassing a unique identifier, age, sex, race, and ethnicity); place (e.g., case's address, including the county and state); time (e.g., date of onset of illness or date of diagnostic laboratory test); clinical illness/ type of infection (e.g., meningitis or culture positive for pneumococcus); and outcome (e.g., hospitalization or death).

(continued)

Table 11–1 (*continued*)

Step	Detailed components of surveillance system development
	• Consider additional data elements—for example, comorbidities, vaccination status, culture source, molecular subtyping, and antibiotic susceptibility.
	• Provide clear instructions, a detailed data dictionary, and simple and clear standard operating procedures and protocols.
	• Consider collecting isolates (from local clinical, state, or national reference laboratories) to characterize pathogen (e.g., antimicrobial susceptibility testing, serotyping, and molecular subtyping).
	• If isolates are collected, collect and submit promptly (e.g., within days to weeks) to prevent isolates from being compromised or discarded by local laboratories.
6. Manage data	• Maintain data in common electronic database wherever possible (instead of paper forms).
	• Automate data entry to minimize data entry errors.
	• When developing database, define database elements and ensure compatibility with other data sources and data standards; incorporate automated data checks and logic edits.
	• Remove identifiers (name, address) prior to transmitting or sharing data with central source as per reporting rules or data privacy practices.*
7. Monitor the system	• Monitor system routinely to assess efficiency from collection of case report to data management.
	• Ensure completeness of reporting, accuracy and quality of data.
	• Audit laboratories via an electronic printout of results or logbooks.
	• Perform internal data checks on database (e.g., automated data entry validation, double data entry, and manual review of data).
	• Provide performance indicators and feedback to all involved in reporting system.

*Note: identifiers might be required for certain data, such as a case of extensively drug-resistant tuberculosis to effectively institute public health interventions across international borders.

the ability to communicate and transfer them between multiple partners. This increased complexity demands careful planning of database development to ensure that information is in a usable format, that access is granted to those who need it while protecting privacy and confidentiality of data, and that multiple databases are truly relational.

In addition to the growing use of the Internet, key trends in data management and information integration in the area of infectious disease surveillance include the need to share surveillance data with multiple levels of public health agencies, the increased integration of data related to a single case from numerous sources and over longer periods, and the need for flexible surveillance systems for new and emerging diseases.

Table 11–2 Examples of Innovative Infectious Disease Surveillance Systems

Name of system	Website and reference
Danish Integrated Antimicrobial Resistance Monitoring and Research Program (DANMAP): surveillance for antimicrobial drug use and antimicrobial resistance in animals, food, and humans in Denmark	www.DANMAP.org (16)
National Antimicrobial Resistance Monitoring System (NARMS) in the United States: collaborative effort by the Food and Drug Admininistration (FDA), U.S. Department of Agriculture (USDA), CDC and State Health Departments to monitor changes in antimicrobial drug susceptibilities of selected enteric bacterial organisms in humans, animals, and retail meats	www.fda.gov/cvm/NARMS_pg.htm (17)
PulseNet: national network of public health and food regulatory agency labs coordinated by CDC that use standardized molecular subtyping with pulsed field gel electrophoresis (PFGE) to detect foodborne outbreaks	www.cdc.gov/pulsenet/ (18)

Expanded Use of the Internet and New Information and Communication Technologies

Public health websites often list the reportable diseases and required timeliness of reporting, provide contact information for public health personnel, and contain reporting forms. Compared with paper-based reporting, Web-based reporting typically is faster and more convenient. In New Jersey, for example, Web-based reporting of infectious diseases reduced the time of data entry on new cases from 28 days to 3 to 5 days after illness onset (19). Databases are often connected to the iInternet, enabling aggregation of data at a central level (e.g., state, national). Use of the Internet is not without challenges, however, including need for a high level of security (e.g., encryption, access restrictions), difficulties using different operating systems at data entry, need for user training, complexities of developing a useful and efficient database and data entry system, and associated costs (20).

Personal digital assistants (PDAs) or handheld computers are a new technology used in both health-care facilities and in the field to increase ease and accuracy of data collection and entry. Compared with paper forms, PDA-based data collections save time, avoid secondary data transfer to an electronic database, and reduce errors normally occurring from the transfer of information from paper forms to electronic databases. PDAs can also incorporate quality checks upon data entry to immediately notify an interviewer for clarification. Data from multiple PDAs can be aggregated into a single database fairly quickly and while in the field, allowing real-time assessment of data quality. However, use of PDAs requires the appropriate information technology support, periodic backups in case of PDA malfunction, and, for people unfamiliar with the technology, more initial training than use of paper forms (*21,22*).

Sharing Information Across Multiple Levels of Public Health Agencies

Nationally reportable infectious disease surveillance data typically are reported locally and then transmitted through state or provincial authorities to a central, national repository. Additional partners and complexity arise when monitoring health-care-associated infections (HAIs). Such complexities have been addressed successfully by CDC's NHSN, which collects data from a sample of health-care facilities across the United States to enable valid estimation of the magnitude of adverse events among patients and health-care personnel and of the adherence to practices that prevent HAI. NHSN allows health-care facilities to share data between a facility and local public health agencies and between facilities in a multihospital system—all while maintaining data security, integrity, and confidentiality. Access to data follows a tiered approach; data may be analyzed on different levels and analysis tailored to the user's needs, as long as the user is permitted access to these data. State public health officials may analyze one or all hospitals in their jurisdiction, whereas hospitals can only access their own data or data within an agreed-upon predefined user group. This system permits recognition of HAI trends and timely recognition of health-care-related safety problems (*23*).

Integration of Data Related to a Single Case From Numerous Sources Over Multiple Periods

Many infectious disease surveillance systems rely on data obtained from numerous sources over time for a single case. These types of systems should accommodate data from multiple sources (clinical, laboratory, epidemiologic) over time, while matching on identifiers unique to each individual case. It is important to ensure de-duplication of records and valid information on individual cases if multiple levels of data entry are used; records must be updated and corrected and staff trained on use of these types of relational databases.

Surveillance for vaccine preventable diseases and for HIV/AIDS illustrates the advantages and complexities of data integration. Influenza surveillance, for example, might include immunization information systems that incorporate immunization status in addition to case and laboratory data. Ideally, such a system should also include data fields for antivirals and the ability to track pandemic influenza countermeasures. In another example, new therapies have changed AIDS into a treatable chronic disease. This has added complexities to HIV and AIDS surveillance, including the need to integrate several sentinel laboratory and clinical events (e.g., first CD4 count, AIDS defining illnesses, date of death) from numerous sources (including multiple providers and laboratories) and multiple states (*24*). This integration requires de-duplication of reports using standardized means of identifying cases common to all reporting jurisdictions.

Flexible Surveillance Systems for New and Emerging Diseases

The emergence of SARS and the worldwide need for rapid detection and response exemplified the importance and challenges of a timely and flexible surveillance system for new infectious agents. In March 2003, CDC's initial surveillance definition for a suspect SARS case incorporated clinical criteria and evidence of an epidemiologic link, defined as potential exposure to a known SARS case. Because SARS-affected countries constituting the epidemiologic link frequently changed, the case definition underwent continual modification. When a new coronavirus was identified as the causative agent 1 month later, laboratory criteria were added to the case definition then refined with development of a convalescent phase antibody test. SARS surveillance was complicated by the need to maintain harmonized international surveillance. These continual changes to the case definition required constant modifications to the reporting system and the associated database. CDC's SARS surveillance was initially paper-based, which increased difficulties of reporting to CDC and delayed timeliness of reports (*25*). These challenges highlight the need for a generic electronic database that would allow for rapid modifications and additions to case definitions, including associated epidemiologic and laboratory parameters.

DATA ANALYSIS AND STATISTICAL METHODS

Analysis of surveillance data begins with a thorough understanding of the underlying dataset and data source, knowing the extent of available information and its inherent limitations or biases. The approach to analysis should be planned logically and proceed from data cleaning to descriptive analyses of person, place, and time, to complex analyses that examine associations or allow for inference, which often require statistical oversight and guidance.

Selection of the analytic methods depends on the goals of the surveillance system, objectives of analysis, and the quality, completeness, and structure of the surveillance database (*see* Chapter 6 for more details; Table 11–3). What conditions are monitored? What is the unit of analysis? How is the baseline determined? If datasets from multiple jurisdictions (e.g., counties, states, or countries) are analyzed, integration requires use of consistent case definitions. Interpreting data is as important as the analysis itself and includes understanding the limits of the surveillance system such as potential underreporting or non-representativeness of the population.

In outbreak detection, "normal" or "baseline" disease rates must be defined first. This is particularly challenging when a disease exhibits seasonality (e.g., influenza), case ascertainment is inconsistent (e.g., modification of case definition), or diagnostic methods change. To determine if a perceived increase (or decrease) in disease is real, surveillance methods must be carefully evaluated to ensure that the observed changes are not an artifact of reporting. Have provider practices changed (e.g., likelihood of blood or stool culture collection in patients with fever or diarrhea)? Have new diagnostics been developed? Do declining disease rates actually reflect a larger surveillance population?

Table 11–3 Examples of Analytic Methods Used With Infectious Disease Surveillance Data

Objective of analysis	*Examples of analytic approach*
Characterize infectious syndrome	• Simple demographic frequencies (e.g., age, race and sex) • Trend analyses (e.g., season and year) • Rates of disease • Prevalence of resistance to antimicrobials • Use of geographic information systems and remote sensing to map cases
Estimate burden of disease in a community	• Incidence rates and prevalence, standardized rates • Case-fatality rates or ratios • Cost-effectiveness studies incorporating costs to healthcare system (e.g., hospitalization and antimicrobials) and community (e.g., days of work lost, deaths and DALYs*)
Identify risk factors for disease	• Descriptive epidemiology • Multivariable regression
Identify etiologic agents/vehicles in infectious disease outbreaks	• Multivariable regression
Identify clusters or epidemics	• Syndrome or pattern recognition by astute clinicians or other public health or safety officials • Visual inspection of surveillance data using graphs, charts, maps • Aberration detection methods (*see* below) using computerized algorithms to identify deviations from baseline disease activity • Network analysis
Monitor impact of public health interventions	• Trend analyses • Cost-effectiveness analyses • Vaccine effectiveness measures
Evaluate or improve quality of surveillance data	• Capture–recapture methods • Multiple imputation (to reduce impact of missing data) • Comparison to alternative surveillance systems or data sources

* DALYs, disability adjusted life years; years of potential life lost because of premature mortality and the years of productive life lost resulting from disability.

Examples of New Approaches to Analysis of Infectious Disease Surveillance Data

Aberration or Outbreak Detection

In response to the threat of bioterrorism events and the subsequent development of syndromic surveillance, which does not rely on specific diagnostic data, computer programs have been developed that review data such as medical records, prescription fill records, and over-the-counter medication sales records to track patient health-seeking behaviors and clinical evaluations (*26,27*). This type of surveillance could be used for non-bioterrorism events as well, such as monitoring for the onset, length, and severity of seasonal influenza. Challenges to the use of such surrogates for diagnostic data are that true increases might be hidden among "noise" and false-positive "signals" are not uncommon.

In the modern food industry, foods produced or grown in one area are often distributed over wide geographic areas and among a variety of populations. Low level bacterial contamination can cause scattered cases of diarrheal diseases. To detect such outbreaks, CDC developed PulseNet, a national network of public health laboratories that use standardized pulsed field gel electrophoresis (PFGE) methods to subtype a variety of bacterial diarrheal pathogens, (e.g., *Escherichia coli* O157:H7 and *Salmonella*). Participating labs can search local and national databases for clusters of indistinguishable PFGE patterns, detecting outbreaks geographically dispersed that otherwise might be missed.

The Salmonella Outbreak Detection Algorithm (SODA) is an outbreak detection tool used in the United States to detect unusual clusters of *Salmonella* by serotype, location and date. SODA, a statistical algorithm, compares current nationally reported *Salmonella* cases to a 5-year historical baseline for that serotype and week. It has been useful for detecting widespread multistate outbreaks, characterizing the etiologic agents and providing a basis on which national trends can be analyzed (*28*).

Multiple Imputation

Missing data are a common problem with many datasets. In active surveillance, missing data fall into the "item nonresponse" category; for an individual case, a variety of variables might be missing but the focus is typically age, race, sex, and outcome (e.g., death). Discarding cases with missing data can lead to inefficient and biased results. A valid and appropriate method of handling missing data is called multiple imputation. Imputation reflects the uncertainty caused by the fact that imputed values are not actual observed values, but allows analysis using complete-data methods. Imputation is one of the preferred methods for handling incomplete data because it can lead to valid inferences. The technique is becoming more routine because of available software analysis programs such as SAS and STATA (*29*).

Geographic Information Systems

Geographic information systems (GIS) is a software program that is "capable of capturing, storing, analyzing, and displaying geographically referenced information" (*30*). A relational database, it integrates data from satellite images or other digitized maps to perform spatial analysis supported by spatial statistics. It has been used increasingly to provide information about the source and spread of infectious disease (*31*).

Recently, global positioning systems (GPS) have been used with PDAs as an innovative method in household surveys to select a probability-based sample; all households in an area can be mapped rapidly, probability-based samples generated relatively quickly, and the same equipment (PDAs) is used to conduct interviews and data entry. This process allows researchers to conduct a rapid, statistically valid survey in an environment with inadequate census information to allow enumeration.

As an example, this process was used in the assessment of insecticide-treated bed net coverage survey as part of a malaria control program in Africa (*21*).

A variety of free and open-source software programs for analysis are now available (Table 11–4). The primary proprietary software packages that are used for epidemiologic analysis of infectious disease surveillance data SAS (*32*), SPSS (*33*), and STATA (*34*).

DATA DISSEMINATION

An important tenet of surveillance is the effective communication of data to control the occurrence of disease, either through policy or practice changes leading to improved prevention and control or through documentation of effective policies and practices. The "what," "who," "how," and "where" of data dissemination need to be considered (*see* Chapter 7).

Table 11–4 Available Free and Open-Source Software for Data Analysis (*35*)

Software	Capacity and functions
Epi Info	Design of data collection forms, data entry with error and logic checking, analysis, graphing, and reporting. http//www.cdc.gov/epiinfo/
EpiDATA Entry and EpiData Analysis (EpiData)	Data collection, entry, analysis, and reporting; data encryption, double-entry; import and export of data. http://www.epidata.dk/
Analysis Software for Word Based Records (AnSWR)	Qualitative and quantitative analysis of text-based data, suitable for collaborative, or group-based analyses. http://www.cdc.gov/hiv/software/answr.htm
CDC EZ-TEXT	Qualitative analysis; no server required; supports questionnaire development and data entry. http://www.cdc.gov/hiv/software/ez-text.htm
CLUSTER	Cluster analysis using techniques that evaluate, time, space, and both time and space clustering, using existing surveillance data. http://www.atsdr.cdc.gov/HS/cluster.html
Open Source Epidemiologic Statistics for Public Health (OpenEpi)	Analysis of person-level and count-level data. http://www.openepi.com/Menu/OpenEpiMenu.htm
WinEpiScope	Wide range of analysis tools specific to a wide variety of study designs. http://www.clive.ed.ac.uk/cliveCatalogueItem.asp?id=B6BC9009-C10F-4393-A22D-48F436516AC4
Computer Programs for Epidemiologic Analyses (PEPI)	Suite of statistical tools. http://sagebrushpress.com/pepibook.html
STD*MIS	Network analysis. http://www.insna.org/INSNA/soft_inf.html.
The Medical Algorithms Project (MAP)	Numerous tools for infectious disease analysis. http://www.medal.org/visitor/www/inactive/ch23.aspx.

Usually, public health departments have the legal authority to use and present infectious disease data in aggregate form. However, the epidemiologist should be aware of which data are proprietary and what restrictions exist. Depending on the initial source of the data, data use agreements might need to be in place. These are formal agreements with outside partners that specify the ownership and use of the data, access to the data, and legal and privacy regulations or requirements. Public health practitioners also need to be aware of regulations specifying reporting certain data to other agencies— for example, reporting of a case of meningococcal disease to a neighboring state, when the case is a resident of that state. Additionally, the WHO 2005 International Health Regulations specify certain conditions and events that need to be reported because they might constitute a public health emergency of international concern (36). Some examples include a case of a new subtype of influenza causing a human infection or a case of poliomyelitis caused by wild-type poliovirus.

It is essential to identify the audience to present the data appropriately. Audiences could include health-care providers, public health professionals, other scientists, legislators, affected populations, or the general public. The data must always be accurate, but the level of detail and complexity should vary by the needs, experience, and training of the audience. Data can be communicated through peer-reviewed scientific publications, surveillance reports such as CDC's *Morbidity and Mortality Weekly Report*, reports for legislators, and information for the public. For the latter two audiences in particular, clear and concise information generally is more effective than that providing excessive detail. In addition to printed reports, venues can include presentations at conferences and postings on websites. Partnering with journalists for lay media is often very successful. Determining the goals of the communication and being cognizant of potential cultural understandings and misunderstandings will make communications more effective.

Uses of Data

There are many examples of carefully collected and analyzed surveillance data being used to establish public health recommendations. Data from GISP on the incidence of ciprofloxacin resistance in gonorrhea led to a change in gonorrhea treatment recommendations (37). Review of obstetric records of women presenting to labor and delivery departments and review of population-based data on invasive group B streptococcal disease from ABCs led to a revision in guidelines for preventing early onset group B streptococcal disease (38,39). Data on invasive pneumococcal disease from ABCs were used to determine the impact of the seven-valent conjugate vaccine and to monitor changes in disease resulting from serotypes not included in that vaccine (40).

Although epidemiologists and public health professionals strive to have complete, accurate data for dissemination, prompt dissemination of preliminary data or data involving only a few cases might have great impact for intervention or policy development. A few cases of intussusception following rotavirus vaccination reported through VAERS led to a rapid evaluation of the possible association of rotavirus vaccine and intussusception and subsequent withdrawal of the first generation rotavirus vaccine (*41*). Three cases of ciprofloxacin-resistant meningococcal disease detected through surveillance in the upper Midwest of the United States led to rapid recommendations to use alternative antimicrobial agents for prophylaxis in eastern North Dakota and northwestern Minnesota (*42*).

Infectious disease data are a crucial part of legislative initiatives for vaccine or other forms of disease prevention and control. Using surveillance data, a number of states recently passed emergency powers acts for the isolation and quarantine in the setting of certain infectious diseases that constitute public health emergencies (*43*).

Infectious disease data have been used to prompt recalls of food or medical products when an implicated item has been associated with disease. Infectious disease data have prompted changes in industry regulations. For example, antibiotic resistance data in enteric pathogens in Denmark led to a ban in the use of antibiotics as growth promoters in food animals (*44*).

An important use of infectious disease data is for the procurement of public health resources. Public health agencies typically depend on allocation of funds at the federal, state, or local level. Presenting data along with the planned public health interventions or objectives is a crucial component of a legislative initiative.

SYSTEM EVALUATION

Monitoring and evaluation are key to developing and maintaining effective surveillance systems for public health activities and response. As described in detail in Chapter 8, monitoring is the routine process of data collection and measurement of progress toward surveillance process and program objectives and analysis of indicators. Evaluation is the use of special studies and study designs to assess relevance, effectiveness, and impact of surveillance. Appropriate evaluation should include an assessment of core activities such as case detection, reporting, analysis and interpretation, and feedback. It should also include an assessment of core system attributes such as sensitivity of the surveillance system, flexibility, and timeliness.

Several elements of monitoring and evaluation, some of which depend on the goals of surveillance, are particularly relevant to surveillance for infectious diseases. Timeliness is critical for outbreak detection, especially systems designed to detect infectious bioterrorism events and diseases of high mortality and infectiousness; in such systems, initial specificity might be sacrificed for sensitivity. In contrast, completeness and accuracy of case ascertainment are particularly important for systems used to guide development of vaccines and to monitor impact of vaccines and other public health interventions. Finally, completeness of pathogen collection and accuracy of laboratory testing are the foundation of most high-quality infectious disease surveillance systems. Public health professionals using laboratory-based surveillance should ensure that appropriate quality assurance and quality control procedures are in place and that proficiency testing occurs on a regular basis.

Examples of Approaches to Monitoring and Evaluation Infectious Disease Surveillance

Case Ascertainment

A recent approach to evaluate completeness of HIV/AIDS case reports was use of capture–recapture methods in nine U.S. study sites in 2002 through 2003. Several reporting sources were used: laboratories, hospitals, private providers, vital statistics departments, local health departments, and HIV-testing and counseling sites. The most common source of HIV/AIDS reports—laboratories—accounted for only 32% to 78% of total reports. Using capture–recapture log-linear models, completeness of HIV infections reported within 1 year and reported up to 6 months after the end of the year was estimated to be 76% and 81%, respectively. Relative to a common method of case validation—active case finding—capture–recapture was a useful and less costly way to assess completeness of reporting routinely (*45*).

Evaluation of Alternative Surveillance Methods

The validity of potential new or alternative surveillance systems should be evaluated by rigorous comparison to an established "gold standard." For example, CDC's resource intensive population- and laboratory-based ABCs surveillance has been used to evaluate two simpler and less expensive systems—sentinel hospital surveillance and routinely produced hospital antibiograms—as alternative surveillance methods for estimating rates of drug-resistant *Streptococcus pneumoniae* (DRSP) infections in the same community. Sentinel surveillance in several large hospitals has been found to be a viable alternative to population-based surveillance in settings where a high degree of accuracy is not necessary; sentinel surveillance can detect large but not small variations in DRSP and is poor at detecting newly emerging resistance (e.g., fluoroquinolone resistance) (*46*). Aggregation of hospital antibiograms was found to be simple and a relatively accurate way to estimate the local levels of penicillin-nonsusceptible pneumococcus but was poor at estimating the proportion of intermediate- and high-level penicillin resistance and resistance to other antimicrobial agents (*47*). Identifying the strengths and weaknesses of varied surveillance systems allow public health personnel to choose the surveillance approach that best fits local needs and available resources.

General Surveillance Evaluation

In 2004, CDC and the Council of State and Territorial Epidemiologists (CSTE) collaborated to develop evaluation standards and an evaluation framework for HIV/AIDS surveillance (*48*). This framework, designed for local and national program evaluation, aims to produce continued quality improvement of HIV surveillance by providing information for training and technical assistance. The guidance includes structural requirements needed to operate an HIV/AIDS surveillance system, process standards, and outcome standards or measurable objectives. Outcome standards also include a minimum level at which data can be used reliably in analyses. The tools enable thorough assessments of whether HIV case data are adequate, reliable, and sufficiently accurate for determining funding and identifying priority populations for interventions and resource allocation (*48*).

Another approach to surveillance system evaluation is an external review. This assessment usually is applied to a larger program or aggregate of several surveillance systems and is most valuable when evaluating the direction and effectiveness of a mature infectious disease surveillance program. Typically, a review committee is formed of both recognized experts in the disease or syndrome under surveillance and persons familiar with practical aspects of surveillance implementation. Questions addressed by the external review committee include:

- Is the surveillance system achieving its stated objectives?
- What are the short-term and long-term goals of the surveillance program and are they relevant to current public health needs? Are they consistent with the sponsoring organization's mission?
- Is the surveillance system maximizing its strengths?
- Are resources appropriated in a manner to optimize success?
- Is the organizational structure of the system effective?
- Are the collection, analysis, interpretation, and dissemination methods effective?
- How can the surveillance system be improved?

A 1998 external review of ABCs surveillance program resulted in establishment of a bank of anonymized bacterial isolates available to basic science and public health researchers via a secure website, expanding the impact and value of the surveillance system. Also, internal communications were improved by a restructuring of annual ABCs investigator meetings, and the overall system strengthened by involvement of additional public health and clinical partnerships.

CONCLUSIONS

Many important steps in planning, implementing, and evaluating an infectious disease surveillance system are common to all surveillance programs, regardless of the disease or risk factor monitored. However, infectious disease surveillance systems are characterized by several unique features: isolate collection and characterization, importance of timeliness for outbreak detection and disease control and intervention, need for flexibility and rapid development in the setting of a new or emerging infections, development and evaluation of vaccines and other disease prevention efforts, and the need to integrate data from an increasing number of sources from diverse public health partners. The globalization of food distribution, new patterns of human–animal interaction, climate change, and growing international travel create greater potential for rapid and extensive disease spread and will continue to challenge public health systems. Development of effective infectious disease surveillance systems requires adherence to the principles of general surveillance development while incorporating—and taking advantage of—the continued advances made in both information technology, infectious disease laboratory techniques, and the basic scientific understanding of infectious disease pathogens.

REFERENCES

1. World Health Organization. The global burden of disease: 2004 update. 2008. http://www.who.int/healthinfo/global_burden_disease/2004_report_update/en/index.html. Accessed March 10, 2009.
2. King LJ. Collaboration in public health: a new global imperative. *Public Health Rep* 2008;123:264–265.
3. M'ikanatha NM, Lynfield R, Julian KG, Van Beneden CA, de Valk H. Infectious disease surveillance: a cornerstone for prevention and control. In: M'ikanatha, Lynfield, Van Beneden, de Valk, eds. *Infectious Disease Surveillance*, 1st ed. Oxford, UK: Blackwell Publishing; 2007:3–17.
4. Russell CA, Jones TC, Barr IG, *et al.* Influenza vaccine strain selection and recent studies on the global migration of seasonal influenza viruses. *Vaccine* 2008;26(Suppl 4):D31–D34.
5. Global influenza surveillance. A World Health Organization (WHO) website. http://www.who.int/csr/disease/influenza/influenzanetwork/en/index.html. Accessed March 11, 2009.
6. Falzon D, Belghiti F. Tuberculosis: still a concern for all countries in Europe. *Euro Surveill* 2007;12(12) pii–3159. http://www.eurosurveillance.org/ViewArticle.aspx?ArticleId=3159. Accessed March 4, 2009.
7. Guris D, Harpaz R, Redd SB, Smith NJ, Papania MH. Measles surveillance in the United States: an overview. *J Infect Dis* 2004;189(Suppl. 1):S177–S184.
8. DeVries A, Lees C, Rainbow J, Lynfield R. Explaining the unexplained: identifying causes of critical illness and death in Minnesota. *Minn Med* 2008;91:34–36.
9. Como-Sabetti K, Harriman KH, Buck JM, Glennen A, Boxrud DJ, Lynfield R. Community-associated methicillin-resistant *Staphylococcus aureus*: trends in case and isolate characteristics from six years of prospective surveillance. *Public Health Rep* 2009;124(3):427–435.
10. Wilder-Smith A, Goh KT, Paton NI. Experience of severe acute respiratory syndrome in Singapore: importance of cases, and defense strategies at the airport. *J Travel Med* 2003;10:259–262.
11. Vaccine Adverse Event Reporting System (VAERS). A Centers for Disease Control and Prevention (CDC) and Food and Drug Administration (FDA) website. http://vaers.hhs.gov/. Accessed March 11, 2009.
12. Gonococcal Isolate Surveillance Project (GISP). Centers for Disease Control and Prevention website. http://www.cdc.gov/std/gisp/. Updated June 4, 2008. Accessed March 11, 2009.
13. Flu activity and surveillance. Centers for Disease Control and Prevention website. http://www.cdc.gov/flu/weekly/fluactivity.htm. Updated March 6, 2009. Accessed March 11, 2009.
14. National Healthcare Safety Network (NHSN) Centers for Disease Control and Prevention website. http://www.cdc.gv/ncidod/dhqp/nhsn.html. Updated May 22, 2008. Accessed March 4, 2009.
15. Active Bacterial Core Surveillance system (ABCs) of the Centers for Disease Control and Prevention website. http://www.cdc.gov/abcs. Updated February 24, 2009. Accessed March 11, 2009.
16. Hammerum AM, Heuer OE, Emborg HD, *et al.* Danish integrated anti-microbial resistance monitoring and research program. *Emerg Infect Dis* 2007;13:1632–1639.

17. Gilbert JM, White DG, McDermott PF. The US national antimicrobial resistance monitoring system. *Future Microbiol* 2007;2:493–500.

18. Swaminathan B, Gerner-Smidt P, Ng LK, *et al.* Building PulseNet International: an interconnected system of laboratory networks to facilitate timely public health recognition and response to foodborne disease outbreaks and emerging foodborne diseases. *Foodborne Pathog Dis* 2006;3:36–50.

19. Centers for Disease Control and Prevention. Progress in Improving State and Local Disease Surveillance–United States, 2000–2005. *MMWR* 2005; 54(33):822–825.

20. M'ikanatha NM, Rohn DD, Welliver DP, McAdams T, Julian KG. Use of the World Wide Web to enhance infectious disease surveillance. In: M'ikanatha, Lynfield, Van Beneden, de Valk, eds. *Infectious Disease Surveillance*, 1st ed. Oxford, UK: Blackwell Publishing; 2007:281–293.

21. Vanden Eng JL, Wolkon A, Frolov AS. Use of handheld computers with global positioning systems for probability sampling and data entry in household surveys. *Am J Trop Med Hyg*, 2007;77(2):393–399.

22. Farley J, Srinivasan A, Richards A, Song X, McEachen J, Perl T. Handheld computer surveillance: Shoe-leather epidemiology in the "palm" of your hand. *Am J Infect Control* 2005;33(8):444–449.

23. National Healthcare Safety Network (NHSN). A Centers for Disease Control and Prevention (CDC) website. http://www.cdc.gov/ncidod/dhqp/nhsn.html. Updated May 22, 2008. Accessed March 30, 2009.

24. Glynn MK, Lee LM, McKenna MT. The status of national HIV Case Surveillance, United States 2006. *Public Health Rep* 2007;122(Suppl 1):63–71.

25. Schrag SJ, Brooks JT, Van Beneden C, *et al.* SARS surveillance in the United States during the emergency public health response, March-July, 2003. *Emerg Infect Dis* 2004;10(2):185–194.

26. Centers for Disease Control and Prevention. Framework for evaluating public health surveillance systems for early detection of outbreaks *MMWR* 2004; 53(RR5):1–11.

27. Hogan WR, Tsui FC, Ivanov O, *et al.* Detection of pediatric respiratory and diarrheal outbreaks from sales of over-the-counter electrolyte products. *J Am Med Inform Assoc* 2003;10:555–562.

28. Public Health Laboratory Information System (PHLIS). A Centers for Disease Control and Prevention website. http://www.cdc.gov/ncidod/dbmd/phlisdata/. Updated December 1, 2005. Accessed March 30, 2009.

29. Rassler S, Rubin DB, Zell ER. Incomplete data in epidemiology and medical statistics. In: Rao CR, Miller JP, Rao DC, eds. *Handbook of Statistics*, Vol 27. Elsevier BV. 2008:569–601.

30. Rogers DJ, Randolph SE. Studying the global distribution of infectious diseases using GIS and RS. *Nat Rev Microbiol* 2003;1:231–237. http://www.nature.com/nrmicro/journal/v1/n3/authors/nrmicro776.html.

31. Seto E, Moore CG, Hoskins RE. Use of geographic information systems and remote sensing for infectious disease surveillance. In: M'ikanatha, Lynfield, Van Beneden, de Valk, eds. *Infectious Disease Surveillance*, 1st ed. Oxford, UK: Blackwell Publishing; 2007: 408–418.

32. SAS website. http://www.sas.com/. Accessed March 30, 2009.

33. SPSS website. http://www.spss.com/. Accessed March 30, 2009.

34. Stata website. http://www.stata.com/. Accessed March 30, 2009.

35. Holmes JH, Rohn DD, Hilbe JM. Software applications for analysis of surveillance data. In: M'ikanatha, Lynfield, Van Beneden, de Valk, eds. *Infectious Disease Surveillance.* 1st ed. Oxford, UK: Blackwell Publishing; 2007:363–366.

36. International Health Regulations. World Health Organization website, 2005 http://www.who.int/csr/ihr/en/. Accessed March 11, 2009.

37. Centers for Disease Control and Prevention. Update to CDC's Sexually Transmitted Diseases Treatment Guidelines, 2006: Fluoroquinolones No Longer Recommended for Treatment of Gonococcal Infections. *MMWR* 2007;56(14):332–336.

38. Schrag SJ, Zell ER, Lynfield R, *et al.* A population-based comparison of strategies to prevent early onset group B streptococcal disease in neonates. *N Engl J Med* 2002;347:233–239.

39. Centers for Disease Control and Prevention. Prevention of Perinatal Group B Streptococcal Disease. *MMWR* 2002;51(RR11):1–22.

40. Centers for Disease Control and Prevention. Invasive pneumococcal disease in children 5 years after conjugate vaccine introduction–eight states, 1998–2005. *MMWR* 2008;57(6):144–148.

41. Murphy TV, Gargiullo PM, Massoudi MS, et al. Intussusception among infants given an oral rotavirus vaccine. *New Engl J Med* 2001;344:564–572.

42. Centers for Disease Control and Prevention. Emergence of fluoroquinolone-resistant *Neisseria meningitidis*–Minnesota and North Dakota, 2007–2008. *MMWR* 2008;57:173–175.

43. Legislation for public health emergencies. Centers for Disease Control and Prevention website. http://www2a.cdc.gov/phlp/legislation.asp. Accessed March 11, 2009.

44. Impacts of antimicrobial growth promoter termination in Denmark. World Health Organization (WHO) website. http://www.who.int/salmsurv/links/gssamrgrowthreportstory/en/ Posted 2003 (WHO reference: WHO/CDS/CPE/ZFK/2003.1). Accessed March 11, 2009.

45. Hall HI, Song R, Gerstle JE, Lee LM. Assessing the completeness of reporting of Human Immunodeficiency Virus diagnoses in 2002–2003: capture-recapture methods. *Am J Epidemiol* 2006;164(4):391–397.

46. Schrag SJ, Zell E, Schuchat A, Whitney CG. Evaluation of sentinel surveillance for drug-resistant *Streptococcus pneumoniae. Emerg Inf Dis* 2002;8(5):496–502.

47. Van Beneden CA, Lexau C, Baughman W, *et al.* Use of aggregated antibiogram data as a method for monitoring drug-resistant *Streptococcus pneumoniae* in the community. *Emerg Infect Dis* 2003;9(9):1089–1095.

48. Hall HI, Mokotoff ED. Setting standards and an evaluation framework for Human Immunodeficiency Virus/Acquired Immunodeficiency Syndrome surveillance. *J Public Health Manag Pract* 2007;13(5):519–523.

12

Public Health Surveillance for Chronic Diseases, Injuries, and Birth Defects

ALI H. MOKDAD, JOSEPH L. ANNEST, ROBIN M. IKEDA, AND CARA T. MAI

Non-communicable diseases, including injuries and chronic conditions such as heart diseases and stroke, are the primary cause of mortality worldwide (*1*). In the United States, chronic diseases have become the principal health challenge. They are the leading cause of death, disability, reduced quality of life, and rising health-care costs. At the turn of the last century, infectious diseases were the leading causes of death in the United States and most of the world (*2*). Several improvements in the health system, however, have led to a decline in death from infectious diseases. The many public health achievements of the 20th century added 25 years of life expectancy in the United States. A series of *Morbidity and Mortality Weekly Report* (*MMWR*) publications focused on the top 10 of these achievements, among them vaccination and control of infectious diseases (*3,4*). These successes shifted the burden of disease in the United States from infectious to chronic diseases.

Because of these epidemiologic shifts, by 2003, chronic diseases accounted for more than 60% of all deaths in the United States (*5*). In addition, unprecedented gains in life expectancy during the 20th century have fundamentally changed the patterns of health and disease, resulting in heavy demands on our systems of public health, health care, and aging services (*6,7*). These problems are compounded by the increased cost of chronic diseases as health-care costs continue to outstrip America's gross domestic product growth. As a result, public health professionals have called for a better balance of resources to prevent and control chronic diseases, emphasizing a public health and a medical care system that puts disease prevention and health maintenance at the forefront of our health activities (*8*).

To prevent and control chronic diseases, there is a need for accurate and timely data to design and implement prevention programs. There is a need for baseline measures for risk factors and disease prevalence to monitor progress toward health goals and objectives. Therefore, to better guide such planning, policy creation, and decision making, improvements are needed in accuracy, timeliness, accessibility, and comparability of surveillance information about chronic diseases in the United States. Data in a public health surveillance system must be collected continually if relevant changes and trends are to be noted quickly enough to be useful. Collecting data and defining epidemiologic measures and other indicators of program progress allow comparability between and within a population over time. Standardizing surveillance methods allows different parties to share knowledge and benefit from experiences in surveillance, prevention, and control of chronic diseases.

Other non-communicable conditions, such as injuries and birth defects, also contribute substantially to morbidity and mortality. In the United States, unintentional injury is the leading cause of death for those ages 1 through 44 years (9). Unintentional injury is also the leading cause of years of potential life lost before age 65. Similarly, homicide and suicide are leading causes of death, accounting for the second and third leading number of deaths for those ages 15 through 34 years. Injuries, including those resulting from unintentional and violence-related circumstances also place a substantial burden on the health-care system. In 2008, an estimated 29,953,000 injured persons were treated in U.S. hospital emergency departments (9). Of these, an estimated 2,236,000 were hospitalized or transferred for specialized medical care. Based on costs in the year 2000, an estimated 50 million injuries that required medical attention resulted in a cost to society of $406 billion, including $80.2 billion in medical costs and $326 billion in productivity losses, including lost wages and benefits and the inability to perform normal household functions (10).

In addition to providing population-based mortality, morbidity, and risk behavior or risk factor data for both injury and violence prevention efforts, injury surveillance systems in the United States have traditionally focused on physical injury resulting when human tissues are acutely exposed to energy in one form or another and sustain some form of damage. Injury surveillance is primarily used to monitor patterns and trends in injuries and risk factors/behaviors by external causes of injury. External cause of injury has two main aspects—the intent of injury and the mechanism of injury, including a wide variety of unintentional (e.g., drowning, falls, poisoning, motor vehicle-related injury) and violence-related (e.g., suicide/self-harm, homicide/assault, intimate partner violence, child maltreatment) injuries. Given the broad range of topics, the relevant surveillance data needs are also multifaceted. Similarly to other non-communicable issues, a myriad of influences might increase or decrease the risk for violence or injury, which further complicates injury surveillance efforts. The social-ecological model has been used to frame these factors and describe how they might interact. The model describes four levels of factors:

- Individual—biologic and personal history factors (e.g., demographic characteristics, attitudes and beliefs, history of aggressive behavior, other risk behaviors);
- Relationship—relationships with family, friends, peers, and others (e.g., supervision by a parent or caregiver, being exposed to friends peers who engage in violence);
- Community—the community context in which social relationships occur (e.g., school, workplace, neighborhoods); and
- Societal—broad societal factors (e.g., cultural norms and beliefs, economic policies, social policies).

Consequently, efforts to develop and improve injury surveillance systems have been underway since the early 1990s (*11*).

Chronic diseases and injuries are leading causes of morbidity and mortality in multiple age groups. In contrast, birth defects are the leading cause of infant mortality in the United States. Birth defects account for one in every five infant deaths, and they also contribute substantially to illness and life-long disabilities. In 2004, hospitalizations for complications associated with birth defects were longer in duration and more than twice as costly as hospitalizations for other conditions. Hospital costs to treat those principally admitted for birth defects totaled $2.6 billion, excluding physicians' fees (*12*).

Birth defects are defined as conditions that: *(1)* result from a malformation, deformation, or disruption on one or more parts of the body; *(2)* are present at birth; and *(3)* have serious, adverse effects on the affected person's health, development, or functioning (*13*). Interest in establishing an on-going monitoring system for birth defects began in the 1960s following the thalidomide exposures of pregnant women in Europe. The Centers for Disease Control and Prevention (CDC) subsequently established the Metropolitan Atlanta Congenital Defects Program in 1967 to detect changes in prevalence of birth defects by employing an active case ascertainment method. Thus began a trend in the United States during the 1970s and 1980s to establish monitoring systems to examine environmental and other exposures for birth defects; more recent surveillance program development in the 1990s and 2000s has focused on collecting data for prevention and intervention activities. The population-based data from birth defects systems are important for: *(1)* monitoring trends and understanding the public health impact of birth defects (e.g., by quantifying morbidity and mortality); *(2)* forming the basis for etiologic and clinical services such as examining the role of maternal obesity and diabetes as risk factors for birth defects; *(3)* identifying children who may need referrals to specialized services in the community; *(4)* providing data on follow-up studies of long-term effects; *(5)* making informed policy decisions; and *(6)* evaluating prevention strategies and actions.

Because health and health risk behaviors can have a great impact on chronic disease, injury, and birth defect morbidity and mortality, it is important to understand the trends associated with these behaviors. Smoking, diet, physical inactivity, and alcohol consumption are the leading causes of death in the United States (*8*). Indeed, preventing the incidence and progression of non-communicable disease and injury through programs that modify risk factors is one of the few strategies available to temper the expected pressures on the health-care system. It is important to achieve a clear balance between the "immediate" and "important" in our public health activities (*14*). Understanding trends in health behaviors is thus critical to prevent non-communicable diseases and prepare for health-care costs, morbidity, and mortality.

Development and on-going maintenance of high-quality surveillance systems for non-communicable conditions emphasizing accuracy, timeliness, accessibility, and comparability are needed to better guide planning, policy development, and decision making. Systematic collection of data in a surveillance system allows for relevant changes, patterns, and trends to be noted. Standardizing case definitions and uniform data elements for epidemiologic measures and other indicators and developing population-based surveillance methods will help provide the basis for comparability between and within populations or communities over time.

This chapter examines how the principles of public health surveillance are applied to non-infectious conditions. We provide examples of systems that have demonstrated innovation or excellence in bringing principles to practice.

SYSTEM DEVELOPMENT AND DATA COLLECTION

Once a need is identified and a public health surveillance system for a non-communicable condition is being developed, the steps considered are similar to any other system. A clear case definition is essential—knowing what the system will cover and ensuring sensitivity and specificity in the case definition will ensure accuracy in the findings of the resulting information. A careful scan of data sources is important; use of existing data where applicable can improve efficiency but must be balanced with cost and effort associated with data ascertainment as well as accuracy of data from such sources. Standardization of data elements is important when ascertainment occurs from existing sources. Often the only option is to plan a new data collection *de novo*, which might entail designing a representative sampling scheme for a survey or record review. A number of non-communicable surveillance surveys in the United States have relied on random digit dialing (RDD) as a survey sampling method, but recent changes in the patterns of land-line and mobile phone usage have caused concerns about representativeness (*15*).

Public health surveillance of behaviors that contribute to chronic diseases, injuries, and even some birth defects in the United States has a long history in the Behavioral Risk Factor Surveillance System (BRFSS). This surveillance system was designed to fill knowledge gaps that existed about the levels of known behavioral risk factors associated with the leading causes of premature mortality among adults: cigarette smoking, alcohol use, physical inactivity, diet, hypertension, and safety restraint use.

The BRFSS was designed as a state-based health surveillance survey. The objective of the BRFSS is to collect both local and state-specific data on health risk behaviors, clinical preventive health practices, and health-care access that are associated with the leading causes of morbidity and mortality in the United States. State health departments requested a state-based surveillance system to ensure state-level data. Data are collected from a representative sample in each state, and the sampling is designed to provide national estimates when all states' data are combined (*15*). Currently, data are collected monthly in all 50 states, the District of Columbia, Puerto Rico, the Virgin Islands, and Guam. More than 414,500 adult interviews were completed in 2008. To facilitate use of data, all BRFSS data, reports, methods, and questionnaires are available at BRFSS web page (*16*).

BRFSS started in 1981 as a point-in-time survey. Beginning in 1984, 15 states participated in an ongoing surveillance system, with their interviews spread out across the whole year. Beginning in 1988, optional, standardized sets of questions on specific topics (optional modules) were made available to states. By 1993, the BRFSS had become a nationwide system, and the total sample size exceeded 100,000 as the system was redesigned, with certain questions asked every year (fixed core) and others asked every other year (rotating core). As part of the 1993 redesign, up to five "emerging" core questions for newly arising topics were included each year for all states. As a result, health departments use the data for a variety of purposes, including identifying demographic variations in health-related behaviors, targeting services, addressing emergent and critical health issues, proposing legislation for health initiatives, measuring progress toward state and national health objectives, and designing evaluations of their programs and policies.

The challenge for BRFSS is effectively managing an increasingly complex surveillance system that serves the needs of multiple programs while adapting to changes in communications technology such as the increased use of cellular telephones and call screening devices, societal behaviors (concerns about privacy and declining participation in surveys), and population diversity (growing number of languages spoken in the United States along with greater cultural and ethnic diversity). To address these challenges, BRFSS maintains an ongoing program to improve the current BRFSS methods by identifying and addressing potential threats to the validity and reliability of BRFSS data. These efforts are critical for improving the quality of BRFSS data, reaching populations previously not included in the survey, and expanding the utility of the surveillance data. Details of all BRFSS improvements and innovations have been described (*15,16*).

Several data collection challenges exist for the BRFSS, including changes in coverage with RDD methods, sampling via the Internet and mobile phone tech- nologies, building a complete sampling frame, and implementing mixed-mode methods. Participation in most RDD telephone surveys is declining, prompting researchers to consider use of alternative survey modes to increase participation. In October and November 2003, a set of experiments was conducted using Internet and mail versions of the BRFSS questionnaire administered to potential respon- dents drawn from the standard BRFSS telephone sampling frame and reverse- matched to identify valid mailing addresses. Telephone survey follow-up was conducted with Internet and mail survey nonrespondents. Results were compared with those from the ongoing computer-assisted telephone interviewing BRFSS. The findings suggest that self-administered modes when used in conjunction with telephone follow-up can improve levels of participation but might also increase differences between respondents and nonrespondents on measures of interest (*17,18*). As a result, overall nonresponse bias might not have been reduced despite increases in response rates.

Advances in electronic record-keeping have allowed researchers to develop and sample from a frame of addresses, which appears to provide coverage that rivals that obtained through RDD sampling methods. BRFSS examined the possibility of using a list of household addresses as a sampling frame (i.e., address-based frames) for surveillance by examining the quality of the frame of addresses. The quality and potential of such frames was promising (*19*). As a result, a pilot study conducted in 2005 compared use of traditional RDD telephone survey methods to an approach using a mail version of the questionnaire completed by a random sample of households drawn from an address-based frame. The findings indicate that the mail survey approach can achieve higher response rates in states with low response rates (<40%) than RDD, particularly when two mailings are sent (20,21). Additionally, the address frame with mail survey design provides access to households with cellular telephones only and offers cost savings over the telephone approach. The address frame seems to provide a potential alternative for RDD (22).

BRFSS conducted a pilot to examine the feasibility of using mixed-mode surveys involving mail surveys with telephone follow-up. The study examined data from a sample of telephone numbers drawn using RDD methods to a sample of addresses drawn using U.S. Postal Service records. The study was conducted in California, Florida, Massachusetts, Minnesota, South Carolina, and Texas. The pilot showed that BRFSS could use a multimode approach for data collection to reduce bias (23,24).

To meet the challenge posed by the growing number of mobile telephone-only households, BRFSS conducted interviews with individuals sampled from known mobile telephone exchanges. The studies were designed to determine the feasibility of conducting BRFSS interviews by mobile telephone, their cost, and the impact on survey estimates of including such interviews. Results clearly showed that BRFSS can reach the mobile phone populations, especially the young age groups that were most likely to be excluded by RDD. In addition, the health behavior of the mobile phone population was different than that of the RDD. Hence, BRFSS concluded that mobile phones should become a routine mode of data collection, although mobile phones pose a major challenge in terms of location and number portability (25).

Another non-communicable risk factor survey in the United States that relies on telephone interview methods is the Injury Control and Risk of Injury Survey (ICARIS). ICARIS, deployed in 1994 in all 50 states and the District of Columbia, was the first national injury-specific risk factor survey system used for surveillance activities to assess injury risk factors and the prevalence of injury prevention counseling. A second ICARIS was conducted, using similar methods, from July 2001 to February 2003 to obtain updated estimates and monitor changes over time. Both of these surveys were cross-sectional RDD telephone surveys. In additional to injury prevention counseling, survey questions covered residential fire and smoke alarm use, bicycle helmet use, sports and recreation safety, motor vehicle safety, falls among the elderly, firearm ownership and storage, dog bites, alcohol consumption, and violence (26–37). These surveys provided much more detail than that obtained on injury-related risk factors in the BRFSS. Following the September 11, 2001 terrorist attacks on the World Trade Center and the Pentagon, a set of questions was added to the second ICARIS to assess the relationship between exposure to these events and post-traumatic stress disorder (38). A second phase of this latter study (ICARIS-2 Phase-2) was conducted from March 2007 to May 2008 in all 50 states and the District of Columbia using methods similar to the earlier studies. The Phase 2 study was conducted primarily to learn about topics for which time and financial limitations prevented inclusion in earlier studies. New topics covered included child supervision, traumatic brain injury and injury and disability, and perpetration of violence. Questions on firearm access and ownership and suicidal ideation, which included in prior surveys, were also asked.

These risk factor surveys face similar issues to BRFSS regarding factors that influence participation rates in telephone interview surveys. The response rate for the second ICARIS (48%) was considerably lower than that of the first ICARIS (56%) using the standard definitions published by the American Association of Public Opinion Research (AAPOR formula RR3) (*39*). There is much debate about the future use of RDD telephone interview for conducting risk factor surveys given the increase use of cellular technology, fewer residential land lines in use, and increased use of blocked calls (*40*).

Another system for injury surveillance began in July 2000 when the National Center for Injury Prevention and Control (NCIPC), CDC in collaboration with the U.S. Consumer Product Safety Commission (CPSC) expanded the National Electronic Injury Surveillance System (NEISS) to collect data on all types and causes of injuries treated in a representative sample of U.S. hospitals with emergency departments (EDs). This system is called the NEISS All Injury Program (NEISS-AIP).

The NEISS-AIP is designed to provide national incidence estimates of all types and external causes of nonfatal injuries and poisonings treated in U.S. hospital EDs. Data on injury-related visits are being obtained from a national sample of 66 out of 100 NEISS hospitals, which were selected as a stratified probability sample of hospitals in the United States and its territories with a minimum of six beds and a 24-hour ED (*41*). The sample includes separate strata for very large, large, medium, and small hospitals, defined by the number of annual ED visits per hospital and children's hospitals. The scope of reporting goes beyond routine reporting of injuries associated with consumer-related products in CPSC's jurisdiction to include all injuries and poisonings. The NEISS-AIP data can be used to: *(1)* measure the magnitude and distribution of nonfatal injuries in the United States; *(2)* monitor unintentional and violence-related nonfatal injuries over time, *(3)* identify emerging injury problems; *(4)* identify specific cases for follow-up investigations of particular injury-related problems; and *(5)* set national priorities. Federal agencies are using this system to conduct special studies of specific injuries or causes of injury (e.g., adverse drug events, medical devices, traumatic brain injury, nontraffic motor vehicle, assaults, intentional self-harm).

NEISS-AIP is providing data on approximately 500,000 cases annually. Data obtained on each case include age, race/ethnicity, sex of the patient, principal diagnosis, primary body part affected, consumer products involved, disposition at ED discharge (i.e., hospitalized, transferred, treated and released, observation, died), locale where the injury occurred, work-relatedness, and a narrative description of the injury circumstances. Also, major categories of external cause of injury (e.g., motor vehicle, falls, cut/pierce, poisoning, fire/burn) and of intent of injury (e.g., unintentional, assault, intentional self-harm, legal intervention) are being coded for each case in a manner consistent with the *International Classification of Diseases, Clinical Modification, Ninth Revision* (ICD-9-CM) (*42*), coding rules and guidelines. NEISS-AIP provides an excellent data source for monitoring national estimates of nonfatal injuries treated in U.S. hospital EDs over time. A limitation of this data system is that it only provides national estimates. These surveillance data are available through Web-based Injury Statistics Query and Reporting System (WISQARS™) and through public use data files at the Interuniversity Consortium for Political and Social Research (ICPSR) (*9,43*).

CDC's work the National Birth Defects Prevention Network (NBDPN) furnishes yet another model for data collection for public health surveillance. This network of state population-based birth defects systems has provided a vehicle for our national understanding of the public health burden of these conditions. For the first time, national estimates for 18 major birth defects of the eye, cleft lip and palate, gastrointestinal system, musculoskeletal system, cardiovascular system, and chromosomes were published using data from population-based surveillance systems that employ active case finding methods (*44*). This method uses abstractors—that is, data collectors who go to the primary data sources such as medical records—to find and confirm cases. Birth certificate data are insufficient as a means of monitoring a wide range of birth defects, and given a lack of a national system for population-based birth defects monitoring, this type of collaborative efforts thus constitutes an important method of gathering and disseminating data.

As the number of multistate data collaborative projects increases, it will be imperative for these birth defects systems to work toward standardized data elements. The NBDPN has published guidelines for conducting birth defects surveillance, and this has provided an important first step toward consistency (*45*). The emphasis now is on developing minimal standards, moving from recommendations of what states "should do" to what states "must" minimally meet to obtain more uniform data. An ongoing challenge is the diversity of systems employing varying methods as well as stipulations attached to various federal and state resource allocations. Nonetheless, agreeing to core standards is key to ensuring data quality, as these collaborations are necessary if we are to move forward in birth defects surveillance and prevention (see Chapter 5).

DATA MANAGEMENT

Sources of data for non-communicable conditions are numerous and variable. Management of data from various sources comes with its own set of challenges, including but not limited to blending different data standards, data with varying degrees of accuracy and reliability, and attaching multiple records for a single incident to the correct case.

CDC National Program of Cancer Registries (NPCR) has found a creative way to deal with data management issues for de-duplication of cases. This is an important task given that the data collected by state cancer registries enable public health professionals to understand and address the cancer burden more effectively. CDC's Division of Cancer Prevention and Control developed Link Plus, a probabilistic record linkage program to support NPCR. Link Plus is a record-linkage tool for cancer registries (*46*). It is an easy-to-use, standalone application for Microsoft® Windows® that can run in two modes: to detect duplicates in a cancer registry database or to link a cancer registry file with external files. Although originally designed to be used by cancer registries, the program can be used with any type of data in fixed width or delimited format. Used extensively across a diversity of research disciplines, Link Plus is rapidly becoming an essential linkage tool for researchers and organizations that maintain public health data.

National injury surveillance provides two examples of data management challenges. The first challenge deals with the dependence of national- and state-based injury mortality and morbidity surveillance on international classification systems for external causes of injuries, commonly called external cause-of-injury-codes (E-codes). Injury mortality surveillance is based on underlying cause of death or external-cause-of-injury codes, using the *International Statistical Classification of Diseases and Related Health Problems, Tenth Revision* (ICD-10) (*47*). Injury morbidity surveillance, including data from hospital discharge and emergency department data systems, is based on external cause-of-injury codes using the ICD-9-CM (*42*). E-codes are defined to capture specific information on the intent and mechanism of injury, as well as the place of occurrence and activity, relevant to the injury circumstances. The injury field has established standard groupings of E-codes in the form of a matrix of intent by mechanism of injury that provide a common framework for presenting injury data by major external cause categories (e.g., motor vehicle traffic, fall, cut/pierce, fire/burn) (*48*). These matrices for ICD-10 and ICD-9-CM have been instrumental in allowing for comparisons across states and among population subgroups. A limitation has been that the completeness and quality of E-coding in state-based morbidity data systems varies substantially among states; also, some states do not currently routinely collect E-codes on injury-related cases (*11*). In response, CDC is leading a national effort to improve the completeness, accuracy, and specificity of E-codes collected in state-based hospital discharge and ED administrative data systems to facilitate their use in designing, implementing, and evaluating state and community level injury prevention programs (*11*). The aim of this effort is to develop action plans to improve (*1*) communication among stakeholders regarding E-codes; (*2*) the collection of E-codes; and (*3*) improve the usefulness of E-coded data for injury prevention efforts.

The second example from injury surveillance illustrates challenges of bringing data from multiple sources on a single case together, connecting the correct information to the correct individual incident or person. National Violent Death Reporting Systems (NVDRS) is a state-based surveillance system that links data from law enforcement, coroners and medical examiners, vital statistics, and crime laboratories to assist each participating state in designing and implementing tailored prevention and intervention efforts. NVDRS defines a death resulting from violence as "a death resulting from the intentional use of physical force or power against oneself, another person, or against a group or community." NVDRS collects information about homicides, suicides, deaths by legal intervention (excluding executions), and deaths of undetermined intent. In addition, information about unintentional firearm injury deaths (i.e., the individual did not intend to discharge the firearm) is collected, although these deaths are not considered violent deaths by the above definition. Deaths are included in this system based on their ICD-10 underlying cause-of-death code (*49*).

NVDRS is incident-based, and each record contains data on all victims and alleged perpetrators (suspects) associated with a given incident. Multiple victims and/or suspects are determined for inclusion into a single incident record by the timing of the violent injuries, rather than the timing of the deaths, and include all persons with fatal injuries occurring within 24 hours of the first fatal injury, along with source documents indicating a clear link among the deaths. Each incident record includes information about victims, suspects, the relationship between the victim and the suspect, circumstances surrounding the death, and the method of injury.

NVDRS demonstrates the importance of linking data from multiple data sources to provide much more detailed information about violent deaths than can be obtained from solely death certificate-based data systems, such as the National Vital Statistics System (NVSS). Seventeen states currently participate in the NVDRS. The goal is to include in the system all 50 states, all U.S. territories, and the District of Columbia. Surveillance data for 16 participating states for 2003 through 2006 are available through WISQARS™ (*9*).

Regardless of ascertainment approaches, many systems rely on data from multiple sources to improve the quality of the collected data and to obtain a better picture of the contribution of these conditions on the individuals and populations. An important step in using multiple administrative datasets is the ability to effectively link the sources to improve the completeness of the data by yielding additional information about the cases collected or verifying data already collected. Although record linkage tools exist to perform this function, they offer limited user-defined parameters and control. An innovative and open source tool, called Fine-grained Record Integration and Linkage Tool (FRIL), was developed and tested using data from CDC's birth defects surveillance program and vital statistics data and yielded 99% precision and 95% recall (*50*). Using a probabilistic linkage approach, this user-friendly tool shows algorithmic decisions that allow users to consider computational issues to enhance accuracy and performance of the linkage process (*50*).

Additionally, birth defects multisource ascertainment methods provide the flexibility to expand case definitions to include health-related conditions of current interest, such as those affecting newborn screening and stillbirth surveillance. Thus, several state birth defects surveillance systems have expanded their case definition to include confirmed newborn screening cases and to collect health outcome data to better understand the impact of these children on the public health system. Challenges with multisource data ascertainment include the lack of data standards and ensuring matching of information to the correct cases in a case-based system. These data management challenges are not insurmountable but require the collaboration of multiple data owners. Relying on infrastructure to expand to other conditions allows better adaptation to communities' changing needs.

DATA ANALYSIS

Typical measures of interest from surveillance systems of non-communicable conditions include prevalence and trends, prevalence ratios, morbidity and mortality, survival probability, quality-of-life indicators, and incidence. Demographic methods (*see* Chapter 6) are of particular use with non-communicable conditions and are often applied to population-based surveillance systems of such conditions. New and innovative analytic methods are needed in several areas—for example, severity scores and composite risk scores. Sampling is often used in non-communicable surveillance methods, making knowledge of and facile skills with sampling weights important for analysts.

The design of chronic disease surveillance systems can be complex and involve multistage sampling. The advances in sampling techniques and software availability have made the analyses of these surveys easier. The BRFSS provides a summary report with data quality and basic analyses that allows researchers to compare their methods to those numbers published on the Internet. Moreover, on its Internet site, BRFSS provides a means to run analyses on a real time basis. The newest innovation is a Web-enabled analyses tool (*16*). This program allows users to run cross-tabulation and logistic regression analysis with no prior knowledge of statistical software for complex survey design. The idea is to increase the data usability and utility. This procedure allows a user to generate frequencies, cross-tabulations, and stratified analyses of BRFSS data. In addition, it allows the user to generate logistic regression models to calculate the effect of one or more predictors, or independent variables, on a dependent variable that has two levels: "at risk" and "not at risk."

There are several examples of innovative methods for analyses of chronic diseases data. The prediction of cancer incidence for future years is a good example. Knowing the potential burden of cancer will guide planning activities for proper public and medical programs, especially resources needed for diagnosis and treatment. Moller et al. have developed models for cancer prediction using statistical models (*51*). Data from cancer registries are used and the methodology accounts for uncertainty in the models assumptions and the random variation of the future number of cases. These models use the classical approach of age–period–cohort for making the cancer incidence prediction. These models have been used widely to predict cancer incidence in many countries.

Some analytic aspects in need of improvement for injury morbidity surveillance include measures of injury severity and injury outcomes. Measuring injury severity based on injury severity score and trauma scoring methods have undergone substantial debate in the injury field, but no agreement has been reached on which method is most valid and reliable (*52*). A method most useful for injury surveillance could be the ICD-based Injury Severity Score (ICISS) (*53*). This method involves calculating a survival risk ratio (SRR) for individual injury diagnosis codes and then assigning a patient's ICISS (survival probability) based on the product of the SRRs associated with all the diagnoses listed on the patient's hospital discharge record. Efforts are underway to develop ICISS thresholds for threat to life and threat to short- and long-term disability associate with injury.

The objective is to define injury indicators that are not affected by changes over time in the utilization of services.

Birth defects surveillance likewise tracks individuals affected with non-communicable conditions. As individuals with birth defects live longer, it has become increasing important to understand the magnitude and survival of these individuals in the United States. Birth defects surveillance systems routinely publish birth prevalence for major birth defects, but prevalence and survival data for other age groups affected with these congenital conditions are sparse. CDC has begun to analyze multistate population-based data to better understand the survival pattern for individuals born with birth defects, such as spina bifida and Down syndrome. More complex analyses of the surveillance data will improve the usefulness of the birth defects surveillance system.

DATA DISSEMINATION AND COMMUNICATION

There are many uses of public health surveillance data. In non-communicable conditions like chronic disease, injury, and birth defects, where cause and effect are often separated by a long period, surveillance data are effectively used for estimating the scope of a problem, examining the geographic distribution of health events, facilitating planning, and evaluating public health programs to promote behavior change or exposure reduction.

Data dissemination and presentation is a key in getting the public health message out. One of the most powerful examples of data dissemination is the use of the obesity maps from BRFSS (Figure 12–1). Published in *JAMA* in 1999 these maps documented visually the rapid rise in obesity in the United States (*54*). The power of these maps has led to the development of many obesity prevention programs. Indeed, these maps showed an epidemic of obesity and called for action.

Injury surveillance has used the Internet as a major vehicle for providing ready access to E-code data by policymakers, program planners, researchers, and the public. CDC has developed and implemented an interactive injury statistics query system that serves this purpose; it is called the WISQARS™ (*9*). WISQARS™ provides data on fatal and nonfatal injuries, including death data from the NVSS and NVDRS, and nonfatal data from NEISS-AIP. There are also numerous state Internet sites that provide useful injury mortality, morbidity, and risk behavior data (*55*).

The NVSS, operated by the National Center for Health Statistics (NCHS), includes all injury-related deaths on the basis of all death certificates filed throughout the 50 states, the District of Columbia, and U.S. territories (*56*). Each year, NCHS releases summary death reports and a multiple-cause-of-death file for use in injury surveillance. The ICD-10 underlying cause (or external cause) of death codes (e.g, each injury-related death is assigned underlying cause code) are used to tabulate injury deaths by external cause groupings. Injury deaths and death rates are then used for examining demographic characteristics and patterns and temporal trends. These national, state, and regional data are available through WISQARS™ from 1981 through 2006, and WISQARS™ is updated every year (*9*).

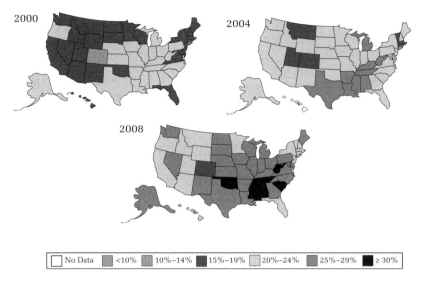

Figure 12–1 Percent of Obese* in U.S. Adults (2000–2008).
Source: Behavioral Risk Factor Surveillance System, CDC.
Note: *BMI ≥30, or ~30 lbs. overwight for 5' 4" person.

In addition to looking at these death data by external cause of injury, the injury field has developed methods for summarizing injury deaths by ICD-10 diagnosis codes. A standard ICD-10 matrix of body region and nature of injury is available (*48*). Currently, methods of using these multiple-cause-of-death data to tabulate the numbers of deaths by injury diagnosis are under much debate (e.g. tabulate deaths based on any mention, total mentions, weighted total mentions, or "as yet undefined" primary diagnosis). This is an important issue for defining and tracking specific injury deaths, such as those resulting from traumatic brain injury, and for estimating the cost of fatal injury by injury diagnosis.

In recent years, birth defects surveillance programs have used data to focus on prevention strategies and link affected children to prevention, medical, and social services. The impetus for this can be attributed to prevention efforts stemming from a 1992 U.S. Public Health Service (PHS) recommendation that all women of child-bearing age should consume 400 mcg of folic acid daily to prevent up to 70% of serious neural tube defects (NTDs)—namely, anencephaly and spina bifida. In a related development, CDC cooperative agreement funding for state birth defects surveillance programs began focusing on occurrent and recurrent prevention efforts as well as linking families of affected children to services within the community.

Following the PHS folic acid recommendation, the Food and Drug Administration issued regulations for folic acid fortification of cereal and grain products in the United States, beginning with optional implementation in 1996 and mandatory compliance by January 1998. Birth defects surveillance systems have been instrumental in documenting the effect of this policy decision. Data from 24 state birth defects surveillance systems documented a 31% decline in the prevalence for spina bifida and 16% for anencephaly (57). This translated to 1,000 fewer NTD-affected pregnancies, declining from 4,000 before folic acid fortification implementation (1995–1996) to 3,000 post-fortification (1999–2000) (58).

Beyond simply identifying the children affected with birth defects, birth defects surveillance programs have started to refer these children to appropriate services to ensure optimal health outcomes. In 2004, of 32 operational birth defects surveillance systems in the United States, 40% indicated that they use surveillance data for referral activities (59). Mechanism for the referral process depends on state legislation and resources and is thus varied. Generally, state birth defects programs direct affected children to state or county services (such as the Maternal and Child Health Title V programs) by referral or notifying families of available programs. These birth defects programs are also working to determine how the public health infrastructure can better serve the needs of families—for example, ensuring that gaps in the service system are identified.

SYSTEM EVALUATION

As with all public health surveillance systems, it is of critical importance that the data collected in and the information disseminated by the system are accurate, valid, and timely. Given the various uses of these data, including making decisions about resource appropriation and allocation, ensuring the data are portraying a valid picture of the health condition is of utmost importance. Evaluation of the system (*see* Chapter 8) must be an integral part of its life-cycle. Many practical and several innovative examples of evaluations of non-communicable public health surveillance systems exist.

The evaluation of surveillance systems is an integral part of their operation. Several methods have been used to evaluate surveillance systems and there are standards for this task. A good example of an ongoing evaluation of a surveillance system is the Registry Certification program by the North American Association of Central Cancer Registries, Inc. (NAACCR). This system is mainly focusing on the completeness, accuracy, and timeliness of the data. Each year, members of the Data Evaluation and Certification Committee evaluate cancer incidence data. Based on this evaluation, the registry staff receive a report containing the results of registry certification evaluation. Based on preset criteria, cancer registries are given either a silver or gold standard ranking. To receive a gold standard, a cancer registry must meet the following criteria: *(1)* has a case ascertainment of 95% or higher; *(2)* has fewer than 3% of reported cancer cases from death certificates; *(3)* has less than 0.1% duplicate case reports; *(4)* has no errors in all data variables used to create incidence statistics by cancer type, sex, race, age, and county; *(5)* has less than 2% of the case reports missing meaningful information on age, sex, and county; *(6)* has less than 3% of the cases missing race; and *(7)* has submitted files for evaluation to NAACCR within 23 months of the close of the diagnosis year under review.

The Agency for Healthcare Research and Quality (AHRQ) has conducted the most comprehensive evaluation of E-codes in states associated with their

Healthcare Costs and Utilization Project (HCUP) (*60*). The HCUP is a system of hospital discharge and ED databases that are updated annually. Participation is voluntary by states that have hospital discharge and ED data systems. The evaluation study, based on 2001 state morbidity data, found that the percentage of injury records with an E-code was 86% in AHRQ's nationally representative database, the HCUP National Inpatient Sample (NIS). For the 33 states represented in the HCUP State Inpatient Databases (SIDs), completeness averaged 87%, with more than half of the states reporting E-codes on at least 90% of injuries. In the nine states also represented in the HCUP State Emergency Department Databases (SEDDs), completeness averaged 93%. In this study, findings also showed that E-coding was more complete in the HCUP NIS than the National Hospital Discharge Survey (NHDS) operated by the National Center for Health Statistics (86% vs. 68%) (*61*). The most likely explanation for this difference in completeness is that the HCUP NIS retains more diagnosis fields than the NHDS for capturing E-codes. The HCUP provides an excellent system for ongoing evaluation of the completeness, accuracy, and specificity of E-codes in state morbidity data systems as national efforts are underway to improve the quality of injury data useful for injury surveillance and prevention program planning and evaluation activities.

CDC has an Injury Indicators Project that provides information on the completeness of E-coding in state hospital discharge data systems (*62*). The most recent annual report provides E-coded data for 33 participating states, and most of these states have evaluated their data systems for completeness of E-coding. The completeness of E-coding of injury-related discharges for these states ranged from 56.3% to 100%, and 19 (57.6%) of these states had completeness of E-coding higher than 90%. The Injury Indicators Project aims to provide a summary of state E-coded data for use in injury surveillance, state comparisons, and priority setting for injury prevention activities.

Because birth defects surveillance systems are established at state and regional levels, individual systems have evaluated their data for completeness, accuracy, and timeliness. The first step in determining the quality of data is to understand the strengths and limitations of the various data sources by comparing them against a "gold standard" source or some other benchmark, such as data generated from national estimates or other systems employing similar ascertainment methods. For example, comparing the prevalence of NTD data collected from birth defects surveillance systems with NTD data from birth certificates, an underestimation of approximately 57% of the cases can be expected (unpublished data).

In addition to evaluating the data quality of a surveillance system, it is also imperative to examine the functions of a surveillance system as they relate to the overall purposes or goals of the program. Logic models provide a useful tool for framing how the data collection system ultimately will be used to ensure that the data are appropriately directed for the desired impact. In the example shown here, a framework for defining surveillance activities and data use has been developed for CDC-funded state birth defects surveillance programs. This conceptual model shows how surveillance data, along with capacity development and data utilization for prevention and referral to services can result in desired outcomes (Figure 12–2).

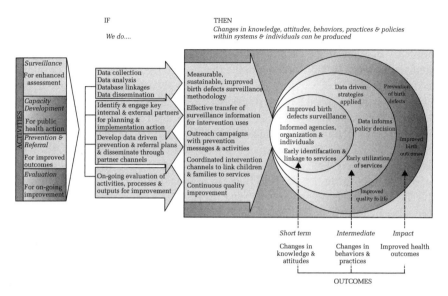

Figure 12–2 Logic Model for the Role and Functions of Surveillance in State Programs Addressing Birth Defects.

CONCLUSION

Given that the burden of non-communicable conditions, including chronic, injury, and birth defects, is the major health challenge and will continue in the near foreseeable future, surveillance of these conditions serves as a powerful tool for public health at the local, state, and national levels. BRFSS is leading the development of alternative modes of data collection to meet the changes in telecommunication (*63*). Lessons learned from injury national surveillance efforts (e.g., improving external cause-of-injury coding, linking data from multiple data sources, utilizing emergency department data) have been helpful to advance the field of injury surveillance and might be useful to improve/enhance public health surveillance systems focused on other topic areas. Surveillance for health conditions such as birth defects and injuries serve an important vehicle in understanding the impact of these conditions on the population, understand possible risk factors, guide public policies, and direct prevention efforts. The continued success and improvements in these surveillance systems are imperative to ensure their survival and utility for monitoring trends and changes in causes, health status, morbidity, and mortality associated with these diseases and conditions.

REFERENCES

1. World Health Organization. *World Health Statistics* 2008. Geneva: WHO Press; 2008.
2. Armstrong GL, Conn LA, Pinner RW. Trends in infectious disease mortality in the United States during the 20th century. *JAMA* 1999;281:61–66.
3. Centers for Disease Control and Prevention. Ten great public health achievements-United States, 1990–1999. *MMWR* 1999;48(12):241–243.

4. Centers for Disease Control and Prevention. Achievements in Public Health, 1990–1999. Changes in the public health system. *MMWR* 1999;48(50):1141–1147.

5. Deaths: Final Data for 2003. Division of Vital Statistics. www.cdc.gov/nch. Accessed March 8, 2010.

6. Schneider EL, Guralnik JM. The aging of America. Impact on health care costs. *JAMA* 1990;263:2335–2340.

7. Clark DO. US trends in disability and institutionalization among older blacks and whites. *Am J Public Health* 1997;87:438–440.

8. Mokdad AH, Marks JS, Stroup D, Gerberding JL. Actual causes of death in the United States, 2000. *JAMA* 2004;291:1238–1245.

9. Centers for Disease Control and Prevention. Web-based Injury Statistics Query and Reporting System (WISQARS™). Atlanta, GA: US Department of Health and Human Services, CDC; 2009. http://www.cdc.gov/injury/wisqars/index.html. Accessed March 8, 2010.

10. Corso P, Finkelstein E, Miller T, Fiebelkorn I, Zaloshnja E. Incidence and lifetime costs of injury in the United States. *Inj Prev* 2006;12:212–218.

11. Centers for Disease Control and Prevention. Strategies to improve external cause-of-injury coding in state-based hospital discharge and emergency department data systems. *MMWR* 2008;57(No. RR-1):1–15.

12. Russo CA, Elixhauser A. 2007. Hospitalization costs for birth defects, 2004. Healthcare Cost and Utilization Project (HCUP). Statistical Brief #24, U.S. Agency for Healthcare Research and Quality, Rockville, MD. www.hcupdoc.net/reports/stat-briefs/sb24.pdf. Accessed March 8, 2010.

13. Centers for Disease Control and Prevention. Improved national prevalence estimates for 18 selected major birth defects—United States, 1999–2001. *MMWR* 2006; 54(51&52):1301–1305.

14. McGinnis JM, Foege WH. The immediate vs the important. *JAMA* 2004;291(10):1263–1264.

15. Mokdad AH, Stroup DF, Giles WH. Public health surveillance for behavioral risk factors in a changing environment: recommendations from the Behavioral Risk Factor Surveillance Team. *MMWR* 2003;52:RR–9.

16. Centers for Disease Control and Prevention, Behavioral Risk Factors Surveillance System. www.cdc.gov/brfss. Accessed March 8, 2010.

17. Link M, Mokdad A. Use of alternative modes for health surveillance surveys: Results from a web/mail/telephone experiment. *Epidemiology* 2005;16:701–704.

18. Link M, Mokdad A. Can web and mail survey modes improve participation in an RDD-based national health surveillance? *J Official Statist* 2006;22:293–312.

19. Link M, Battaglia M, Giambo P, Frankel M, Mokdad A, Rao S. 2005. Assessment of address frame replacements for RDD sampling frames. *Proceedings Am Statist Assoc Survey Methodol Section.* (CD-ROM), Alexandria, VA, 2005.

20. Link M, Battaglia M, Frankel M, Osborn L, Mokdad A. Comparison of address-based sampling (ABS) versus random-digit dialing (RDD) for general population surveys. *Public Opin Q* 2008;72:6–27.

21. Link M, Battaglia M, Frankel M, Osborn L, Mokdad A. 2005. Effectiveness of address-based sampling frame alternative to RDD: BRFSS mail survey experiment results. *Proceedings Federal Committee Statist Methodol Research Conference.* (CD-ROM), 2005, Arlington, VA.

22. Link M, Battaglia M, Frankel M, Osborn L, Mokdad A. Address-based versus random-digit dialed surveys: comparison of key health and risk indicators. *Am J Epidemiol* 2006;164:1019–1025.

23. Battaglia M, Link M, Frankel M, Osborne L, Mokdad A. 2007. Incorporating a multi-modality design into a random-digit-dialing survey. *Proceedings Am Statist Assoc, Survey Methodol Section* (CD-ROM), Alexandria, VA, 2007.

24. Link M, Battaglia M, Frankel M, Osborne L, Mokdad A. 2007. Comparing mixed-mode address-based surveys with random digit dialing for general population surveys. *Proceedings Am Statist Assoc, Survey Methodol Section* (CD-ROM), Alexandria, VA, 2007.

25. Link MW, Town M, Mokdad AH. 2007. Telephone number portability and the prevalence of cell phone numbers in random digit-dialed telephone survey samples. *Internat J Public Opin Res* 19:504–511.

26. Boyd R, Stevens J. Falls and fear of falling: burden, beliefs, and behaviours. *Age Ageing* 2009;38(4):423–428.

27. Dellinger A, Chen J, Vance A, Breiding M, Simon T, Ballesteros M. Injury prevention counseling for adults: have we made progress? *J Fam Community Health* 2009;32(2):115–122.

28. Shults M, Kresnow M, Lee K. Driver- and passenger-based estimates of alcohol-impaired driving, 2001–2003. *Am J Prev Med* 2009;356(6):515–522.

29. Boyd R, Dellinger A, Kresnow M. Alcohol-impaired driving and children in the household. *J Fam Community Health* 2009;32(2):167–174.

30. Simon T, Kresnow M, Bossarte R. Self-reports of Violent Victimization among U.S. Adults. *Violence Vict* 2008;23(6):711–726.

31. Boyd R, Kresnow M, Dellinger A. Adult seat belt use: does the presence of children in the household make a difference? *Traffic Inj Prev* 2008;9(5):414–420.

32. Gilchrist J, Sacks J, White D, Kresnow M. Dog Bite: Still a Problem? *Inj Prev* 2008;14;296–301.

33. Jieru Chen J, Kresnow M, Simon T, Dellinger A. Injury prevention counseling and behavior among U.S. children: results from the second injury control and risk survey. *Pediatrics* 2007;e958–e965.

34. Basile K, Chen J, Lynberg M, Saltzman L. Prevalence and characteristics of sexual violence victimization among US adults, 2001–2003. *Violence Vict* 2007;22(4);437–438.

35. Ballesteros MF, Kresnow M. Prevalence of residential smoke alarms and fire escape plans in the U.S.: results from the second injury control and risk survey (ICARIS-2). *Public Health Rep* 2007:122(2):224–231.

36. Basile K, Swahn M, Jieru Chen J, Saltzman L. Stalking in the United States: recent national prevalence estimates. *Am J Prev Med* 2006;31(2):172–175.

37. Lynberg M, Kresnow M, Simon T, Arias I, Shelley G. Telephone survey respondent's reactions to questions regarding interpersonal violence. *Violence Vict* 2006;21(4):445–459.

38. Chen J, Kresnow M, Simon TR, Dellinger A. Injury-prevention counseling and behavior among U.S. children: results from the second injury control and risk survey. *Pediatrics* 2007;119:e958–e965.

39. The American Association for Public Opinion Research. 2008. *Standard Definitions: Finals Dispositions of Case Codes and outcome Rates for Surveys. 5th edition.* Lenexa, Kansas: AAPOR.

40. Link MW, Kresnow M. The future of random-didit-dial surveys for injury prevention and violence research. *Am J Prev Med* 2006;31(5):444–450.

41. US Consumer Product Safety Commission. NEISS All Injury Program: sample design and implementation. Schroeder T, Ault K, preparers. Washington, DC: US Consumer Product Safety Commission, 2001.

42. Centers for Disease Control and Prevention. Clinical Modification, (ICD-9-CM). In: *International Classification of Diseases*, 6th ed. 9th rev. Hyattsville, MD: US Department of Health and Human Services, CDC; 2008. http://www.cdc.gov/nchs/datawh/ftpserv/ftpicd9/ftpicd9.htm.

43. Centers for Disease Control and Prevention. National Electronic Injury Surveillance System—All Injury Program (NEISS-AIP) data. Atlanta, GA: US Department of Health and Human Services, CDC; 2008. http://www.icpsr.umich.edu/NACJD and key word "NEISS". Accessed March 8, 2010.

44. Centers for Disease Control and Prevention. Improved National Prevalence Estimates for 18 Selected Major Birth Defects—United States, 1999–2001. *MMWR* 2006; 54(51&52):1301–1305.

45. National Birth Defects Prevention Network (NBDPN). In: Sever LE, ed. *Guidelines for Conducting Birth Defects Surveillance*. Atlanta, GA: National Birth Defects Prevention Network, Inc.; June 2004.

46. Centers for Disease Control and Prevention. National Program of Cancer Registries. Link Plus. http://www.cdc.gov/cancer/npcr/tools/registryplus/lp.htm.

47. World Health Organization. *International Statistical Classification of Disease and Related Health Problems, Vol. 1.* 10th Rev. Geneva, Switzerland: World Health Organizations; 1992.

48. Centers for Disease Control and Prevention. Injury data and resources. Hyattsville, MD: US Department of Health and Human Services, CDC; 2008. http://www.cdc.gov/nchs/injury.htm. Accessed March 8, 2010.

49. Paulozzi LJ, Mercy J, Frazier L, Annest JL. CDC's National Violent Death Reporting System: background and methodology. *Inj Prev* 2004;10:47–52.

50. Jurczyk P, Lu JJ, Xiong L, Cragan JD, Correa A. Fine-grained record integration and linkage tool. *Birth Defects Res A Clin Mol Teratol* 2008;82(11):822–829.

51. Moller B, Fekjaer H, Hakulinen T, *et al*. Prediction of cancer incidence in the Nordic countries up to the year 2020. *Eur J Cancer Prev* 2002;11(Suppl 1):S1–S96.

52. Centers for Disease Control and Prevention. Discussion document on injury severity measurements in administrative datasets. Hyattsville, MD: US Department of Health and Human Services, CDC; 2004. http://www.cdc.gov/nchs/data/injury/DicussionDocu.pdf. Accessed March 8, 2010.

53. Davie G, Cryer C, Langley J. Improving the predictive ability of the ICD-based Injury Severity Score. *Inj Prev* 2008;14:250–255.

54. Mokdad AH, Serdula MK, Dietz WH, Bowman BA, Marks JS, Koplan JP. The spread of the obesity epidemic in the US. *JAMA* 1999;282:1519–1522.

55. State and Territorial Injury Prevention Directors' Association. Consensus recommendations for injury surveillance in state health departments. Marietta, GA: State and Territorial Injury Prevention Directors' Association; 2007. http://www.stipda.org/displaycommon.cfm?an=8. Accessed March 8, 2010.

56. Kung HC, Hoyert DL, Xu JQ, Murphy SL. Deaths: Final Data for 2005. *National Vital Statistics Reports*; vol 56 no 10. Hyattsville, MD: National Center for Health Statistics. 2008.

57. Williams LJ, Mai CT, Edmonds LD, *et al*. Prevalence of spina bifida and anencephaly during the transition to mandatory folic acid fortification in the United States. *Teratology* 2002;66:33–39.

58. Centers for Disease Control and Prevention. Spina bifida and anencephaly before and after folic acid mandate—United States, 1995–1996 and 1999–2000. *MMWR* 2004;53(7):362–365.

59. Farel AM, Meyer RE, Hicken M, Edmonds LD. registry to referral: using birth defects registries to refer infants and toddlers for early intervention services. *Birth Defects Res A Clin Mol Teratol* 2003;67(9):647–650.

60. Coben, JH, Steiner, CA, Barrett, M, Merrill, CT, Adamson, D. Completeness of cause of injury coding in healthcare administrative databases in the United States, 2001. *J Internat Society Child Adolesc Inj Prev* 2006;12(3):199–201.

61. Barrett M, Steiner C, Coben J. Healthcare Cost and Utilization Project (HCUP) E Code Evaluation Report. 2004. HCUP Methods Series Report # 2004-06 ONLINE. April 14, 2005. U.S. Agency for Healthcare Research and Quality. http://www.hcup-us.ahrq.gov/reports/methods.jsp. Accessed March 8, 2010.

62. Johnson RL, Thomas RG, Thomas KE, Sarmiento K. State Injury Indicators Report: Fourth Edition— 2005 Data. Atlanta, GA: Centers for Disease Control and Prevention, National Center for Injury Prevention and Control; 2009. http://www.cdc.gov/injury/indicators2005.html.

63. Mokdad AH. The behavioral risk factor surveillance system: Past, present and future. *Ann Rev Public Health* 2009;30:43–54.

13

Surveillance for Determinants of Population Health

ROY GIBSON PARRISH II, SHARON M. McDONNELL,
AND PATRICK L. REMINGTON

INTRODUCTION AND PURPOSE

Health-related surveillance was initially applied to diseases and specifically to acute communicable diseases. In his 1963 article on surveillance, Langmuir described a system for the surveillance of malaria, poliomyelitis, influenza, and hepatitis (*1*). His approach remains the basis for communicable disease surveillance conducted in the United States and other countries. As the major causes of morbidity and mortality shifted from acute communicable diseases to injuries and chronic conditions,[1] the need for information about these conditions, their causes, and strategies to prevent them increased, and surveillance systems for them were developed. In 1993 McGinnis and Foege emphasized the importance of behaviors and risk factors by directing attention away from diseases as the "causes" of death to a set of risk factors for disease and injury that were considered to be more basic causes of death[2] (*3*). In addition to monitoring acute and chronic diseases and injuries, surveillance systems now monitor health behaviors and other risk factors associated with these diseases.[3]

---

[1] In 1900 the five leading causes of death in the United States were (*1*) pneumonia (all forms) and influenza; (*2*) tuberculosis (all forms); (*3*) diarrhea, enteritis, and ulceration of the intestines; (*4*) diseases of the heart; and (*5*) intracranial lesions of vascular origin. In 1998 they were (*1*) diseases of the heart; (*2*) malignant neoplasms; (*3*) cerebrovascular diseases; (*4*) chronic obstructive pulmonary disease and allied conditions; and (*5*) accidents and adverse effects (*2*).

[2] McGinnis and Foege, and more recently Mokdad et al., presented evidence that five behavioral factors and four environmental "agents" caused half of the mortality in the United States (*3,4*). The five factors and the percentage of all deaths caused by them in 2000 (in parentheses) are tobacco (18%), poor diet and physical inactivity (17%), alcohol consumption (4%), sexual behavior (1%), and illicit drug use (1%). The four agents and the percentage of all deaths in 2000 caused by them are microbial agents (3%), toxic agents (2%), motor vehicles (2%), and firearms (1%) (*4*). Reducing the prevalence of these factors forms the basis for many of the preventive actions recommended by Healthy People 2010 for improving health in the United States, and current public health surveillance for determinants focuses on these factors (*5*).

[3] In this chapter we use "diseases" to refer to both diseases and injuries.

Work over the past 35 years has also established the potency of cultural,[4] social, and economic forces on morbidity and mortality at both individual and community levels[5] (7–17). These forces, which include social isolation, cohesion,[6] hierarchy, education, community efficacy, income, and wealth, work beyond the level of the individual and emerge at the societal level as the cultural, social, economic, and political environment in which individuals live. Addressing these societal forces with political, legal, and environmental strategies can shape behavior and health outcomes in a positive way, as exemplified by marked reductions in tobacco use, lead poisoning, and motor vehicle fatalities, following the implementation of public health policies and laws.

Positive social forces lead to the production of health in at least two ways. First, social connections and community cohesion and efficacy enhance individual adaptability, resilience, and well-being by buffering the harmful effects of chronic stress and counterbalancing better-known behavioral and biomedical risk factors (e.g., poor diet, smoking, lack of exercise, and hypertension). They decrease the risk of illness and mortality and increase the likelihood of recovery from illness for both individuals and populations (7,19,20). Second, because real and perceived inequalities and inequities[7] in the societal distribution of education, wealth, and power create chronic stress and erode immunologic function, personal or community measures that increase social equality and equity are linked to better population health outcomes (21–24).

The purpose of this chapter is to describe an ecological or determinants approach to health production, identify important health determinants, enumerate guiding principles and basic approaches for monitoring these determinants, and describe practical applications of these principles to their surveillance. We end the chapter with recommendations for improving surveillance for health determinants.

---

[4] "... culture should be regarded as the set of distinctive spiritual, material, intellectual and emotional features of society or a social group, and that it encompasses, in addition to art and literature, lifestyles, ways of living together, value systems, traditions and beliefs" (6).

[5] For example, prospective studies have shown increases in age-adjusted mortality in males and females (RR: 2.6–4.0) related to the level of social integrations after controlling for other risk factors and baseline health status (7).

[6] "Social cohesion refers to the extent of connectedness and solidarity among groups in society. ... A cohesive society is also one that is richly endowed with stocks of social capital. Social capital is defined as those features of social structures—such as levels of interpersonal trust and norms of reciprocity and mutual aid—that act as resources for individuals and facilitate collective action. ... Social cohesion and social capital are both collective, or ecological, dimensions of society, to be distinguished from the concepts of social networks and social support, which are characteristically measured at the level of the individual" (18).

[7] "Inequality and equality are dimensional concepts, simply referring to measurable quantities. Inequity and equity, on the other hand, are political concepts, expressing a moral commitment to social justice. Health inequality is the generic term used to designate differences, variations, and disparities in the health achievements of individuals and groups. A straightforward example of health inequality is higher incidence of disease X in group A as compared with group B of population P. ...Health inequity refers to those inequalities in health that are deemed to be unfair or stemming from some form of injustice. ...The crux of the distinction between equality and equity is that the identification of health inequities entails normative judgment premised upon (a) one's theories of justice; (b) one's theories of society; and (c) one's reasoning underlying the genesis of health inequalities" (ref. 21; pp. 647–648).

FACTORS INFLUENCING HEALTH: DEFINITIONS AND MODELS

Health[8] and disease are not randomly distributed in populations: at the population level the people most likely to be sick and die of cardiovascular diseases in 2009 (the poor and the socially isolated or disadvantaged) are essentially the same as those that died of tuberculosis or cholera in 1809 (27). To maximize health, epidemiologists and social scientists must look for the root causes, or "cause of causes"—the factors that lead populations and individuals toward or away from health and well-being—rather than focusing only on specific diseases and behaviors. In this chapter, we will use "health determinant" to refer to "the range of personal, social, economic, and environmental factors which determine the health status of individuals or populations" (28). This definition is strikingly broad, encompassing societal level inequalities, such as income and poverty, as well as individual behaviors, such as the use of seat belts and tobacco. This term encompasses other similar terms, such as risk factors, influencing factors, direct and indirect contributing factors, and causal factors.[9] It challenges us to create systems to monitor and better understand the complex multidimensional relationships of the determinants of health and disease.

Most diseases and injuries result from the convergence and interplay of many determinants. For example, even an infectious disease such as salmonellosis, which appears to result from a single cause, *Salmonella typhimurium,* results from many determinants, including inadequate oversight of chicken farms because of lax policies or enforcement, environmental conditions favoring the growth of salmonella, infection of chickens with salmonella, contamination of eggs with salmonella, the education level of those cooking eggs, inadequate cooking of eggs to kill bacteria, quantity of contaminated eggs ingested, and host susceptibility.

Figure 13–1 depicts a simplified causal pathway involving three determinants (causes) and one outcome to illustrate potential relationships and interactions of determinants. The outcome might be positive (improved health) or negative (disease, injury, or increased susceptibility to disease or injury). Figure 13–2 (a causal web) elaborates on Figure 13–1 by showing a causal pathway with *multiple* levels of determinants and their complex interactions (29,30). The dynamic interaction of "distal determinants" (such as poverty and social isolation) with physiological responses (such as hypertension) by way of intermediate or more "proximal determinants" (such as diet and chronic stress) creates an increasingly complex system. Ultimately, these myriad determinants and their interactions result in health outcomes, such as hypertensive heart disease and stroke.

Numerous authors have developed graphical models to depict the interactions of health determinants (31–35). The value of these models is not simply academic, as they demonstrate different conceptualizations and, therefore, understandings of the pathways to health and disease. The structure and comprehensiveness of the model

---

[8] The WHO definition of health is "a state of complete physical, mental and social well-being and not merely the absence of disease or infirmity" (25). The WHO goal of *health for* all is described in the Ottawa Charter for Health Promotion (26).

[9] Note that a determinant may be both the effect of a cause and the cause of another effect.

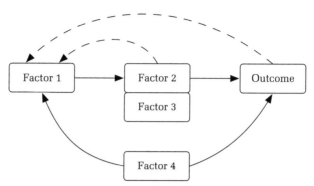

Figure 13–1 Simple causal diagram showing the relationship of several factors to an outcome.

Note: Factor 1 is more *distal* (i.e., occurs earlier, is more "upstream") in the causal pathway than factor 2, which is more *proximal* (i.e., occurs later, is more "downstream"). The dashed arrows represent feedback, which could be either positive or negative, between factors or between the outcome and causal factors. Factor 3 interacts with factor 2, and factor 4 is a potential confounder of the relationship between factor 1 and the outcome. For additional information on causal diagrams, see (*36*) and (*37*).

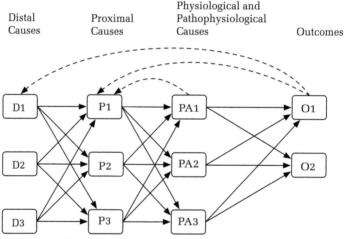

Figure 13–2 A causal web showing various levels of causality. Feedbacks from outcomes to preceding causes might also exist. For example, individuals or societies might modify their behaviors or policies based on health outcomes. (Dashed lines illustrate examples of feedback.) Adapted from (*30*).

that is selected and used—explicitly or implicitly—by researchers, public health practitioners, and policymakers and the relationships and interactions of its elements will influence decisions about the focus of surveillance, data needed for surveillance, analyses of these data, and actions taken based on surveillance findings.

Figure 13–3 applies this causal framework to determinants of lung cancer. It illustrates how seemingly distant determinants, such as culture, impact the occurrence

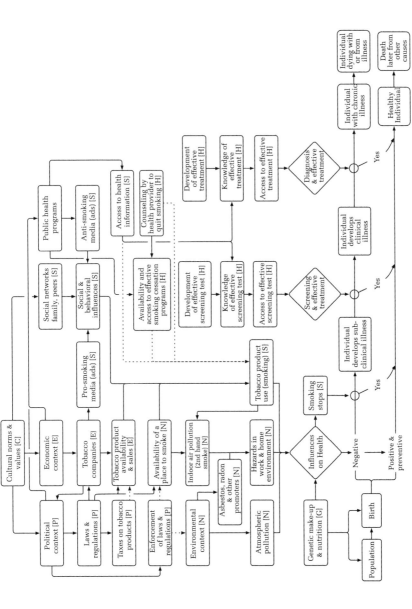

Figure 13-3 C = Cultural influences, E = Economic influences, G = Genetic & nutritional influences, H = Health care influences, N = Environmental influences, P = Political & governmental influences, S = Social & behavioral influences

of a specific disease within members of a population; at any given point in time, the production of health—or disease—in individuals occurs within an environment and a context that either fosters it or impedes it. Figure 13–3 also highlights the complexity, multiple levels, and interactions of determinants. The prevalence of smoking in a population—the most important behavioral determinant of lung cancer—is the coalescence of influences from many sectors, including the agricultural, advertising, public policy, economic, and health sectors. Because smoking causes a host of diseases, this example is also relevant to other smoking-related cancers, emphysema, chronic bronchitis, and cardiovascular and cerebrovascular disease.

To be most effective, health promotion actions must "address the full range of potentially modifiable determinants of health—not only those which are related to the actions of individuals, such as health behaviours and lifestyles, but also factors such as income and social status, education, employment and working conditions, access to appropriate health services, and the physical environment"[10] (*28*). These societal factors create the living conditions that impact health.

SURVEILLANCE FOR DETERMINANTS OF HEALTH: PRINCIPLES

Like disease surveillance, surveillance of determinants involves continued watchfulness over their "distribution and trends."[11] The temporal and geographic *scales* for monitoring different determinants vary, as they do with different diseases. Unlike disease surveillance and its reliance on outcome data, surveillance for determinants requires data on factors that *cause* those outcomes. Many determinants have their origin and influence at the level of populations or societies rather than individuals, and the most effective strategies for addressing them are at the population level. These characteristics of determinants require the use of different, and occasionally additional, *sources* and *methods* for obtaining data than those typically used for disease surveillance, as well as different methods of analysis and interpretation.

Determinants As "States" and Measuring Their Prevalence

Many health determinants represent *states* or *conditions* rather than events, and surveillance for such determinants focuses on *prevalence* rather than incidence.[12] Surveillance for these determinants uses estimates of their prevalence at different points, typically from repeated surveys. Depending on the determinant, its ease of measurement, and its likely time-scale for change in response to interventions

---

[10] The decline in cigarette smoking in the United States is associated with increases in high school and college graduation rates, restrictions on marketing and sales of cigarettes, increases in taxation of cigarettes, and decreased agricultural subsidies for growing tobacco. These strategies aimed at the larger population are as important as programs targeting individuals' health behaviors and lifestyles.

[11] In 1963, Langmuir defined disease surveillance as "the continued watchfulness over the distribution and trends of incidence (of a disease) through the systematic collection, consolidation, and evaluation of morbidity and mortality reports and other relevant data" (*1*).

[12] Surveillance for *chronic* diseases often uses data on disease prevalence as well as disease incidence.

or other factors,[13] its prevalence should be measured periodically at appropriate intervals—usually not exceeding 2 to 3 years. Recently, methods to "continuously" measure the prevalence of certain determinants in a defined population have been developed to provide information about changes in prevalence on a more frequent basis (*5,38,39*).

Distribution of Determinants and the Role of Inequity in Health Production

How a health determinant is distributed within a population and its subpopulations is a measure of population health equity (or fairness) and is as important as its overall level within the population. From an epidemiologic perspective, an association between an unequally distributed determinant and a similarly distributed health outcome suggests a role for the determinant in causing the health outcome. From a health perspective, greater inequalities in the distribution of social determinants of health, such as education, occupation, and income—particularly when their distribution is perceived as inequitable—are associated with greater health inequalities even after controlling for health-related behaviors (*12,17,24,40*). The relationship of a measure of income inequality in a population—for example, the Gini coefficient—to the population's mortality rate and self-rated health exemplifies this relationship (*12*). From a policy perspective, public health programs that address only the levels of health determinants in a population might not alter their distribution and fall short of their goal. Finally, having long-term trend data on the distribution of health determinants and the extent of inequalities is critical to monitoring the impact of policies and other interventions designed to address these inequalities.

Three Approaches to Health Determinant Surveillance

Surveillance for health determinants within a population or geographic area can be approached in at least three ways: *(1)* surveillance for an individual determinant, such as seat belt use or prevalence of smoking; *(2)* surveillance for a group of conceptually similar determinants, such as behavioral risk factors, environmental pollutants, or economic measures; and *(3)* surveillance for a set of determinants chosen to represent the major categories of health determinants for a given population.[14] The first approach is useful for tracking the effect of targeted interventions, usually those directed at individual behaviors or specific environmental agents. The second approach is useful for efficiently characterizing a category of

---

[13] The prevalence of a health determinant may change over short time scales (e.g., unemployment rate, air quality, diet, and blood pressure), long time-scales (e.g., social networks, housing availability, and BMI), or very long time-scales (e.g., topography, political system, and discrimination). Collecting data for a specific determinant should be done with a clear understanding of the time-scale over which it is likely to change. Too short an interval between data collections wastes resources and may result in frustration with the lack of success of interventions; too long an interval may miss significant change—or lack of change—that could have implications for whether to institute or continue a particular intervention strategy.

[14] The categories of determinants include the cultural, social, economic, political, natural, and built environments; individual and group behaviors (lifestyles), biological characteristics, and the availability of health and social services.

determinants for which similar prevention and control measures might be applied. The Behavioral Risk Factor Surveillance System (BRFSS), described below, is an example of this approach. The third approach measures determinants at multiple levels and is used to gain a comprehensive view of the health of a population, to predict future burden of disease, and to monitor the impact of multifaceted strategies to produce health. The Health Poverty Index in the United Kingdom exemplifies a comprehensive approach.

SURVEILLANCE FOR HEALTH DETERMINANTS: CURRENT PRACTICE

To provide a broad perspective from which to make policy decisions, implement interventions, and evaluate the effectiveness of interventions, surveillance should target important health determinants at all levels in the causal web. It should also address national, regional, and local needs and the needs of those population subgroups most likely to experience health disparities. Currently, however, surveillance of health determinants in the United States and many other countries is uncoordinated and uneven, scattered over different sectors and disciplines, and reliant on a patchwork of different data sources. Developing a comprehensive, coherent, cohesive, and useful system of surveillance for health determinants would yield significant benefits for population health—and individual health care—but will require an enduring commitment of resources and effort that should not be underestimated. Nevertheless, examples exist to guide governments and the public health community as they move forward with the development and implementation of such surveillance systems: the WHO framework for health equity surveillance, the United Kingdom's health poverty index, the United States' BRFSS, state and county health rankings in the United States, and King County's Communities Count.

WHO Framework for Health Equity Surveillance

In 2008, the WHO's Commission on Social Determinants of Health (CSDH) issued *Closing the Gap in a Generation: Health Equity through Action on the Social Determinants of Health*. This landmark report recommended that "National governments establish a national health equity surveillance system, with routine collection of data on social determinants of health and health inequity" (ref. *23*; p. 180). The report also provided an example of "a framework for health equity surveillance," which includes social, political, environmental, and economic determinants of health (Table 13–1). The CSDH recognized that current data on social determinants in many countries are scattered over a "multitude" of data systems and hoped that a health equity surveillance system would "bring together in one place data on a broad range of social determinants of health." In building such a system, the Commission recommended that countries take a series of actions: *(1)* establish routine health statistics systems where

Table 13–1 Items for Possible Inclusion in a Comprehensive National Health Equity Surveillance Framework, World Health Organization, 2008

HEALTH INEQUITIES

Include information on:

Health outcomes stratified by:

  –Sex

  –At least two socio-economic stratifiers (education, income/wealth, occupational class)

  –Ethnic group/race/indigeneity

  –Other contextually relevant social stratifiers

  –Place of residence (rural/urban and province or other relevant geographical unit)

Distribution of the population across subgroup

  –Summary measure of relative health inequity: measures include the rate ratio, the relative index of inequality, the relative version of the population attributable risk, and the concentration index

  –Summary measure of absolute health inequity: measures include the rate difference, the slope index of inequality, and the population attributable risk

HEALTH OUTCOMES

Mortality (all cause, cause specific, age specific)

Early childhood development

Mental health

Morbidity and disability

Self-assessed physical and mental health

Cause-specific outcomes

DETERMINANTS, WHERE APPLICABLE, INCLUDING STRATIFIED DATA

Daily living conditions

Health behaviors

  –Smoking

  –Alcohol

  –Physical activity

  –Diet and nutrition

Physical and social environment

  –Water and sanitation

  –Housing conditions

  –Infrastructure, transport, and urban design

  –Air quality

  –Social capital

Working conditions

  –Material working hazards

  –Stress

Health care

  –Coverage

  –Health-care system infrastructure

Social protection

  –Coverage

  –Generosity

(*continued*)

Table 13–1 (*continued*)

Structural drivers of health inequity
    Gender
        –Norms and values
        –Economic participation
        –Sexual and reproductive health
Social inequities
    –Social exclusion
    –Income and wealth distribution
    –Education
Sociopolitical context
    –Civil rights
    –Employment conditions
    –Governance and public spending priorities
    –Macroeconomic conditions

CONSEQUENCES OF ILL-HEALTH
Economic consequences
Social consequences

Source: Reference *23*, p. 182.

they do not currently exist; *(2)* improve routine health statistics so that health and mortality trends are available for men and women and for different age and social groups; *(3)* increase the quality, frequency, comparability, and completeness of surveys used as the source of routine health statistics; and *(4)* provide "sufficient long-term core funding" to a central agency to coordinate the surveillance system.

Health Poverty Index

In response to the United Kingdom's National Health Service Plan, the Department of Health funded the development of the *Health Poverty Index* to assess the degree of health inequality by geography and cultural identity. The resulting index is composed of 8 indicators of *root causes* of health, 7 indicators of *intervening factors*, and 10 indicators of an area's *situation of health* (Table 13–2). A majority of the indicators represent determinants of health and include measures of regional and household wealth; work, recreational, and home environments; available resources for education, health care, and social care; and access to health and social care services. There are also 4 indicators of health status. Regional and local data are used to construct these indicators and a health poverty index for each ethnic minority group in each of the Local Authority Districts in England (*41*). A Web-based tool produces both graphs and tables that allow the comparison of the Health Poverty Index for a geographic area at different time-points, for two areas at the same time-point, for two ethnic groups in the same area, and for the same ethnic group in two different areas (Fig. 13–4).

Table 13–2 Indicators and Sub-indicators Used in the Health Poverty Index, Department of Health, United Kingdom, 2008

Root causes	Regional prospects	Gross value added per capita
		Change in job supply
		Educational resources
	Local conditions	Social capital
		Education quality
	Household conditions	Income
		Wealth
		Human capital
Intervening factors	Resources to support health	Local government resources
		Preventive care resources
	Healthy areas	Recreation facilities
		Effective preventive health care
	Behaviors and environments	Lifestyle
		Home environments
		Work and local environments
Situation of health	Resources for health and social care	Health-care resources
		Social care resources
	Appropriate Care	Effective primary care
		Access to secondary care
		Access to social care
		Quality of social care
	Health status	Psychological morbidity
		Health capital
		Physical morbidity
		Premature mortality

Source: Reference *41.*

Behavioral Risk Factor Surveillance System

In 1984, the U.S. Centers for Disease Control and Prevention (CDC) established the BRFSS to monitor health risk behaviors, preventive health practices, and access to health care for a representative sample of households in each participating state. In 2008, all states, the District of Columbia, and three U.S. territories had their own BRFSS. In addition to state-level data, the BRFSS can provide data for selected metropolitan statistical areas, and several states conduct their own county-level BRFSS to produce estimates for at least some of their counties. The BRFSS uses telephone interviews, with a core set of standard questions administered by all states and optional modules and state-added questions on various topics to meet local needs. Optional modules include intimate partner violence, hypertension awareness, and indoor air quality. In 2009, the BRFSS introduced a "social context" module, which is being used by 12 states, the District of Columbia, and 20 communities. The module consists of eight questions intended to assess civic engagement and food, housing, and job security. The BRFSS is the only available source of state-level data on health-related behaviors for many states and has proven useful for identifying emerging health problems, establishing and tracking health objectives, developing and evaluating public health policies and programs, and supporting health-related legislative efforts (5).

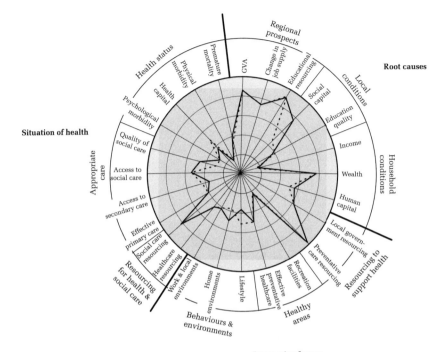

Figure 13–4 The solid line represents data for the Indian ethnic group; the dashed line represents data for the white ethnic group. For each indicator, a score of zero (the center of the diagram) indicates the best situation in terms of health poverty, and a score of one (the outermost circle) the worst situation. In other words, an area, time period, or ethnic group with a score nearer zero for a particular indicator has lower levels of health poverty in that domain than another area, time period, or ethnic group with a score nearer one. *Source:* Adapted and redrawn from (*41,42*).

State and County Health Rankings

Ranking[15] the health of nations, states, and counties is intended to compel action. The United Health Foundation's annual *America's Health Rankings* monitors and ranks health at the state level using 22 measures of health determinants and outcomes: 3 measures of health policies, 6 of community environment, 3 of personal behavior, 3 of clinical care, and 7 of health outcomes.[16] Since its inception in 1990, the rankings have evolved as new research findings and data have become available. For example, in 2007 a calculation of "preventable hospitalizations" was incorporated using data from the Dartmouth Atlas of Health Care. In 2008, the rankings added a measure of health inequality, based on the variation in mortality

---

[15] Rankings are usually based on a composite, standardized measure derived from valued health indicators.

[16] Although categorized by the United Health Foundation as measures of health determinants, three, and possibly four, of these measures are outcome measures that serve as proxies for health determinants: violent crime rate, occupational fatality rate, infectious disease (AIDS, TB, hepatitis) incidence rate, and rate of preventable hospitalizations.

rates among counties within each state. The annual report provides a profile of each state with its ranking by year since 1990 and estimates the influence that each state's current health determinants are expected to have on that state's future overall rank (43).

The Population Health Institute at the University of Wisconsin has developed and published annual rankings for all Wisconsin counties since 2003. The *Wisconsin County Health Rankings* rank each county using four categories of health determinants: health care, health behaviors, socioeconomic factors, and physical environment. Health determinants and health outcomes are measured and ranked separately for each county (44). The rankings have been favorably received by local health officials, generated considerable media attention, engaged a broad array of partners, and provoked action by some counties to improve their rankings (45,46).

King County's Communities Count

In the early 1990s, citizens and health officials in King County, Washington, created a commission to engage members of the public, elected officials, and county employees to develop a vision of a healthy community and a method for assessing progress toward the vision. Communities Count, the program that emerged from this collaboration, developed a set of social and health indicators (Table 13–3), which have been tracked over the past 10 years and used to inform the design and evaluation of programs to improve community health in King County. Communities Count uses existing data from various sources[17] and enriches these data with qualitative data from community telephone surveys and from focus groups composed of population subgroups under-represented in the telephone surveys. Two central features of Communities Count are its sustained effort to engage the community in all aspects of the project and its decision to allow indicators to evolve over time to reflect changes in the environment and community priorities (47–49). Engaging its constituents to ensure that Communities Count meets their needs has created and maintained interest in and support of the system.

SURVEILLANCE FOR HEALTH DETERMINANTS: MOVING FORWARD

Any agency or organization implementing surveillance for health determinants at the national or local level should proceed in a thoughtful, orderly fashion. Table 13–4 provides steps for creating or updating a surveillance system (*see* Chapter 3; ref. 50). What follows is an explanation—based on lessons learned in many countries and localities—of selected steps in this sequence that are particularly relevant to establishing and conducting surveillance for health determinants. These steps can

---

[17] Sources of data include the U.S. Census Bureau, Seattle-King County Department of Public Health, other King County agencies, the Washington Assessment of Student Learning, Child Protective Services, the Washington Association of Sheriffs and Police Chiefs, and local jurisdictions within King County.

Table 13–3 Social and Health Indicators Included in Community Counts, King County, Washington, United States, 2008

Basic Needs and Social Well-Being
– Adequate food
– Affordable housing
– Living wage income and poverty
– Income distribution
– Social support
– Freedom from discrimination

Positive Development through Life Stages
– Family-friendly employment benefits
– Parent/guardian involvement in child's learning
– Quality, affordable child care
– School readiness
– Academic achievement
– Risk and protective factors in youth
– Participation in life-enriching activities

Safety and Health
– Perceived neighborhood safety
– Crime
– Violence in the home
– Motor vehicle injuries and deaths
– Infant mortality
– Teen births
– Stress
– Tobacco and alcohol use
– Physical activity and weight
– Limitation in daily activities
– Health insurance and access

Community Strength
– Neighborhood social cohesion
– Involvement in community organizations
– Community service

Natural and Built Environment
– Ease of access to shops and services
– Transportation choices
– Pollution in neighborhoods
– Air quality
– Water quantity and quality
– Land cover
– Farmland

Arts and Culture
– Participation in arts and culture
– Presence of arts organizations
– Employment in arts and culture
– Funding for arts and culture

Source: Reference *48.*

Table 13–4 Recommended Steps for Establishing Surveillance for Health Determinants

1. State the problem to be addressed by the surveillance system.
2. Understand the setting in which surveillance will occur.
3. Clarify the purpose of the surveillance system and the use of its findings.
4. Formulate the topic and content of the surveillance.
5. Define the scope of surveillance (geographic area, population, and time period)
6. Determine what specific information is needed about each health determinant.
7. Determine how quickly information is needed.
8. Identify the resources that are available for conducting surveillance, including compiling any data that will be needed.
9. Select the sources and the method of collecting data for surveillance based on the purpose, content, scope, and setting of surveillance.
10. Conduct a pilot test to determine whether source and method can provide the data needed for surveillance.
11. Collect the data.
12. Compile, process, and analyze the data.
13. Interpret the data.
14. Communicate the findings of surveillance.
15. Ensure that those who want to use the findings receive them.
16. Evaluate usefulness of data that are collected and the findings that are produced to those who use them.

Source: Adapted from references *50,51.*

be adapted and phased to accommodate local interest, data sources, and resources. Several steps not discussed below are addressed in other chapters of this book.

State the problem to be addressed and the goals to be met with the information gained from the surveillance system (step 1). Typically, the problem to be addressed by surveillance for health determinants is the suboptimal level and unequal and unfair distribution of health within a population. The goal is forward-looking: to create conditions that will improve health and well-being in the population. Articulating the expected contribution of surveillance to meet this goal can build enthusiasm and serve as a call to generate resources for surveillance. Typically, the goal of surveillance is the production of information for understanding the problem, guiding policy and interventions intended to address the problem, and tracking progress toward resolution of the problem. Periodically evaluating the surveillance system's contribution to meeting overall health-related goals will increase the likelihood that the surveillance system will be useful and sustained.

Understand the setting (step 2). The setting is the overall physical, socio-cultural, economic, and political environment in which information will be gathered and used. The elements of the setting most important to conducting surveillance will depend on the particular problem, place, time, and population under surveillance. For example, whether the setting is low-resource, post-disaster, secure, urban, partisan, rural, or technologically advanced will affect the methods chosen for surveillance. The presence of basic infrastructure, such as electricity, transportation, and human resources, and their reliability and organization will also impact the nature and success of surveillance efforts. These and other factors affect the capacity to collect and interpret information and can cause surveillance methods to vary considerably among and within countries. An indication that surveillance for health determinants can be established and maintained in a given setting is the presence of an infrastructure that regularly collects routine population and health statistics (e.g., data on population size, births, and deaths). Another positive sign is the extent to which a society views *health* as the product of numerous societal forces rather than as solely the product of its health-care system; such a society is more likely to have the political will and leadership and the technical means to implement surveillance for health determinants.

Formulate the topic and content of surveillance (step 4). Using knowledge of the setting, the population under surveillance, and the social, economic, and environmental determinants most likely to impact the targeted population's health, one next selects the key health determinants to be monitored. It is important to select or adapt a model of health that depicts the current understanding of important health determinants and their relationships to each other and to the goal of improved population health. Such a model can assist in identifying and organizing potential measures of health and disease and in choosing a final set of indicators from these measures (*see* step 6 below), while maintaining a focus on the overall health situation and its root causes. Adapting a model involves negotiation among those who are affected by the problem, those who will be conducting surveillance, and those who will be responsible for addressing the problem. The results of the process should be clearly summarized and then actively communicated and "marketed" to all affected parties.

Determine what specific information (e.g., measures or indicators) is needed to track each health determinant (step 6). For each determinant selected, one next chooses a *manageable* number of indicators that are clearly defined and relevant to the setting and the population.[18] For example, "civic engagement or participation" is often chosen as an indicator of the "social environment." Civic engagement measures *participation* in *(1)* a broad range of civic organizations that community members believe contribute to the quality of public life, such as Alcoholics Anonymous, hospitals, shelters, and parks and *(2)* electoral activities, such as voting (*52*). Indicators must be clearly defined, measurable, and understandable when presented to constituents.

Adhering to three principles for selecting indicators will ensure that the indicators are maximally useful: *(1)* The final list of indicators should reflect the production of health over the entire life span, from childhood to the end of life. For example, the percent of postpartum mothers and families that receive a home visit by a care provider within 3 to 4 days postpartum reflects a health system that is supportive of families, children, and parents. Similarly, indicators of the social integration of the elderly reflect not only the level of their overall integration in society but also the health of a population group that manifests lack of social integration with increased loss of function, morbidity, and mortality. *(2)* The indicators should reflect all major types of determinants, such as environment,

---

[18] One of the great risks to successful surveillance comes from trying to track too many indicators. The process for selecting indicators must be strategic and disciplined, with good facilitation and wise, committed partners.

social policies, and education—and their interactions—to ensure that no major influences on health are overlooked. *(3)* The indicators should include information about the medical system to ensure that public health officials working at all jurisdictional levels can speak knowledgeably about costs and other concerns associated with medical care, such as inadequate access to appropriate care and, conversely, over-reliance on medical care to produce health. Including information on medical care, as exemplified by the United Health Foundation and Wisconsin rankings mentioned earlier, serves to engage public health in efforts to reform care and to facilitate advocacy for better medical programs and outcomes.

Select the source of information and the method of collection based on purpose, content, scope, and setting (step 9). A major challenge in developing a surveillance system for health determinants in most countries, including the United States, is deciding whether (and how) to use data from an existing source, augment an existing source, or develop a new source. To decide, first determine whether existing sources have sufficient data to meet the purposes of surveillance. Some countries, states, and localities create inventories of relevant data that can inform them about a wide variety of health determinants. For example, the state of Virginia has compiled a listing of data sources to support monitoring of health equity *(53)*. Matching and linking different data sources is another option. The Health Poverty Index, the United Health Foundation and Wisconsin rankings, and the King County Indicators, described earlier, provide important lessons about compiling existing data to track health determinants.

If existing sources cannot meet surveillance data needs, it might be possible to augment an existing system to do so. Adding questions to the BRFSS on social determinants, increasing the number of survey respondents to provide county level estimates, and oversampling population subgroups (such as ethnic minorities) are examples of this approach. Finally, if augmenting an existing system cannot provide needed data, it might be necessary to establish a new data collection system, although cost and political resistance can present considerable hurdles.

Population censuses and surveys, environmental sampling, and reanalysis of administrative data are the principal methods for obtaining data about health determinants. A complete census of a population has the advantage of providing information for all geographical levels and population subgroups. It also provides denominator data for the calculation of rates and a sampling frame for population surveys. Birth registration and, occasionally, death registration can provide information on some health determinants as can school-based administrative and health records.[19]

Population-based surveys, such as the BRFSS and the General Social Survey, typically collect data on more than one determinant, and some survey designs rotate questions over time to collect data on an even larger number of determinants. Surveys can be repeated to provide estimates of the temporal trend of determinants. Environmental sampling can provide information on the geographic and

---

[19] The Family Educational Rights and Privacy Act (FERPA) (20 U.S.C. § 1232g; 34 CFR Part 99) is a Federal law that protects the privacy of student education records and might limit access to these records. FERPA allows schools to disclose records, without consent, to appropriate officials in cases of health and safety emergencies. See http://www.ed.gov/policy/gen/guid/fpco/ferpa/index.html for additional information on FERPA and procedures for obtaining school records.

temporal distribution of air, water, and soil pollutants. To provide comparable data for different locations and different times, the methods used for sampling populations and the environment should be standardized and validated.[20]

Community, state, or national legal, economic, and administrative data can provide useful, low-cost information on determinants. Secondary analyses of these data can be used to monitor the presence and potential impact of economic policies or taxes on income distribution and certain behaviors; the sale of specific products, such as alcohol and tobacco products, that are linked with specific proximal determinants, such as alcohol consumption and smoking; and the distribution of income, wealth, and poverty. Data on the use of health care or social services might be available from administrative records kept by providers of these services, as demonstrated by their use in syndromic surveillance systems originally designed to more effectively monitor the use of urgent care and emergency services.

Traditionally, health- care providers and health-care records have been the principal source of information for public health surveillance systems. Information collected by health-care providers from patients about illnesses, risk factors, environmental exposures, family history, and genetic risks has been the foundation of public health reporting and surveillance, and is the basis for notifiable disease reporting, cancer registries, birth and death records, and hospital discharge data. The usefulness of data from health care-related interviews could be improved substantially if information on a selected set of robust indicators about social determinants of health were gathered. For example, including four to five short validated questions about perceived social class (or sense of control), isolation, education, and community efficacy could enhance the physician's ability to predict individual health risk. This same information could be used during the investigation of outbreaks or community health problems by public health practitioners to provide useful contextual information about the forces that create and sustain outbreaks, as well as how to mitigate the effects of these forces. For example, based on lessons learned from the 1993 Chicago heat wave, better information on the built environment, social support, and community efficacy could lead to more effective preventive interventions in certain situations that could halve morbidity and mortality (57).

Qualitative methods, including market research techniques using small, focused samples; observational methods; or case studies, can be used to obtain information on health determinants meaningful to a community. Jointly designed and conducted qualitative data collections and analyses might energize and guide community stakeholders and health programs more effectively than the estimates available from random samples drawn from larger geographic areas that are used for state and national population surveys. In addition, qualitative methods can be useful for better understanding a particular determinant as it relates to health, and as a source of ideas for questions for population surveys or sites for environmental sampling.

Table 13–5 provides an overview of systems in the United States that monitor specific health determinates or that provide data that could be used for this purpose.

---

[20] The U.S. National Center for Health Statistics and the U.S. Census Bureau formally develop and evaluate the questions and questionnaires used in their surveys (54,55), and the U.S. Environmental Protection Agency uses standardized, approved methods for sampling and analyzing air and water (56).

Table 13–5 Major National and State Data Systems Used to Monitor Determinants of Health, United States, 2009

Data System (Acronym)	Topic	Data Collection			Geographic coverage		
		Approach	Method	Frequency	National	State	Local
Air Quality System (AQS)(58)	air quality	monitoring stations	air sampling and analysis	ongoing			x[1]
American Community Survey (ACS)(59)	personal characteristics[2], housing, education, employment, income	population survey	mailed questionnaire	annually	x	x	x[3]
American Housing Survey (AHS)(60)	housing and neighborhood quality; housing type, size, and costs; equipment and fuels; household composition; tenure	household survey	personal and telephone interviews	every 2 years	x		x[3]
Behavioral Risk Factor Surveillance System (BRFSS) (5)	behavioral risks, health status, health-care access, preventive practices	population survey	telephone interview	annually	x	x	x[3]

(continued)

Table 13-5 (*continued*)

Data System (Acronym)	Topic	Data Collection		Frequency	Geographic coverage		
		Approach	Method		National	State	Local
Current Population Survey (CPS)(*61*)	personal characteristics, employment, occupation, income, poverty, education, other[4]	household survey	personal and telephone interviews	monthly	x		
Decennial Census (DC) (*62*)	personal characteristics	census	personal interview	every 10 years	x	x	x
Economic Census (EC) (*63*)	businesses in the United States and their characteristics, revenues, employment	census	mailed questionnaire	every 5 years	x	x	x[3]
General Social Survey (GSS)(*64*)	personal characteristics, housing, education, employment, occupation, income, beliefs, opinions, attitudes[5]	population survey	personal interview	annually	x		
Medical Expenditure Panel Survey (MEPS) (*65*)	access to health care, health-care quality and cost, health insurance coverage	population survey health-care provider survey insurance provider survey	personal interview telephone interview	every 2 years	x		

Survey	Content	Type	Method	Frequency			
Monitoring the Future Study (MTF) (66)	attitudes about and use of alcohol, illicit drugs, and tobacco	student survey	school-based, self-administered questionnaire	annually	x		x^3
National Crime Victimization Survey (NCVS)(67)	crime	household survey	telephone and personal interviews	annually	x		
National Health Care Surveys (NHCS) (68)	health-care cost, quality, patterns of delivery, staffing	provider and facility surveys	provider completed form abstraction of medical records	annually	x		
National Health and Nutrition Examination Survey (NHANES) (69)	environmental, social, family, economic, occupational, housing, behavioral, dietary, anatomical, physiological, metabolic, and genetic factors; health conditions	population survey	personal interview, physical exam, and laboratory tests	every 2 years	x		
National Health Interview Survey (NHIS)(70)	personal characteristics, behaviors, health care, health conditions	household survey	personal interview	annually		x	

(continued)

Table 13–5 (*continued*)

Data System (Acronym)	Topic	Data Collection			Geographic coverage		
		Approach	Method	Frequency	National	State	Local
National Survey on Drug Use and Health (NSDUH) (71)	alcohol, illicit drug, and tobacco use and treatment for use; personal characteristics	household survey	personal interview	annually	x	x	
National Profile of Local Health Departments (NPLHD) (72)	local public health agencies	agency survey	mailed questionnaire	periodically (approximately every 3 years)			x
National Survey of Family Growth (NSFG) (73)	personal characteristics; sexual and reproductive history; adoption; marital and relationship history	household survey	personal interview	periodically (approximately every 2 years)	x		
School Health Policies and Programs Study (SHPPS) (74)	school health policies and programs	administrative data, school district and school-based survey	mailed questionnaire telephone and personal interviews	periodically (approximately every 6 years)	x	x	
State Tobacco Activities Tracking and Evaluation System (STATE) (75)	tobacco use, sales, taxes, programs, tobacco control legislation	data warehouse	secondary data collected from various sources	continuous		x	

STORET (76)	water quality	monitoring groups	water sampling and analysis	continuous			x
Survey of Consumer Finances (SCF)(77)	wealth, income, pensions, personal characteristics	population survey	personal interview	every 3 years	x		
Youth Risk Behavior Surveillance System (YRBSS) (78)	health-related behavior	student survey	school-based, self-administered questionnaire	every 2 years	x	x	

---

[1] Data are collected and available for specific geographic locations (e.g., lake, pond, river, well) or monitoring stations, which may be specified by their address or latitude and longitude.

[2] Personal characteristics include age, sex, race, ethnicity, marital status, household relationships.

[3] Data are collected and available for one or more metropolitan areas.

[4] The CPS has a several supplements, which periodically collect information on housing, health, health insurance, food security, hunger, child support, fertility, unemployment insurance, volunteer activities, tobacco use, and other topics.

[5] There is a core set of topics covered in each GSS and topics that change each year. In addition, the GSS contains topical modules, which collect information at one or more points in time on a variety of topics, including social networks, mental health, religion, culture, altruism, health status, intergroup relations, participation in groups and organizations, information society, and work environment. The GSS is also a member of the International Social Survey Program.

Most systems provide national and occasionally regional estimates from representative samples of the U.S. civilian population and use personal interviews, telephone interviews, or mailed questionnaires to collect information. Most are repeated yearly and provide annual data. Several systems provide state or local data and estimates, including AQS, ACS, BRFSS, CPS, DC, STATE, STORET, and YRBSS.[21] Many of the surveys maintain a core set of questions to provide temporal trends about specific determinants and supplement these questions with questions on other topics that are administered on a one-time or occasional basis. Most of the systems produce reports summarizing their findings, and many make datasets available for analysis by other interested parties. Data from the systems are used for a variety of purposes from informing policy and directing resources to enforcing laws.

Communicate the findings of surveillance (step 14). In addition to reports and scientific publications, government agencies and other groups have used innovative approaches to make their findings more attractive and useful to various audiences, including policy developers, community organizers and planners, and program evaluators. These approaches increasingly use the Internet and include the U.S. Census Bureau's Web site, DataPlace (*79*), CDC WONDER, and state Web-based data query systems (*80*). Gapminder World is a remarkable visualization tool that provides international data on a variety of determinants and outcomes and "unveils the beauty of statistical time series by converting boring numbers into enjoyable, animated and interactive graphics" (*81*).

Various indicators, indices, and summary measures have been developed for presenting health determinants in a form useful to policymakers and the public. Examples include the Health Poverty Index, described earlier, and the Human Development Index, which is composed of life expectancy at birth; adult literacy; combined gross enrollment in primary, secondary, and tertiary level education; and gross domestic product per capita (ref. *80*, p. 225). In 2005, the European Union released a compendium of public health indicators that includes demographic and socio-economic factors and health-related behaviors (*82*). The Community Health Status Indicators presents estimates of health status and determinants for each U.S. county using data compiled from federal agencies. Each county's demographic profile and health status at a single point in time is compared with a set of peer counties (*83*).

CHALLENGES FOR FUTURE WORK

Conducting surveillance for health determinants is a rapidly evolving area in public health, and public health practitioners face challenges as they move forward.

Is surveillance for determinants the correct paradigm? Surveillance has traditionally focused on individual diseases. Surveillance systems arise and decline in response to outbreaks of specific diseases or the appearance of new diseases. Given the diversity and breadth of health determinants, their complex interactions, and the long time-frame required to bring about needed change in some of them, we might need to take a more comprehensive, sustained approach

---

[21] Acronyms for these systems are explained in Table 13–5.

to monitoring them. Working with other sectors and academic disciplines—such as coordinating surveys and other methods for gathering data on multiple determinants, rather than focusing on individual determinants—might be more appropriate.

The relationships between health outcomes and health determinants are complex with uncertainty about the nature and extent of causal relationships. As exemplified in Figure 13–3, models of causality for chronic diseases such as lung cancer are complex, with great variability in our understanding of specific determinants and their interrelationships. Lack of agreement about the nature and extent of these relationships can make it difficult to establish surveillance for certain determinants. For example, whereas few would disagree about the importance of monitoring smoking rates in a surveillance system of lung cancer risk, little consensus exists about whether—and how—to monitor other factors in the model, such as rates of smoking in movies, peer pressure, or supportive social networks.

In the United States and some other countries, "health" has become a province belonging solely to experts within the medical system. In public and media discussions about health, views of "health" are often reduced to "medical care," and health is viewed as solely a product of the medical system. Broadening the definition of health in popular culture to include population health and societal factors that influence it, as well as deputizing partners in multiple sectors, would bring more actors and resources to monitoring a broader spectrum of health determinants.

Few incentives exist in public health programs to include health determinants. Categorical funding in the United States at the national and state levels encourages surveillance to be limited to specific diseases (or exposures) with few incentives to take a more comprehensive view of health and its determinants. For example, state-based tobacco control programs often focus on proximal behavioral risks and provide funds to collect information on rates of smoking, efforts to quit, or exposure to environmental tobacco smoke. These programs might not see the utility of collecting data on more distal determinants, such as social connectedness, education level, or adverse childhood events, although their influence on smoking and other behavioral risks is well-established.

Few examples exist for monitoring a broader array of health determinants in the community health improvement process. Standard methods exist for the use of surveillance data in community health assessments, one of the first steps in the community health improvement process (*36*). When assessing needs and public health burden, most of these methods focus on the burden of disease rather than on a more comprehensive view of health and its determinants. Health planners might be reluctant to focus resources on problems that they believe lie outside of the health care or public health sector, such as education or income security.

RECOMMENDATIONS FOR IMPROVING SURVEILLANCE OF HEALTH DETERMINANTS

To address these and other challenges, public health practitioners—in collaboration with partners in medical care, community development, and other key sectors—should first *incorporate data on a wider range of health determinants, such as social isolation, civic engagement, and community cohesion, into existing surveillance systems, particularly those that provide data at state and local levels.* This would enrich available data while also providing actionable information about health determinants at the community level. The addition of the social context module to the 2009 BRFSS serves as a welcome example of the kind of effort that is needed. Similarly, validated questions and other tools that can be used during clinical visits and in outbreak investigations for gathering data on a comprehensive set of health determinants should be developed and field-tested. Efforts should be made to incorporate these validated tools in the routine workflows of key partners, including clinicians and public health epidemiologists. Beyond providing an additional source of data for surveillance, having such data would allow more robust analyses of clinical interventions and disease outbreaks, as well as assisting clinicians and epidemiologists to better understand their role in the broader health context. For public health agencies, information on specific health determinants would improve the value of existing surveillance systems to chronic disease control efforts, outbreak investigations, and the community health improvement process.

Second, public health practitioners should *examine strategies for presenting and using these new data to support programs focused on the root causes of population health problems.* This will require care and political sensitivity. Few policymakers are familiar with such data or research showing the importance of the social determinants of health. Compelling and eye-catching ways of presenting data about social and behavioral determinants, such as Gapminder World, are needed to motivate policymakers and other constituents to expand their view of health beyond medical care and individual behaviors.

Third, *vision, strong leadership, and long-term strategies will be needed for coordinating and integrating existing sources of data into a comprehensive and sustainable system for the surveillance of health determinants.* The WHO's Commission for the Social Determinants of Health has provided a vision, and it is now up to governments and policymakers to provide the leadership, and public health practitioners to provide the long-term strategies for realizing this goal.

Acknowledgement   The authors acknowledge the careful review and helpful suggestions of Daniel J. Friedman, Marilyn Metzler, Nene Riley, and the editors in the preparation of this chapter.

REFERENCES

1. Langmuir AD. The surveillance of communicable diseases of national importance. *N Engl J Med* 1963;268:182–192.

2. U.S. Department of Health and Human Services, National Center for Health Statistics. Historical Data. National Center for Health Statistics Website. http://www.cdc.gov/nchs/datawh/statab/unpubd/mortabs/hist-tabs.htm. Accessed May 4, 2008.

3. McGinnis JM, Foege WH. Actual causes of death in the United States. *JAMA* 1993;270:2207–2212.

4. Mokdad AH, Marks JS, Stroup DF, Gerberding JL. Actual causes of death in the United States, 2000. *JAMA* 2004;291:1238–1245.

5. U.S. Department of Health and Human Services, Centers for Disease Control and Prevention. Behavioral Risk Factor Surveillance System. Centers for Disease Control and Prevention Website. http://www.cdc.gov/brfss/. Updated Apr 29, 2008. Accessed May 3, 2008.

6. United Nations Educational, Scientific and Cultural Organization. Universal Declaration on Cultural Diversity. http://www.unesco.org/education/imld_2002/unversal_decla.shtml. Accessed May 3, 2008.

7. House JS, Landis KR, Umberson D. Social relationships and health. *Science* 1988;241(4865):540–545.

8. Berkman LF, Syme L. Social networks, host resistance, and mortality: a nine-year follow-up study of Alameda County residents. *Am J Epidemiol* 1979;109:186–204.

9. Berkman LF, Kawachi I, eds. *Social Epidemiology.* New York: Oxford; 2000.

10. Cassel J. The contribution of the social environment to host resistance. *Am J Epidemiol* 1976;104:107–123.

11. Christakis NA, Fowler JH. The collective dynamics of smoking in a large social network. *N Engl J Med* 2008;358(21):2249–2258.

12. Kawachi I. Income inequality and health. In: Berkman LF, Kawachi I, eds. *Social Epidemiology.* New York: Oxford; 2000:76–94.

13. Link BG, Phelan J. Social conditions as fundamental causes of disease. *J Health Social Behavior* 1995; Extra Issue:80-94.

14. Marmot MG, Davey-Smith G, Stansfeld SA, *et al.* Health inequalities among British civil servants: the Whitehall II study. *Lancet* 1991;337:1387–1393.

15. Marmot M, Wilkinson RG, eds. *Social Determinants of Health*, 3rd ed. Oxford: Oxford; 2006.

16. Sapolsky R. Sick of poverty. *Scientific Am* 2005;Dec:92–99.

17. Wilkinson R, Marmot M, eds. *Social Determinants of Health: The Solid Facts*, 2nd ed. Copenhagen: WHO; 2003. http://www.euro.who.int/document/e81384.pdf. Accessed May 4, 2008.

18. Kawachi I, Berkman L. Social cohesion, social capital, and health. In: Berkman LF, Kawachi I, eds. *Social Epidemiology.* New York: Oxford; 2000:174–190.

19. Berkman LF, Leo-Summers L, Horwitz R. Emotional support and survival after myocardial infarction. *Ann Intern Med* 1992;117:1003–1009.

20. Mookadam F, Arthur HM. Social support and its relationship to morbidity and mortality after acute myocardial infarction. *Arch Intern Med* 2004;164:1514–1518.

21. Kawachi I, Subramanian SV, Almeida-Filho N. A glossary for health inequalities. *J Epidemiol Commun Health* 2002;56:647–652.

22. Saplosky R. The influence of social hierarchy on primate health. *Science* 2005; 308:648–652.

23. World Health Organization, Commission on Social Determinants of Health. *Closing the Gap in a Generation: Health Equity Through Action on the Social Determinants of Health.* Geneva: WHO; 2008:178–185.

24. Marmot M. Social determinants of health inequalities. *Lancet* 2005;365: 1099–1104.

25. World Health Organization. Preamble to the Constitution of the World Health Organization as adopted by the International Health Conference, New York, 19-22 June, 1946; signed on 22 July 1946 by the representatives of 61 States (Official Records of the World Health Organization, no. 2, p. 100) and entered into force on April 7,1948.

26. World Health Organization. Ottawa Charter for Health Promotion, 1986. Geneva: WHO; 1986. http://www.euro.who.int/AboutWHO/Policy/20010827_2. Accessed May 4, 2008.

27. Link BG, Phelan JC. McKeown and the idea that social conditions are fundamental causes of disease. *Am J Public Health* 2002;92:730–732.

28. World Health Organization. Division of Health Promotion, Education and Communications (HPR) and Health Education and Health Promotion Unit (HEP). Health Promotion Glossary. Geneva: Switzerland; 1998. http://www.who.int/hpr/NPH/docs/hp_glossary_en.pdf.

29. Krieger N. Epidemiology and the web of causation: has anyone seen the spider? *Soc Sci Med* 1994;39(7):887–903.

30. Murray CJL, Ezzati M, Lopez AD , Rodgers A, Vander Hoorn S. Comparative quantification of health risks: Conceptual framework and methodological issues. *Population Health Metrics* 2003;1:1. http://www.pophealthmetrics.com/content/1/1/1. Accessed Apr 23, 2008.

31. Lalonde M. *A New Perspective on the Health of the Canadians*. Ottawa: Ministry of National Health and Welfare; 1974.

32. Evans RG, Stoddart GL. Producing health, consuming health care. *Soc Sci Med* 1990;31:1347–1363.

33. Evans RG, Stoddart GL. Consuming research, producing policy. *Am J Public Health* 2003;93:371–379.

34. Institute of Medicine. *The Future of the Public's Health in the 21st Century.* Washington, DC: National Academy Press; 2003:52.

35. Krieger N. Ladders, pyramids and champagne: the iconography of health inequities. *J Epidemiol Community Health* 2008;62:1098–1104. http://jech.bmj.com/cgi/content/abstract/62/12/1098#otherarticles.

36. Institute of Medicine. *Improving Health in the Community: A Role for Performance Monitoring.* Washington, DC: National Academy Press; 1997. http://www.nap.edu/catalog.php?record_id=5298. Accessed February 1, 2008.

37. Greenland S, Pearl J, Robins JM. Causal diagrams for epidemiologic research. *Epidemiology* 1999;10(1):37–48.

38. U.S. Department of Health and Human Services, National Center for Health Statistics. National Health and Nutrition Examination Survey, 2007-2008: Overview. National Center for Health Statistics Website. http://www.cdc.gov/nchs/data/nhanes/nhanes_07_08/overviewbrochure_0708.pdf. Accessed April 23, 2008.

39. Smith PJ, Hoaglin DC, Battaglia MP, *et al.* National Center for Health Statistics. Statistical methodology of the National Immunization Survey, 1994–2002. *Vital Health Stat* 2005;2(138):1–56.

40. Lynch J, Kaplan G. Socioeconomic position. In: Berkman L, Kawachi I, eds. *Social Epidemiology.* New York: Oxford; 2000:13–35.

41. Dibben C, Watson J, Smith T, *et al.* The Health Poverty Index. The NHS Information Centre Website. http://www.hpi.org.uk. Accessed Mar 14, 2009.

42. Dibben C, Watson J, Smith T, *et al.* The Health Poverty Index, 2008. The National Health Service Information Centre. Leeds, UK. http://www.hpi.org.uk/. Accessed May 24, 2009.

43. United Health Foundation. *America's Health Rankings—2008 Edition.* Minnetonka: United Health Foundation; 2008. http://www.americashealthrankings.org/2008/index.html. Accessed March 14, 2009.

44. Taylor KW, Athens JK, Booske BC, O'Connor C, Jones NR, Remington PL. 2008 Wisconsin County Health Rankings: Full Report. Madison, WI: University of

Wisconsin; 2008. http://www.pophealth.wisc.edu/UWPHI/pha/wchr/2008/fullReport.pdf. Accessed March 14, 2009.

45. Peppard PE, Kindig DA, Dranger E, Jovaag A, Remington PL. Ranking community health status to stimulate discussion of local public health issues: the Wisconsin County Health Rankings. *Am J Public Health* 2008;98(2):209–212.

46. Rohan AMK, Booske BC, Remington PL. Using the Wisconsin County Health Rankings to catalyze community health improvement. *J Public Health Management Practice* 2009;15(1):24–32.

47. Horsley K, Ciske SJ. From neurons to King County neighborhoods: partnering to promote policies based on the science of early childhood development. *Am J Public Health* 2005;95(4):562–567.

48. Public Health–Seattle & King County. Communities count: social and health indicators across King County 2008. Seattle: Public Health–Seattle & King County; 2008. http://communitiescount.org/index.php. Accessed March 17, 2009.

49. Communities Count Website. http://communitiescount.org/index.php. Accessed March 17, 2009.

50. Parrish RG, McDonnell SM. Sources of health-related information. In: Teutsch SM, Churchill RE, eds. *Principles and Practice of Public Health Surveillance,* 2nd ed. New York: Oxford University Press; 2000:30–75.

51. Abramson JH. *Survey Methods in Community Medicine,* 4th ed. Edinburgh: Churchill Livingston; 1990.

52. Zukin C, Keeter S, Andolina M, Jenkins K, Delli Carpini MX. *A New Engagement? Political Participation, Civic Life, and the Changing American Citizen.* New York: Oxford University Press; 2006.

53. Virginia Department of Health. Health Equity Statistics. Virginia Department of Health Website. http://www.vdh.virginia.gov/healthpolicy/healthequity/statistics.htm. Updated August 15, 2008. Accessed March 16, 2009.

54. U.S. Department of Health and Human Services, National Center for Health Statistics. Working paper series: cognitive methods. National Center for Health Statistics Website. http://www.cdc.gov/nchs/products/pubs/workpap/workpap.htm. Updated January 11, 2007. Accessed May 5, 2008.

55. U.S. Department of Commerce, Census Bureau. Census Bureau standard: pretesting questionnaires and related materials for surveys and censuses. Washington, DC: US Census Bureau, 2003. http://www.census.gov/srd/pretest-standards.pdf. Accessed May 5, 2008.

56. U.S. Environmental Protection Agency. Test method collections. Environmental Protection Agency Website. http://www.epa.gov/OSA/fem/methcollectns.htm. Updated December 14, 2007. Accessed April 29, 2008.

57. Klinenberg E. Heat Wave: *A Social Autopsy of Disaster in Chicago.* Chicago: University of Chicago; 2002.

58. U.S. Environmental Protection Agency. Air Quality System (AQS). Environmental Protection Agency Website. http://www.epa.gov/ttn/airs/airsaqs/. Updated December 19, 2007. Accessed April 29, 2008.

59. U.S. Department of Commerce, Census Bureau. American community survey. Census Bureau Website. http://www.census.gov/acs/www/. Updated March 26, 2008. Accessed April 29, 2008.

60. U.S. Department of Commerce, Census Bureau. Current Housing Reports, Series H150/05, American Housing Survey for the United States: 2005. Washington, DC: U.S. Government Printing Office; 2006. http://www.census.gov/hhes/www/housing/ahs/ahs.html. Updated January 25, 2008. Accessed May 3, 2008.

61. U.S. Department of Commerce, Census Bureau. Current Population Survey. Census Bureau Website. http://www.census.gov/cps/. Updated October 18 2007. Accessed April 29 2008.

62. U.S. Department of Commerce, Census Bureau. United States Census 2000. Census Bureau Website. http://www.census.gov/main/www/cen2000.html. Updated April 7, 2009. Accessed May 24, 2009.

63. U.S. Department of Commerce, Census Bureau. 2007 Economic Census. Census Bureau Website. http://www.census.gov/econ/census07/. Updated May 7, 2009. Accessed May 24, 2009.

64. National Opinion Research Center. General Social Survey. National Opinion Research Center Website. http://www.norc.org/GSS+Website. Accessed April 29, 2008.

65. U.S. Department of Health and Human Services, Agency for Healthcare Research and Quality. Medical Expenditure Panel Survey. Agency for Healthcare Research and Quality Website. http://www.meps.ahrq.gov/mepsweb/. Accessed May 24, 2009.

66. University of Michigan, Institute for Social Research. Monitoring the Future. Monitoring the Future Website. http://monitoringthefuture.org/. Updated May 4, 2009. Accessed May 24, 2009.

67. U.S. Department of Justice, Bureau of Justice Statistics. Crime and victims statistics. Bureau of Justice Statistics Website. http://www.ojp.usdoj.gov/bjs/cvict.htm. Updated August 29, 2008. Accessed May 24, 2009.

68. U.S. Department of Health and Human Services, National Center for Health Statistics. National Health Care Surveys. National Center for Health Statistics Website. http://www.cdc.gov/nchs/nhcs.htm. Updated March 14, 2008. Accessed May 3, 2008.

69. U.S. Department of Health and Human Services, National Center for Health Statistics. National Health and Nutrition Examination Survey. National Center for Health Statistics Website. http://www.cdc.gov/nchs/nhanes.htm. Updated December 27, 2007. Accessed May 3, 2008.

70. U.S. Department of Health and Human Services, National Center for Health Statistics. National Health Interview Survey. National Center for Health Statistics Website. http://www.cdc.gov/nchs/nhis.htm. Updated April 16, 2008. Accessed May 3, 2008.

71. U.S. Department of Health and Human Services, Substance Abuse and Mental Health Services Administration, Office of Applied Studies. National Survey on Drug Use & Health. Office of Applied Studies Website. http://www.oas.samhsa.gov/nhsda.htm. Updated December 30, 2008. Accessed May 24, 2009.

72. National Association of County and City Health Officials. 2005 National profile of local health departments. Washington: NACCHO; 2006. http://www.naccho.org/topics/infrastructure/documents/NACCHO_report_final_000.pdf. Accessed May 4, 2008.

73. U.S. Department of Health and Human Services, National Center for Health Statistics. National Survey of Family Growth. National Center for Health Statistics Website. http://www.cdc.gov/nchs/NSFG.htm. Updated May 14, 2009. Accessed May 24, 2009.

74. U.S. Department of Health and Human Services, Centers for Disease Control and Prevention, National Center for Chronic Disease Prevention and Health Promotion. SHPPS: School Health Policies and Programs Study. Healthy Youth! Website. http://www.cdc.gov/HealthyYouth/shpps/index.htm. Updated January 16, 2009. Accessed May 24, 2009.

75. U.S. Department of Health and Human Services, Centers for Disease Control and Prevention. State Tobacco Activities Tracking and Evaluation (STATE) System. Centers for Disease Control and Prevention Website. http://apps.nccd.cdc.gov/state-system/. Accessed May 24, 2009.

76. U.S. Environmental Protection Agency. STORET. Environmental Protection Agency Website. http://www.epa.gov/STORET/. Updated January 31, 2008. Accessed May 5, 2008.

77. Federal Reserve Board. Survey of Consumer Finances. Federal Reserve Board Website. http://www.federalreserve.gov/PUBS/oss/oss2/scfindex.html. Updated March 28, 2008. Accessed May 3, 2008.

78. US Department of Health and Human Services, Centers for Disease Control and Prevention, National Center for Chronic Disease Prevention and Health Promotion. YRBSS: Youth Risk Behavior Surveillance System. Healthy Youth! Website. http://www.cdc.gov/HealthyYouth/yrbs/index.htm. Updated April 2, 2009. Accessed May 24, 2009.

79. KnowledgePlex. DataPlace. KnowledgePlex Website. http://www.dataplace.org/. Accessed May 4, 2008.

80. Friedman DJ, Parrish RG, eds. State web-based query systems. *J Public Health Management Practice* 2006;12(2):109–195.

81. Gapminder Foundation. Gapminder world. Gapminder Website. http://www.gapminder.org/. Accessed May 4, 2008.

82. United Nations Development Programme. Human *development report 2007/2008*. New York: Palgrave Macmillan; 2007. http://hdr.undp.org/en/. Accessed April 28, 2008.

83. European Union. Public health indicators for Europe: context, selection, definition. Final report by the ECHI project, phase II. Brussels: European Union; 2005. http://www.healthindicators.org/ICHI/general/startmenu.aspx. Accessed April 28, 2008.

84. U.S. Department of Health and Human Services. Community Health Status Indicators. U.S. Department of Health and Human Services Website. http://www.communityhealth.hhs.gov. Accessed March 10, 2009.

85. Greenland S, Brumback B. An overview of relations among causal modeling methods. *Intern J Epidemiol* 2002;31:1030–1037.

14

Public Health Surveillance for Preparedness and Emergency Response

Biosurveillance for Human Health

DANIEL M. SOSIN AND RICHARD S. HOPKINS

INTRODUCTION

Concern for increasing vulnerability to emerging infectious diseases led to the Institute of Medicine's influential 1992 review on this topic (*1*). The increasingly realistic threat of mass casualties from weapons of mass destruction—biological, chemical, radiological, explosive, or nuclear—added to the sense of population vulnerability after 2001 (*2*). Recent hurricane seasons, wildfires, earthquakes, and tsunamis emphasized persistent human vulnerability to natural disasters. Global interconnectedness through rapid international travel and trade increases opportunities for the transmission of emerging infectious diseases (*3*) and for terrorism (*4*). In the face of these threats, interest in public health monitoring of population exposures and disease has increased. There is also increased interest in improving individual patient medical care by providing timely information to clinicians that reflects the current community situation (*5*). Exchange of data and information between the health-care system and public health is expected to improve both population and individual patient health care (*5*).

Monitoring the health of a population in support of preparedness and emergency response stretches the boundaries of public health surveillance. What we call "biosurveillance" in this chapter addresses the use of surveillance and investigation methods in public health emergencies that may have distinctive features:

(1) The event may occur in the context of a terrorism threat;
(2) The agent in an event might be novel, so surveillance limited to known clinical syndromes or specific diagnoses might miss an emerging event;
(3) The mode of transmission of the agent might be novel, so patterns of disease occurrence in the community might not resemble those typically associated with contaminated food or water, or with transmission

The findings and conclusions in this report are those of the authors and do not necessarily represent the official position of the Centers for Disease Control and Prevention.

in schools, daycare facilities, long-term care facilities, and other familiar settings;

(4) The agent might be familiar but the context might be novel—for example outbreaks in the aftermath of a natural disaster;

(5) The event might develop rapidly, because of multiple introductions, widespread population susceptibility, high transmission rates, or a short incubation period;

(6) Delays in obtaining laboratory results to confirm and characterize the causative agent or in piecing together epidemiologic information spread across multiple systems and stakeholders might result in significant human impact; and/or

(7) The size of the event might be very large, so that health-care facilities might be unable to keep up with the volume and intensity of care needed and inflexible surveillance mechanisms will be ineffective.

In this context, population health monitoring is expected to be faster, bigger, and better: *faster* in that effective mitigation depends on how quickly an event can be identified, the exposed population can be recognized and treated, and the exposure contained; *bigger* because of the potential for incidents of catastrophic scale; and *better* because the resources of multiple organizations and expertise of multiple disciplines must be applied together to achieve the goal of early detection and event characterization.

DEFINITIONS

The term *biosurveillance* as used in this chapter includes both the systematic and routine monitoring of population health for acute events and targeted follow-up investigations. These two activities are needed in tandem to verify a threat or event and to establish acute situation awareness for effective response. Biosurveillance is a function in the practice of public health and does not include data collection for the purpose of research. The U.S. Homeland Security Council defined biosurveillance in the Homeland Security Presidential Directive-21 (HSPD-21) as "the process of active data gathering with appropriate analysis and interpretation of biosphere data that might relate to disease activity and threats to human or animal health—whether infectious, toxic, metabolic, or otherwise, and regardless of intentional or natural origin—in order to achieve early warning of health threats, early detection of health events, and overall situational awareness of disease activity (6)." Additionally, the Pandemic and All-Hazards Preparedness Act established the need for "a near-real-time electronic nationwide public health situational awareness capability through an interoperable network of systems to share data and information to enhance early detection of, rapid response to, and management of, potentially catastrophic infectious disease outbreaks and other public health emergencies that originate domestically or abroad (7)."

Situation awareness is a state of understanding resulting from the availability of effective information products and the training and experience to interpret them.

Situation awareness has been defined as "the perception of elements in the environment within a volume of time and space, the comprehension of their meaning, and the projection of their status in the near future (8)." A common operating picture is a single display of information used to support situation awareness for decision making when anticipating an event and continuing through response and recovery. An effective common operating picture should display information from multiple sources, including surveillance systems, media, and professional networks. A common operating picture should be dynamic, populated with real-time data, and enhanced through methods of data and information visualization.

When an adverse public health event is detected, public health investigation is initiated to verify the signal or cue, explore the nature of the impediment to health, devise strategies to counteract it, and assess the effectiveness of those strategies to improve response. Biosurveillance as used by Wagner "encompasses both detection and characterization" and "involves a positive feedback loop: when the continuous collection and analysis of surveillance data identifies an anomalous number of sick individuals (or single case of a dangerous disease), investigators collect additional information that feeds back into the analytic process, resulting in better characterization of the event (9)." Public health surveillance contributes to biosurveillance but is itself not sufficient to meet the information needs across all phases of an event (i.e., pre-event, detection, response, recovery).

HSPD-21 goes further to define epidemiologic surveillance as the human-health component of biosurveillance. The term *syndromic surveillance* has been used to capture only some of this scope. Syndromic surveillance is the ongoing, systematic collection, analysis, interpretation, and application of real-time (or near-real-time) indicators for diseases and outbreaks that allow for their detection before public health authorities would otherwise note them. Syndromic surveillance emphasizes timeliness and applies automated analysis and visualization tools to screen non-specific indicator data in electronic form so as to detect unexpected patterns that warrant investigation (10). The definition of biosurveillance used here is consistent with what is referred to as "epidemic intelligence" by the European Centre for Disease Control, encompassing all activities related to the early identification of health hazards, including the functions of public health surveillance—both structured and unstructured—and epidemiologic investigation with the goal to recommend public health control measures (11). "Epidemic intelligence" was earlier used by Langmuir to reflect the role of epidemiology in rendering disaster and epidemic aid services during a biological warfare attack (12). Given the limitations of all of these terms, however, biosurveillance is used in this chapter to reflect the human health-related component of the term biosurveillance as used in HSPD-21.

PURPOSES

Biosurveillance in the context of human health is the science and practice of managing health-related data and information for early warning of urgent threats and hazards, early detection of events, and rapid characterization so that effective actions can be taken to mitigate adverse health effects. The biosurveillance life-cycle includes planning to establish critical information requirements, collection and management of data and information, analysis and interpretation of all sources of information, the dissemination of actionable findings, and then evaluation and further planning to reset the cycle. Biosurveillance is intended to allow a wide array of decision makers to put resources and capabilities in place to prevent and mitigate the adverse impact of all-hazards population health events of significant concern. The wide and thoughtful use of information technology as well as new digital information sources and analytic techniques, holds the potential to accelerate recognition of health threats and improve the accuracy of assessments. With greater availability of real-time digital health information, it is possible to create and maintain a comprehensive picture of the health of a jurisdiction or of the nation and detect aberrations in normal disease patterns faster and more accurately. Early warning seeks to identify hazards in the environment before they cause harm to people. Early detection establishes the presence of disease in human populations at the earliest time possible so that countermeasures will have the greatest likelihood of success. Event characterization supports decision making about targeted countermeasures and response actions. Ongoing biosurveillance activities provide information needed to assess the effectiveness of countermeasures so that they may be continued, modified, or stopped.

SYSTEM REQUIREMENTS

The purposes of a surveillance system establish the priority requirements of the system (13). Biosurveillance purposes, and hence requirements, adjust to the phases of an incident (Fig. 14–1).

In the absence of a specific threat, baseline surveillance is expected to run quietly in the background to detect hazards in the environment or any unusual pattern of disease or behavior that warrants further investigation. A system designed for early warning must balance the sensitivity required to detect significant conditions at the earliest possible time with the costs of comprehensive systems and the cost of repeated responses to alarms that prove to be nonsignificant. Collecting, managing, and analyzing these data responsibly consumes resources, so not all possible data sources can be examined routinely. Similarly, resources are necessary to respond and there are opportunity costs of not attending to other public health matters, so not all alerts can be investigated fully.

Once there is a credible threat, biosurveillance must transition into a heightened state of vigilance. This might result from a high-profile planned event (e.g., National Special Security Event), specific intelligence or recognition of a deliberate attack or highly communicable disease in another jurisdiction, or an impending natural disaster. In the presence of a threat, the predictive value positive (PVP) of an alert in a surveillance system is higher (because the prior probability is higher), and the costs of more complete biosurveillance and a lower response threshold are warranted by specific conditions. Response to a credible threat might include more frequent collection or analysis of routine surveillance data and expansion of the types and sources of data collected. Data elements collected within routine

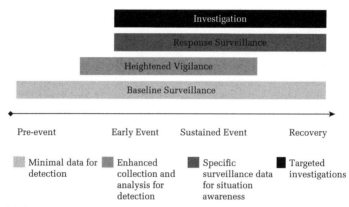

Figure 14–1 Data needs for phases of biosurveillance.

data sources can be expanded (e.g., collect radiology data from hospital sources that did not submit those data routinely), new systems of data collection can be implemented for a limited period, and additional analyses can be carried out with existing data sources (e.g., new queries of free-text emergency department visit chief complaints to monitor conditions not usually under surveillance).

Drop-in surveillance conducted at health facilities during high-profile political or sports events is an example of heightened vigilance for an elevated threat, as is surveillance for visits at health-care facilities after natural or man-made disasters or in refugee situations (*14*). As the availability of electronic health information exchange increases, such as jurisdictions where ESSENCE (*15*), NC-Detect (*16*), or BioSense (*17*) are in routine use and have high population coverage, manual drop-in surveillance will become unnecessary as long as the health-care system continues to function.

The third phase of biosurveillance occurs when an outbreak or other acute health event is detected in a community and the emergency response infrastructure transitions to a response mode. Biosurveillance is now looked to for insight on what is needed and where to meet the health needs of the population. In contrast to the traditional public health surveillance approach described throughout this textbook, in a biosurveillance context there is no clear demarcation between case-finding, descriptive epidemiology, more formal investigations, and collection in the field of data about the implementation and effectiveness of interventions. From a security and emergency response perspective, the entire information supply chain must be managed. Ongoing collection, analysis, and reporting of data must be integrated with targeted data collection to investigate specific aspects of an event so that there is a smooth transition between phases. A case-control study within the affected population might be necessary to identify sources of infection, modes of transmission, or risk factors that need to be addressed to protect health. Special studies or analyses may also be needed to assess effectiveness and modify control measures. The term *biosurveillance*, as used today, focuses on all health-related information needs irrespective of one-time or ongoing nature.

The outbreak phase can be divided further into two functional periods: early and sustained. During the early outbreak period, the high number of unknown factors drives a need to investigate through specific data collection efforts to clarify and characterize the risk by time, place, and person attributes. When many of the key factors of exposure and population risk are understood, the outbreak moves into a less dynamic phase of sustained management, and routine collection, analysis, and reporting regain importance to support the response. For example, once targeted laboratory and epidemiologic investigations have determined the characteristics of the agent (e.g., subtyping of the agent to identify cases or tests to establish the agent sensitivity to available antimicrobials), the laboratory and epidemiologic variables of interest can be narrowed. Finally, biosurveillance transitions again in the recovery phase where health data urgency lessens and monitoring for late effects and possible changes in the agent and its prevalence is necessary on top of routine surveillance.

Within limits, developing and improving public health surveillance for the wide range of conditions and events that do not rise to the level of emergencies or disasters is necessary to maximize the likelihood of early detection and characterization of an emergency. Skills and techniques learned and honed in responding to events such as widespread *Salmonella* contamination of food products or pandemic influenza will be extremely useful in a bioterrorism or other large event. Some of the capacity likely to be needed for large and rare events can, however, only be tested and trained on during exercises or simulations.

SYSTEM PERFORMANCE

Successful biosurveillance capability must achieve the following functional requirements:

- Case Detection—Discovery of a single instance of a disease. A front-line biosurveillance activity, it is typically accomplished as a byproduct of routine medical or veterinary care, laboratory work, or via an astute observer.
- Event Detection—Continuous analysis of frequency data to detect unusual patterns of conditions that may signal an outbreak or event. Clusters are commonly detected by people who are not formally part of the public health system but bring a potential outbreak to public health attention.
- Signal Validation—Validation and confirmation processes ensure that clusters, signals, and other such cues represent acute public health events that require a response. These might be labor and time intensive.
- Event Characterization—The range of processes that establish the causative agent, source, route of transmission, and other characteristics of an event. These characteristics guide effective response actions, including the treatment of victims and control measures to prevent additional cases.
- Notification and Communication—Processes, including notifiable disease reporting, that ensure that those with a need and authority to know have

the information (event details as well as response guidance) they need as soon as possible and that all users understand their responsibilities for use and management of the information.

- Quality Control and Improvement—Ensuring data management, including protecting the privacy and confidentiality of biosurveillance data and monitoring the system through performance measurement to confirm that objectives are being met.

The foundation of disease and outbreak detection is the reporting relationship between health-care providers (including physicians, laboratories, and hospitals) and the local public health system. The health-care system addresses all health hazards, it provides nationwide geographic coverage, and it produces the most precise health-related information for individuals that is subsequently aggregated and analyzed for population health situation awareness. Case-based surveillance is a cornerstone of public health surveillance. It is accomplished by implementing clear and consistent criteria and requirements for reporting cases. Critical sources of case-based surveillance include, but are not limited to, direct communications from clinicians and affected individuals, investigations by public health officials, and reports of laboratory data. In the near future, data contained in electronic health records may also contribute to case reporting. These sources of data can provide specific information about case-patients and/ or pathogens (e.g., genomic subtype data) that is often required to take public health action. In the United States, the state is the locus of public health authority and regulates what conditions must be reported and within what time intervals (18). The historical limitation of this method has been that it requires knowledge of the criteria for case reporting, recognition that the criteria have been met, and active effort to report this information by professionals outside the public health system. The quality of case reporting of notifiable diseases varies considerably by condition and by jurisdiction, and it tends to be incomplete and delayed (16), two attributes that seriously hamper detection and situation awareness for urgent threats.

Effective event detection depends on overcoming limitations of early case detection—particularly for new threats or presentations too common to put under case-based routine surveillance (e.g., viral respiratory illness). Statistical tools enhanced through software applications and visualization tools (e.g., mapping) have facilitated the regular, automated analysis and early identification of nascent disease clusters. Since 2001, these tools have become more sophisticated, expanding from process control algorithms for detecting temporal clusters to include other regression models, time-series methods, and scan statistics to add a geographic component to aberration detection (19). Near-real-time electronic laboratory reporting is being applied to improve timeliness and completeness of case ascertainment (18).

Case and event detection and characterization necessitate capabilities at the state and local levels where follow-up investigation can take place, domain knowledge can be incorporated for accurate interpretation, information quality feedback loops can be executed, and, ultimately, effective response actions can be taken. Close working relationships, resourcing, and training support are needed to ensure that a robust and effective biosurveillance capability resides at the state and local levels.

Across the previously described phases of an incident, the biosurveillance system attributes of greatest importance are extreme timeliness, sensitivity (i.e., the percentage of all events intended to be captured that are captured by the system), predictive value of positive and negative results (i.e., the likelihood that a positive or negative system result is correct), and the integration of information across response organizations and disciplines to improve the timeliness and quality of response. There is generally a tradeoff among timeliness, sensitivity, and PVP in the performance of any one system. Improving one of these attributes usually requires compromises in one or both of the others. It is possible to improve all three at once by modifying fundamental system characteristics—for example, by improving the inherent timeliness of data transmission, improving the quality of the data collected (adding certain lab results to chief complaint data from emergency departments or incorporating results of improved rapid bedside or office testing), or improving the algorithms used to detect anomalies.

DATA SOURCES

Laboratory-based testing and surveillance provide a critical foundation for effective biosurveillance practice. The value of laboratory information lies in its diagnostic specificity and key role in identifying cases and events of public health significance. The intent of electronic reporting of positive or abnormal results from laboratories to epidemiology services is to improve timeliness, accuracy, completeness, and availability of laboratory data for use by those who need the information for investigation and decision-making. Electronic data transfer from clinical laboratories to public health has been shown to improve the timeliness of event detection and increase the number of reports received (20). Analysis of surveillance data in Florida has shown that implementing electronic laboratory results reporting from clinical laboratories to public health authorities would make a substantial difference for salmonellosis, shigellosis, and hepatitis A although it would yield little if any improvement in timeliness of case reports of meningococcal disease, because cases currently are often reported before laboratory results are reported out (21).

Traditional surveillance picks up cases of diseases of public health significance earlier when cases are reported on clinical suspicion. Some states (e.g., Florida) have clarified requirements for clinicians and laboratories to immediately report cases of certain high-priority diseases (e.g., those resulting from potential bioterrorism agents) whenever they are suspected, without waiting for a final diagnosis (22). Other states have required laboratories to make an immediate telephonic or electronic case report or to consult the state public health laboratory immediately when an order or specimen for selected priority diseases is received (e.g., California, Florida) (23). Additionally, exposure surveillance and registries might be implemented to track long-term health effects following potentially toxic exposures (24).

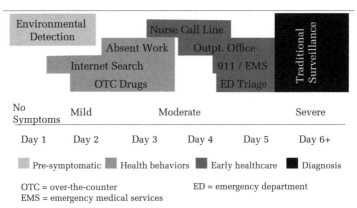

Figure 14–2 Stylized detection timeline by data type. OTC, over-the-counter; EMS, emergency medical services; ED, emergency department.

Expanding data types beyond those for traditional case-based surveillance might support earlier detection and more complete situation awareness of disease outbreaks but requires further evaluation. Ease of access through electronic tools has opened public health surveillance to a diversity of clinical, commercial, and public data sources, but not all are inherently useful. Experience has demonstrated that types of data closest to clinical diagnosis (e.g., laboratory data or office visits for respiratory disease) are more specific and therefore have higher predictive value than those less directly linked to health events (e.g., absenteeism, Internet behavior, or purchase behaviors) (25). These latter health-related data tend to come with less specificity and less reliability of positive and negative findings but might be earlier indicators of disease than health-care markers. Data removed from clinical diagnosis include environmental tests for exposure to threat agents; health-related behaviors such as product purchases, absenteeism, and health queries; and early clinical indicators such as diagnostic test orders and results, and presenting complaints and preliminary diagnoses (Fig. 14–2).

Surveillance data have long been collected using a wide range of media (paper, voice, electronic) with much of the information available in free-form text or other unstructured formats (e.g., images) that can be interpreted by a person but not readily manipulated by a computer. Outbreaks are detected by clinicians, teachers, school nurses, family members, people who attended group events like weddings or restaurant meals, nursing home staff, and a wide variety of ordinary citizens. Unstructured data are pieces of information that are not organized or integrated in a database structure designed for quantitative analyses. As technology has progressed and as more information is recorded onto digital media, it is possible to build a more comprehensive picture of health situation awareness. Health information can be found in unstructured data throughout public health and health-care organizations. Key pieces of information that would provide context for a case report (such as the name of a restaurant) might lie in an epidemiology investigator's phone call and case notes, e-mails sharing information about consultations or investigations, outbreak listings, posts to a state-level health alert

network, consumer complaint logs, surveillance system reports, or other potentially readable media that are not yet readily searchable or computer-synthesized.
Similarly valuable information might reside in emergency department triage
nurse notes or free-text chief complaints or in the narrative portions of electronic
medical records or poison control center data systems.

Unstructured data found in the private sector and in Internet-based sources can
be used to augment public health and health care information. Resources such as
the Global Public Health Intelligence Network (GPHIN) (26) that continuously
search global news media sources and health and science websites give health-
care professionals additional insights into incidents of relevance in their community and around the world. This system gathers information in nine languages 24
hours per day, 7 days per week. Many public health workers subscribe to services
that monitor U.S. or state-level media for items of public health interest. Rigorous
research and experience are needed to develop this capability, as well as additional technologies, tools, and skilled analysts to validate and apply the findings.

The ability to collect and integrate diverse biosurveillance data rapidly, reliably, and securely and to share health-related information among public health,
health-care, and other response entities is valued particularly in the context of
urgency and health security. Because the responsibility for public health emergency response is shared across levels of government and professional practice,
and across scientific disciplines, the timely exchange of reliable and actionable
information is essential. Advances in technology and epidemiologic science offer
the potential to support situation awareness and communication networks that
lead to earlier awareness of hazards and events, real-time monitoring as events
unfold, enhanced connectivity to the evidence, and greater access to knowledgeable public health and health-care professionals to reduce impacts. The integration
or fusion of health-relevant information includes the methods, tools, and analytic
capabilities of the workforce to pull together different information resources and
create analytic synergy for actionable health information.

CHALLENGES

Complex health emergencies occur within a system of community services.
Public health practitioners must plan and respond effectively as part of a multidisciplinary, multipurpose team. Biosurveillance represents a new health information paradigm for public health that seeks to integrate and efficiently manage
urgent health and health-related data and information across a range of applications over the course of an emergency for the purpose of timely and accurate population health situation awareness. The following challenges serve as a reminder
of the principles that must be addressed thoughtfully to achieve effective systems
of biosurveillance.

- *Clarity of Purpose*: Successful surveillance systems have clear objectives and are designed to meet those objectives (27). If clarity of purpose
  is not maintained, there is a tendency to collect more information than

necessary and a concomitant degradation in the quality of and appropriate use of the data. Clarity of purpose among system operators and users can enhance quality improvement and confidence about the value of the biosurveillance endeavor.

- *Value.* Sustained commitments to biosurveillance require return on investment. Authoritative consultation with public health on matters that affect individual patient care can support improved reporting quality. Assuring that data collected come back in a time and form for use in the clinical environment can also support improvement in timeliness and quality of those data. Similarly, national situation awareness must be of value to state and local public health to sustain the efforts involved in producing national biosurveillance.

- *Completeness*: Sensitivity for detection of public health emergencies is highly reliant on thorough coverage of the population and completeness of reporting. The greater the penetration of biosurveillance systems into a community, the more completely the data will represent the health of the community and the more quickly and completely outbreaks will be detected and tracked. Redundancies in systems, as long as recognized and accounted for, can minimize the impact of reporting gaps in individual systems.

- *Collection Burden*: Workload requirements on data providers are a significant impediment to timeliness and quality. Reporting and collection should be automated wherever possible. Data that are not needed should not be collected. Quality of data entered into automated systems also depends on data providers (e.g., clinicians and laboratories) appreciating the uses of the data and their value.

- *System Architecture*: The structure and management of data need to be planned. Flexibility must be prioritized to assure maximal opportunity to explore and learn from integrated information resources. Mechanisms to enhance the safe and effective use of surveillance repositories (e.g., dedicated staff assigned at clinical levels to analyze data for decisions made there) should be considered. Federated system architectures can allow partners in a surveillance enterprise to view data derived from each other's systems in ways that are transparent to the users without needing to move the data to a new physical location. Such systems still need explicit agreements among the partners as to how much detail they will make accessible and to whom and how partners may act on or make public statements about data that came from other partners.

- *Legal and Ethical Issues*: The state is the locus of public health authority in the United States and operates within a delicate balance between individual privacy and collective good. Although advances in information technology make it possible to more efficiently leverage nationwide biosurveillance data assets and analytic capabilities, the privacy contract that public health agencies have with their populations (as reflected in state laws and the public's trust) must be protected.

- *Role Delegation*: Public health actions happen at the local level and are highly dependent on relationships nurtured at the local level. Improved availability of biosurveillance data across levels of government will require explicit delineation of roles and responsibilities to assure that public health authorities are being exerted at the appropriate levels. Person-level information is necessary for guiding local public health actions, but each level of government removed from the local level usually requires less personal detail and less sensitive data. If increased availability of data at higher levels of government or outside government results in interpretations independent of the local context, then actions inconsistent with local intentions can be taken that are wasteful or can undermine the public health response system.

- *Analytic Discipline*: Quality data and effective notification routines must be matched with analytic rigor. Robust automated analysis routines must be complemented by quality epidemiologic analyses to validate and interpret signals and respond appropriately. Additionally, in times of heightened threat, customized supplemental analyses will be necessary. Data should be analyzed and interpreted routinely and frequently by time, place, and person. Furthermore, the analysis and interpretation should be integrated across all the systems with relevant data. Achieving this is highly dependent on human integrative skills.

- *Distributed Analysis*: In most existing surveillance systems, considerable noise is removed from case and event reports before they are passed to the federal level. Transmission of case data and other surveillance data streams can be faster if local- and state-level validation and data cleaning are bypassed, but analysts at the national level will then have data of lower quality and reliability. The increase in timeliness might not compensate for the loss of quality and local contextual knowledge. A distributed analysis model allows complementary roles: local users understanding local context and state and national users seeing larger patterns.

- *Response Discipline*: By design, more robust biosurveillance will demand greater investment in public health investigation to validate and respond to incidents that would not otherwise have been discerned by current systems. Disciplined routines of investigation and continuously adapting detection algorithms will be needed to minimize the negative impact on public health resources. Increasing the accessibility of quality health information in queryable electronic format will improve the efficiency of investigations as well.

- *Personal Relationships*: Technology, standard operating procedures, and laws all have a role in biosurveillance, but the success of the effort hinges on personal relationships. Without trust and mutual value, technical and legal impediments will arise to lessen the quality and ultimately the utility of the data collected. Those who make decisions based on biosurveillance must have trust and confidence in the systems producing it. Personal relationships around the collection and interpretation of data should be valued and supported, rather than depending strictly on technology, rules, and laws.

- *Evaluation*: Limited direct evidence has been published to establish the effectiveness of enhanced surveillance systems for prospective early detection of all but the largest seasonal outbreaks (e.g., influenza and viral gastroenteritis) (*28*). The role of biosurveillance in providing situation awareness during events is also evolving. These gaps in our knowledge reinforce the importance of systematic ongoing evaluation of these emergency preparedness surveillance systems and the need to share results through the peer reviewed biomedical literature (*29*).

CONCLUSIONS

Containing the spread of disease in an intensely interconnected world requires vigilance for signs of an outbreak, rapid validation of its presence, and swift characterization so that resources and response strategies can be employed effectively. Greater information sharing and strengthened collaborations among public health, health-care, animal, plant, and environmental health communities along with partnerships with private sector organizations addressing common goals will produce more informed situation awareness to prevent, protect, and mitigate health threats and hazards.

More robust biosurveillance will arise from a combination of improved reporting of notifiable disease cases, lab results, and suspicious clinical presentations; improved analysis and decision-support tools; and expanded types of data that improve timeliness and population coverage. Biosurveillance must be flexible as the requirements transition from baseline monitoring through elevated threat levels and phases of event response and recovery. A layered approach that scales to the circumstances is most likely to align with resources and stakeholder support.

Active evaluation is needed as biosurveillance evolves and we explore new tools and data sources. We must capture the lessons of the best systems to understand what architecture and data elements yield most utility. Evaluation might show that some approaches have limited usefulness or none at all. Evaluation guidance is increasing, but more experience must be shared in a systematic fashion from state and local public health departments (*30*).

Biosurveillance has costs, including the direct cost of initiating and running the system; the costs of storing, analyzing, and responding to the data; potential costs to privacy and liability from misuse or disclosure; and opportunity costs. More biosurveillance is not always better. Careful planning and reflection are needed in concert with social norms at all levels of government to establish the most appropriate biosurveillance strategy.

REFERENCES

1. Lederberg J, Shope RE, Oaks SC Jr, eds. Institute of Medicine. *Emerging Infections: Microbial Threats to Health in the United States.* Washington, DC: National Academy Press; 1992.
2. Homeland Security Presidential Directive 10 (HSPD-10). National Security Presidential Directive 33 (NSPD-33). *Biodefense for the 21st Century.* Washington, DC: The White House; 2004. http://www.whitehouse.gov/homeland/20040430.html Accessed January 15, 2009.

3. Knobler S, Mahmoud A, Lemon S, Pray L, eds. Institute of Medicine. The Impact of Globalization on Infectious Disease Emergence and Control: Exploring the Consequences and Opportunities: Workshop Summary. National Academy Press. Washington, DC: 2006. http://www.nap.edu/catalog.php?record_id=11588#toc Accessed January 15, 2009.

4. Shelley L. The globalization of crime and terrorism. eJournal USA: Global Issues. 2006; 11(1):42–45. http://www.america.gov/publications/ejournalusa.html#globalization. Accessed January 15, 2009.

5. Kukafka R, Ancker JS, Chan C, et al. Redesigning electronic health record systems to support public health. *J Biomed Informat* 2007;40(4):398–409.

6. Homeland Security Presidential Directive/HSPD-21. Washington, DC: The White House; October 18, 2007. http://www.whitehouse.gov/news/releases/2007/10/20071018-10.html. Accessed January 15, 2009.

7. The Pandemic and All-Hazards Preparedness Act of 2006 (PL 109-417), 120 Stat. 2831 (2006).

8. Endsley MR. Design and evaluation for situation awareness enhancement. In: *Proceedings of the Human Factors Society 32 Annual Meeting.* Santa Monica, CA: Human Factors Society, 1988:97–101.

9. Wagner MM. Chapter 1: Introduction. In: Wagner MM, Moore AW, Aryel RM, eds., *Handbook of Biosurveillance.* Boston, MA: Elsevier Academic Press; 2006: 3–12.

10. Sosin DM. Syndromic surveillance: the case for skillful investment. *Biosecurity Bioterrorism: Biodefense Strategy, Practice, Science* 2003;1(4):247–253.

11. Paquet C, Coulombier D, Kaiser R, Ciotti M. Epidemic intelligence: a new framework for strengthening disease surveillance in Europe. *Eurosurveillance* 2006;11(12):212–214.

12. Langmuir AD, Andrews JM. Biological warfare defense. 2. The Epidemic Intelligence Service of the Communicable Disease Center. *Am J Pub Health* 1952;42(3):235–238.

13. Centers for Disease Control and Prevention. Updated guidelines for evaluating public health surveillance systems: recommendations from the Guidelines Working Group. *MMWR* 2001;50(No. RR-13).

14. Centers for Disease Control and Prevention. Syndromic Surveillance for Bioterrorism Following the Attacks on the World Trade Center—New York City, 2001. MMWR 2002;51(Special Issue): 13–15. http://www.cdc.gov/mmwr/PDF/wk/mm51sp.pdf. Accessed January 15, 2009.

15. Lombardo JS, Burkom H, Pavlin J. ESSENCE II and the Framework for Evaluating Syndromic Surveillance Systems. In: Syndromic Surveillance: Reports from a National Conference, 2003. *MMWR* 2004;53(Suppl):159–165. http://www.cdc.gov/mmwr/pdf/wk/mm53su01.pdf. Accessed January 15, 2009.

16. http://www.ncdetect.org/NC_DETECT_summary.pdf. Accessed January 15, 2009.

17. Bradley CA, Rolka H, Walker D, Loonsk J. BioSense: Implementation of a National Early Event Detection and Situational Awareness System. In: Syndromic Surveillance: Reports from a National Conference, 2004. *MMWR* 2005;54(Suppl):11–19. http://www.cdc.gov/mmwr/pdf/wk/mm54su01.pdf. Accessed January 15, 2009.

18. Birkhead GS, Maylahn CM. State and local public health surveillance. In: Teutsch SM, Churchill RE, eds. *Principles and Practice of Public Health Surveillance.* New York, NY: Oxford University Press; 2000:253–286.

19. Farrington P, Andrews N. Outbreak detection: Application to infectious disease surveillance. In: Brookmeyer R, Stroup DF, eds. *Monitoring the Health of Populations.* New York: Oxford University Press; 2004:203–231.

20. Effler P, Ching-Lee M, Bogard A, Ieong MC, Nekomoto T, Jernigan D. Statewide system of electronic notifiable disease reporting from clinical laboratories: comparing automated reporting with conventional methods. *JAMA* 1999;282(19):1845–1850.

21. Kite-Powell A, Hamilton JJ, Hopkins RS, DePasquale JM. Potential effects of electronic laboratory reporting on improving timeliness of infectious disease notification—Florida, 2002–2006. *MMWR* 2008;57:1325–1328.

22. Florida Administrative Code 64D-3.029(2).

23. Florida Administrative Code 64D-3.031(2). California Administrative Code title 17, sections 2505(j), 2551, and 2614.

24. Brackbill RM, Thorpe LE, DiGrande L, *et al.* Surveillance for World Trade Center disaster health effects among survivors of collapsed and damaged buildings. In: Surveillance Summaries, April 7, 2006, *MMWR* 2006;55(SS-2):1–18.

25. Buckeridge DL. Outbreak detection through automated surveillance: a review of the determinants of detection. *J Biomed Informat* 2007;40(4):370–379.

26. Mykhalovskiy E, Weir L. The Global Public Health Intelligence Network and early warning outbreak detection: a Canadian contribution to global public health. *Can J Pub Health* 2006;97(1):42–44.

27. Sosin DM, Hopkins RS. Monitoring disease and risk factors: surveillance. In: Pencheon D, Guest C, Meltzer D, Gray JAM, eds. *Oxford Handbook of Public Health Practice.* Oxford, UK: Oxford University Press; 2006:112–118.

28. Beuhler JW, Sosin DM, Platt R. Evaluation of surveillance systems for early epidemic detection. In: M'ikantha N, de Valk H, Lynfield R, Van Beneden CA, eds. *Infectious Disease Surveillance.* London, UK: Blackwell Publishing; 2007:432–442.

29. Centers for Disease Control and Prevention. Framework for evaluating public health surveillance systems for early detection of outbreaks; recommendations from the CDC Working Group. *MMWR* 2004;53(No. RR-5):1–13.

30. Watkins RE, Eagleson S, Hall RG, Dailey L, Plant AJ. Approaches to the evaluation of outbreak detection methods. *BMC Public Health* 2006; 6: 263. http://www.pubmedcentral.gov/picrender.fcgi?tool=pmcentrez&blobtype=pdf&artid=1626088. Accessed January 15, 2009.

15

Healthcare Quality and Safety
The Monitoring of Administrative Information Systems and the Interface with Public Health Surveillance

JAMES F. MURRAY AND CHESLEY RICHARDS

INTRODUCTION

Public health surveillance is the ongoing systematic collection, analysis, and interpretation of health-related data essential to the planning, implementation, and evaluation of public health practice, closely integrated with the timely dissemination of these data to those who need to know with an application to prevention and control. The monitoring of health care quality is a rapidly expanding and evolving discipline that faces significant challenges but also tremendous potential for improving the public's health. Increasingly, a variety of government and private sector organizations collect and use data on health care quality to accomplish aims and with methods similar to those of public health surveillance. In this chapter, a discussion of current methods for monitoring of health care quality that has existed primarily among organizations focused on clinical care is followed by examples of evolving public health surveillance efforts to guide patient safety initiatives. Although monitoring for health care quality and surveillance for patient safety have not been traditional foci for public health agencies and practitioners, public health departments increasingly will be called on to expand these surveillance activities; to articulate which activities—including types of data acquisition and analyses—qualify to operate with the latitude accorded by legislation to public health surveillance; and to become part of the joint enterprise of many organizations accountable for the quality and safety of health-care services delivered to populations within their jurisdictions.

HOW IS HEALTH CARE QUALITY DEFINED?

Ernest Codman is credited with introducing a concern on health care quality by an introspective assessment of surgical practice at Massachusetts General Hospital (*1,2*). Various definitions and measurements of quality were proposed in the ensuing years. Today, a commonly cited definition of quality comes from the Institute of Medicine (IOM):

> "Quality of care is the degree to which health services for individuals and populations increase the likelihood of desired health outcomes and are consistent with current professional knowledge. (*3*)"

Drawing on work since Codman, Avedis Donabedian produced an exhaustive treatise on health care quality with definitions, a taxonomy, and a set of examples that described and categorized the previous work on the issue (*4–6*). Donabedian institutionalized three fundamental concepts for measuring quality: structure, process, and outcomes.

Structure addresses the question "How is the care organized?" A few examples the components of "structure" include:

- the credentials of the providers based on their training and experience;
- the capital resources available for providing care (e.g., equipment within surgical suites; availability of an electronic medical record or other health information technology); and
- access (e.g., institutional hours of availability and call centers).

Process answers the question "What actions or activities were taken, and how were they taken?" Examples of attributes of "process" include:

- clinical processes (e.g., screening for breast cancer, immunization rates, and performing lab tests); and
- administrative processes (e.g., communication, customer service, and making appointments).

Finally, recent efforts have put a large emphasis on achieving outcomes: "What are the impacts and results of the care provided"? Outcomes are complex and the most difficult to measure. Examples are:

- long-term outcomes such as mortality, morbidity, and functional or health status of the population. (These are defined as long term because they often are not exhibited or measurable until some time after the delivery of relevant care.); and
- intermediate outcomes that assess whether biomarkers such as lipid levels and blood pressure are within the limits recommended by clinical guidelines. (These measures are good but imperfect predictors of the long term outcomes above.)

The basic concepts captured by Donabedian have been complemented and extended by the IOM. In 2001, the IOM offered the following as the important constructs for measuring quality (*7*):

- safe: avoiding injuries to patients from the care that is intended to help them;
- effective: providing services based on scientific knowledge to all who could benefit, and refraining from providing services to those not likely to benefit;

- patient-centered: providing care that is respectful of and responsive to individual patient preferences, needs, and values;
- timely: reducing waits and sometimes harmful delays for both those who receive and those who give care;
- efficient: avoiding waste, including waste of equipment, supplies, ideas, and energy; and
- equitable: providing care that does not vary in quality because of personal characteristics.

Within the last 20 years the efforts to define and measure quality have been connected to quality improvement techniques pioneered in the service and manufacturing sectors. This joining of health care with industrial quality demonstrated that the health care quality can be measured and improved using a systems approach. Thus, quality measurement has evolved from an analytical exercise to an increasing catalyst for change.

The definition and measurement of quality continue to evolve. Another important concept has been to define and measure quality as underuse, misuse, or overuse. Underuse occurs when necessary and appropriate care is not provided in all of the situations where it is indicated. An example of underuse would be immunization or screening (e.g., lab tests in diabetics for cholesterol and HgA1C) that fall below acceptable rates in a population. The concept of misuse is when care is given that is inappropriate or given in an incorrect manner. Examples would be unnecessary lab tests or poor medication management where inappropriate drugs are prescribed. Finally, the concept of overuse implies more utilization that optimal. Examples include necessary lab tests performed more frequently than required or medication given when it is unnecessary.

WHO IS HELD ACCOUNTABLE FOR QUALITY?

Over the past five decades, accountability for health care quality has mirrored the evolution of quality measurement in the United States. In the 1950s, the principal foci of accountability for and measurement of quality were hospitals and other institutions, such as nursing homes, professional societies, state professional licensing agencies, with leadership especially from selected innovative health plans, such as Kaiser Health Plan on the West Coast and HIP in New York City. During the 1980s, with the rise of health maintenance organizations and managed care, health plans came under scrutiny and began to be held accountable for quality. Current efforts have shifted to physicians, who are the principal agents for deciding the allocation of medical services to patients and who perform most of the high cost and high medical impact procedures, such as surgery, endoscopy, and endovascular procedures. Most recently, system issues such as health-care-associated infections or medical product safety have become an accountability focus in public health.

STANDARDIZATION AND COLLABORATION ON QUALITY MEASURES

During the 1990s there was an unprecedented growth in the development and application of quality measures. This came from not only from the National Committee on Quality Assurance (NCQA) and the Joint Commission on Accreditation of Hospitals, but many health plans, medical professional societies, advocacy groups (such as the American Heart Association), and academic researchers undertook the development and implementation of quality measures. This plethora of measures, many assessing similar concepts and constructs, created a situation where it was impossible to make comparisons because of the "apples and oranges" nature of the quality measures. This dramatically impeded decisions on who provided the best quality as well as effective actions to improve quality. To address this issue an IOM panel released a report entitled "Performance Measurement: Accelerating Improvement" (8). It stated:

> The committee fully recognizes that many public- and private-sector initiatives have made substantial progress in developing, implementing, and reporting on measures of provider performance. These efforts have yielded a laudable array of assets for performance measurement. However, the committee believes a well-functioning national system that can meet the need for performance measurement and reporting is unlikely to emerge from current voluntary, consensus-based efforts, which are often fragmented and lack a consistent connection to explicit, overarching national goals for healthcare improvement. In short, while recent efforts offer some promise, the committee believes a bolder national initiative is required.
>
> The current approach to quality measurement in the United States is unlikely to evolve on its own into an effective national system for performance measurement and reporting...

The IOM called on Congress for the establishment of a "National Quality Coordination Board" (NQCB) to address these issues. To avoid government involvement and potential regulations, a "voluntary" consensus emerged that the National Quality Forum (NQF) would serve the role of the proposed NQCB. The NQF is a private, not-for-profit organization created to develop and implement a national strategy for health care quality measurement and reporting (9). The mission of the NQF is to improve the U.S. health-care system through the endorsement of consensus-based national standards for measurement. This is realized by the public reporting of health-care performance data that provides meaningful information about whether care is safe, timely, beneficial, patient-centered, equitable, and efficient. Their largest and most powerful stakeholder is the Centers for Medicare and Medicaid Services (CMS), which gives NQF considerable influence.

CMS plays a leading role in the development, endorsement, and standardization of quality measures (10). CMS is the single largest insurer in the country in terms of both population covered and expenditures. Their various quality initiatives touch every aspect of the U.S. health-care system and focus on publicly reporting quality measures for health plans, physicians, nursing homes, home health agencies, hospitals, and kidney dialysis facilities.

WHO PERFORMS QUALITY MEASUREMENT?

The Joint Commission on Accreditation of Hospitals was founded in 1951 by the American College of Physicians, the American Hospital Association, the American Medical Association , and the Canadian Medical Association (11). It was given the mission to measure health care quality—specifically the quality of care provided by hospitals—and to accredit those deemed worthy. The demand for this accreditation coincided with the rise of health-care insurance. Purchasers asked, "How can I ensure that I am purchasing good care?" This same question remains a catalyst in the evolution of quality measurement.

The NCQA is a nonprofit organization created to measure the quality of HMO and other managed care plans (12). NCQA was formed in 1979 by the HMO industry and housed in their trade organization until it became independent in 1990. The spin-off of the NCQA was driven by purchasers with the same question of value. Managed care offered an attractive cost proposal, but the question of quality persisted: how could purchasers ensure that they were getting good quality? The NCQA provided two important products and services. The first was the accreditation of managed care health plans akin to what the Joint Commission did for hospitals. NCQA review was and still is voluntary, but plans seek accreditation because of the requirement by larger purchasers. The second important product of the NCQA was an independent set of quality measures known as the Health Plan Effectiveness and Data Information Set (HEDIS). HEDIS is a set of standardized performance measures designed to give purchasers and consumers information to compare the quality of managed health-care plans. The quality measures in HEDIS are related to many significant public health issues such as cancer, heart disease, smoking, asthma, and diabetes. HEDIS includes a standardized survey of consumers' experiences knows as the Consumer Assessment of Health Plan Satisfaction (CAHPS). CAHPS evaluates plan performance in areas such as customer service, access to care, and claims processing. Currently, HEDIS is evolving to be applicable to physicians' groups and to provide the same quality measures as for health plans.

A common feature between government and private sector efforts in quality measurement and public health surveillance is the dissemination of data to a variety of stakeholders with a focus on affecting improvements in health. In quality measurement efforts, however, the focus has been on measuring and improving the quality of health care with an expected subsequent improvement in health among patients in health plans or receiving care by health-care providers. Public health surveillance, on the other hand, has traditionally focused on measuring and tracking disease as a means of selecting and targeting prevention interventions most effectively, some of which might be related to improvements in the quality of health-care services, such as in the avoidance of health-care-associated infections (HAIs).

WHO USES HEALTH CARE QUALITY DATA?

Purchasers

Purchasers, because of their fiduciary responsibility for the selection and management of health-care benefits for their employees and retirees, are a major catalyst for and supporter of quality measurement and improvement. Purchasers can be divided into two main categories: private and public (i.e., governmental). Their interests and efforts are closely aligned but not identical.

For private purchasers, such as employers, a growing number are developing health benefit management strategies based on value—that is, a combination of quality and cost. Many large employers require NCQA accreditation and HEDIS information as a condition for offering a managed care plan to employees (13,14). In addition, employers often provide "healthcare report cards," usually based on HEDIS, to help their employees in their selection of a health plan or physician (15).

In addition to their individual efforts, employers have combined forces within coalitions to increase their leverage to measure and improve quality. Through strength in numbers, coalitions demand the reporting of quality measures and demonstrable improvements on quality in their contracts with plans and providers. They use a variety of methods that often incorporate the Joint Commission and NCQA accreditation and certification as well as NQF endorsed measures. Some notable examples of leading coalitions are the New York Business Group on Health, the Buyers Health Care Action Group in Minnesota, and the Pacific Business Group on Health. One example of a purchaser collaborative effort used by these coalitions is a tool called eValue8. eValue8 was developed by the National Business Coalition on Health as a standardized "request for information" that collects and scores quality information for the use of value-based purchasing. Coalitions not only use such information when deciding which plans to offer to their employees but also report the information to their employees.

The most notable governmental user is CMS. CMS has initiated a number of programs that set precedents and standards for how quality measure can be used to improve quality, addressing various clinical settings within the health-care system (16). They are:

- Nursing Home Quality Initiative (2002): reporting of post-acute and chronic care quality measures within nursing homes;
- Home Health Quality Initiative (2003): reporting of quality measures relating to improvements in patient functionality;
- Hospital Quality Initiative (2003): voluntary reporting of a starter set of 10 hospital quality measures. (The Medicare Modernization Act provided a financial incentive for hospitals to report these measures, and the Deficit Reduction Act of 2005 expanded the set of measures and increased the amount of the financial incentive.);
- End-Stage Renal Disease Quality Initiative (2004): measures of quality for dialysis facilities; and
- Physician-Focused Quality Initiative (2004): reporting of measures of the quality of ambulatory care (e.g., the quality of care for chronic diseases and

preventive services provided in doctors' offices), and supporting the physicians' adoption and effective use of information technology to collect the necessary data and report the measures. (The providers receive a premium incentive on their Medicare reimbursement for reporting these measures. There is currently no effort to assess or act on the actual results though it was included in recent Medicare legislation. It is been considered an effective start to engaging physicians in the measurement and reporting of quality.)

These CMS initiatives have established a strong foundation and platform for quality measurement and have significantly increased the interest and efforts to measure quality in all part of the U.S. system.

Building on these initiatives, CMS is exploring the potential of Pay-For-Performance (P4P) programs as a catalyst to improving the quality of care within Medicare (17). P4P is the concept of financial rewarding providers and institutions for achieving certain thresholds of quality on a variety of measures. P4P programs are being implemented in hospitals, physician groups, health plans, and nursing homes. These programs are testing a wide variety of measures as well as structures and processes for the financial rewards. For example, the Physician Quality Reporting Initiative discussed previously is one of the CMS P4P program. Physicians who successfully report a set of quality measures from July 1 to December 31, 2007, can earn a bonus payment equal to 1.5% of total their total allowed Medicare charges for the 6-month period.

Health Plans

It is now commonly accepted that health plans will both collect and act on assessments of the quality of care being delivered by the plan and by the providers within the plan. In a recent survey of 252 HMOs covering 91% of all HMO enrollees, greater than 90% of the plans collected and acted on quality information using seven HEDIS measures (11). The assessments were: (1) Did the plan collect data on a measure?; (2) Did they target the measure for quality improvement programs; and (3) Did they demonstrate improvement on the measure over time (Table 15–1). In the Landon study, the collection of quality measurement data was good (i.e., ranged from 92.1% to 99%), but the efforts to target the measure for quality improvement and achieving improvement over time were somewhat less effective. However, the study generally shows that quality measures have been powerful incentives and catalysts for performance-improvement programs (18). This shows that the Deming principle of "that which gets measured gets managed" holds true.

Providers

Physicians are increasingly using quality of measures to improve care. The Landon study (18) documented significant effort to collect quality information and make improvements at the level of the individual physician. The study assessed four actions being taken by the health plans at the physician level: (1) Are they collecting quality data at the physician level?; (2) Are they providing feedback to the

Table 15–1 HMO Data Collection on Quality Measures in 252 U.S. Health Maintenance Organizations in 2005 *(18)*

Measure	% HMOs that collect data	% HMOs targeting measure for improvement	% HMOs demonstrating improvement in measure
Patient satisfaction	99.2	92.6	74.0
Breast cancer screening	98.3	93.0	45.5
Antidepressant medication management	91.3	84.3	47.5
Hypertension control	92.1	68.6	58.3
Appropriate use of asthma medications	95.0	87.6	81.4
Diabetes care	98.8	97.5	93.0
Cholesterol management	92.1	83.1	73.1

physicians on their performance?; *(3)* Are the using they results in a P4P to reward the physicians for good quality; and *(4)* Are the plans making the data publicly available through the use of report cards? (*See* Table 15–2.)

Efforts at the physician level are still in the early stages of acceptance and use; they were not at the same level as the health plans. However, the ultimate success for both plans and physicians requires shared accountability with a systemic view and approach to the measurement and improvement of quality. The accountability and ability of the health plan to improve quality on its own is limited. Without shared accountability and joint efforts between plans and providers to improve care, neither will be able to achieve their full potential to improve the quality of care.

Consumers

Studies have shown that consumers will use the following information when selecting a health plan *(19–21)*:

- quality,
- cost to the consumer,
- benefit packages (i.e., covered services) offered to the member,
- availability of preferred physicians, and
- administrative requirements of the health plan (i.e., the health plan's policies and procedures on what you have to do to get the care you need).

The goal is to allow individuals to select the best health plan based on the above criteria. What has been lacking is an incentive to drive consumer use of this information. There are recent efforts to make consumers an active part of the health-care decisions by the introduction of "Consumer-Directed Health Plans" that give individuals more autonomy and responsibility for the care they seek. The most common structure of such plans is coverage with a high deductible

Table 15–2 Health Plan Quality Data on Physician Performance in 252 U.S. Health Maintenance Organizations in 2005 (*18*)

Measure	% Health plans collecting data on the measure	% Health plans providing feedback	% Health plans using pay for performance	% Health plans using physician report cards
Patient satisfaction	56.2	47.1	27.3	17.8
Breast cancer screening	77.7	67.4	35.1	23.6
Antidepressant medication management	53.7	38.4	17.4	13.6
Hypertension control	50.4	37.6	14.5	12.8
Appropriate use of asthma medications	79.8	68.6	33.1	21.5
Diabetes care	81.4	72.3	40.5	25.2
Cholesterol management	68.2	58.3	28.9	19.0

(e.g., $2000) that is offset partially by the availability of a spending account (i.e., a pool of money under the control of the person or family that covers some or all of the deductible). The goal is to make consumers more cost and quality-sensitive because they now have a greater stake in what they purchase and from whom they purchase. As a result, it is expected that the consumer will be driven to seek and use the type of information mentioned above.

MEASURING QUALITY FOR PREVENTIVE, ACUTE, AND CHRONIC CARE

HEDIS is an example of how quality can be measured across the domains of preventive, acute, and chronic care in the acute care setting. The 2008 reporting year list of measures for the HEDIS "Effectiveness of Care" illustrate several important points (Table 15–3). HEDIS assesses different quality measures, using the health plan as the unit of accountability. There are differences in accountability as not all plan types are held accountable for all measures. The decision on accountability is made, in part, based on the demographics contained within that plan type. For example, Medicare plans are not held accountable for childhood quality measures. Commercial and Medicaid plans are not held accountable for measures that are targeted for the elderly under a Medicare plan. The HEDIS measures were developed for the acute care setting. To assign accountability, the responsible party has to have a sufficient degree of control and responsibility for the target measures and population within that setting. When this occurs, there is an implicit joint accountability. The beta-blocker measure is an example where the

Table 15–3 List of HEDIS Measures and Applicability to Alternative Financing Plans, United States, 2008

HEDIS 2008 Measures	*Applicable to*			
Effectiveness of care measures	*Medicaid*	*HMO/ POS plans*	*Medicare*	*Preferred provider org. plans*
Childhood immunization status	X	X		X
Adolescent immunization status	X	X		X
Appropriate treatment for children with upper respiratory infection	X	X		X
Appropriate testing for children with pharyngitis	X	X		X

HEDIS 2007 measures	*Applicable to*			
Effectiveness of care measures	*Medicaid*	*HMO/ POS plans*	*Medicare*	*Preferred provider org. plans*
Inappropriate antibiotic treatment for adults with acute bronchitis	X	X		X
Colorectal cancer screening			X	X
Breast cancer screening	X	X	X	X
Cervical cancer screening	X	X		X
Chlamydia screening in women	X	X		X
Osteoporosis management in women who had a fracture			X	X
Controlling high blood pressure	X	X	X	X
Beta-blocker treatment after a heart attack	X	X	X	X
Persistence of beta-blocker treatment after a heart attack	X	X	X	X
Cholesterol management for patients with cardiovascular conditions	X	X	X	X
Comprehensive diabetes care	X	X	X	X

(continued)

Table 15–3 (*continued*)

HEDIS 2007 measures	Applicable to			
Effectiveness of care measures	*Medicaid*	*HMO/ POS plans*	*Medicare*	*Preferred provider org. plans*
Use of appropriate medications for people with asthma	X	X	X	X
User of spirometry testing in the assessment and diagnosis of chronic obstructive pulmonary disease (COPD)	X	X	X	X
Follow-up after hospitalization for mental illness	X	X	X	X
Antidepressant medication management	X	X	X	X
Follow-up care for children prescribed attention-deficit/ hyperactivity disorder (ADHD) medication	X	X		X
Glaucoma screening in older adults	X	X	X	X
Use of imaging studies for low back pain	X	X	X	X
Disease modifying anti-rheumatic drug therapy in rheumatoid arthritis	X	X	X	X
Annual monitoring for patients on persistent medications	X	X	X	X
Drugs to be avoided in the elderly			X	X
Potentially harmful drug–disease interactions in the elderly			X	X
Medical assistance with smoking cessation	X	X	X	X
Flu shots for adults ages 50–64				X
Flu shots for older adults			X	X
Pneumonia vaccination status for older adults			X	X
Medicare Health Outcomes Survey			X	X
Management of urinary incontinence in older adults			X	X

(*continued*)

Table 15–3 (*continued*)

HEDIS 2007 measures	Applicable to			
Effectiveness of care measures	Medicaid	HMO/ POS plans	Medicare	Preferred provider org. plans
Physical activity in older adults			X	X
Fall risk management			X	X
Osteoporosis testing in older women			X	X
Satisfaction with the experience of care				
CAHPS* 4.0H Adult Survey	X	X		X
CAHPS 3.0H Child Survey	X	X		
Children with chronic conditions	X	X		

The full specifications for these measures are available from the National Committee for Quality Assurance. At the time of publication, HEDIS 2008 was the most current version of the accountability measurement set. (NCQA, HEDIS 2008).
*CAHPS = Consumer Assessment of Health care Providers and Systems.

health plan, the physician, and the hospital can all be held accountable. All parties have taken on a significant role in ensuring patients have a script for a beta-blocker medication when they are discharged after an acute myocardial infarction. As a result, this measure has been the most successful quality measure to date.

These are only a few of the questions and analyses that could be applied to the HEDIS set. As one examines the list of HEDIS measures, it is clear that it does not measure all aspects of care or the overall performance of the health-care system. It was never intended to do so, but it is a good example of selective measures of preventive, acute, and chronic care. Many of the concepts and methods that are used to develop HEDIS have been adopted by the NQF and other quality measure developers.

QUALITY IMPROVEMENT DRIVEN THROUGH QUALITY MEASUREMENT

One of the most effective demonstrations of the power of quality measurement to achieve change was the HEDIS beta-blocker measure. In 1996, the NCQA introduced a quality measure to assess the rate of beta-blocker use within 7 days of hospital discharge for myocardial infarction (MI). The failure to prescribe beta-blockers was a problem that caused significant mortality and morbidity as well as additional resource utilization (e.g., hospital readmissions). When the NCQA released the first results in 1997, the average health plan use of beta-blockers in post-MI patients was at 62%. Ten years later, the NCQA 2006 report on the State of Healthcare Quality showed that the use of beta-blockers after a heart attack was at 94.3% of eligible patients in 2003, 96.2% in 2004, and 96.6% in 2005 (22).

This measure was reported for the last time in 2007 when the NCQA showed that the national average had reached 97.7%, with little to no variation in performance among health plans. It is now a retired measure. It was the measurement and reporting of quality results that catalyzed action to improve care to a level where measurement was no longer necessary. We propose that the success in the measure has partly resulted from the acceptance of shared accountability and improvement efforts between all parties that could affect positive change.

PUBLIC HEALTH SURVEILLANCE FOR HEALTH-CARE SAFETY AND QUALITY ISSUES

Quality measurement and associated quality improvement efforts have many features in common with more traditional public health surveillance, including the ongoing nature of data collection, data analysis, and interpretation, as well as a focus on improving services. Some public health agencies—especially those responsible for the provision of preventive and primary care—may utilize data such as HEDIS or quality measures submitted for Medicaid or Medicare beneficiaries. However, the focus of quality measurement data tends has been focus on health-care services, whereas public health surveillance historically has had a primary focus on the detection of specific diseases (i.e., notifiable conditions) or particular health conditions that reflect opportunities for prevention in the health-care setting (such as HAI) or in the community (such as lead poisoning or a foodborne infection). Public health surveillance for patient safety and emerging diseases have become increasingly important as the demand for quality and the increased costs of preventable health-care-associated morbidity and mortality have come to light. Two examples of public health surveillance efforts in the health-care setting are surveillance for healthcare associated infections and surveillance for medical product safety problems.

HEALTH-CARE-ASSOCIATED INFECTIONS

Approximately 1.7 million hospital-associated infections occur each year, resulting in $27 billion to $33 billion (23) in excess health-care costs and an associated 99,000 deaths (24). With mounting evidence that these infections can be prevented and high levels of consumer and legislative interest in HAI prevention, state health departments increasingly have been tasked to conduct and support surveillance for HAIs in hospitals and other health-care settings. In January 2009, the Department of Health and Human Services (HHS) released an HHS Action Plan to Prevent Healthcare-Associated Infections (Action Plan) (25). The Action Plan was developed by the HHS Office of Public Health and Science (OPHS), the Centers for Disease Control and Prevention (CDC), CMS, the Agency for Healthcare Research and Quality, and other HHS Offices and agencies. By June 2009, 20 states used CDC's National Healthcare Safety Network (NHSN) as the tool for reporting and NHSN participation has grown from 300 hospitals nationally to approximately

2100 hospitals in 2.5 years. In late 2009, HHS and CDC provided substantial funding to state health departments to build the workforce, training, and tools necessary to rapidly scale up to meet this new public health surveillance work (26).

NHSN is a secure, internet-based surveillance system used by health-care facilities to track, analyze, and interpret data on HAIs (22). Employing these data, facilities can evaluate interventions, share successes with other facilities, and test new methods for preventing HAIs in hospitals and other health-care facilities. With focus areas including patient safety and health-care personnel safety, NHSN has been a surveillance system used by a variety of health-care facilities, including acute care hospitals, ambulatory surgery centers, long-term care facilities, and rehabilitation hospitals.

Using NHSN, as well as its predecessor, the National Nosocomial Infection Surveillance (NNIS) system, intensive care units in participating hospitals have demonstrated 40% to 50% reductions in central line-associated bloodstream infections resulting from methicillin-resistant *Staphyloccus aureus* between 1997 and 2007 (Fig. 15–1; ref. 27). With newly added features, states can compare data collected and analyzed by type of hospital, get specific training in "hot topics" such as inpatient influenza vaccination, and compare interventions and outcomes with similar institutions.

Historically, HAI surveillance using NNIS and NHSN was based on a voluntary, confidential reporting model using standard definitions and surveillance methods and with data collection and entry by infection control professionals. These data not only were useful for national public health surveillance but were also used for quality improvement at the local hospital level (28). The recent shift toward public reporting of HAI data using NHSN coordinated by state health departments has offered both opportunities and challenges (29). Public reporting and state health department involvement have shifted NHSN toward greater emphasis on public health action and accountability; however, some will question whether the publicly reported data in NHSN collected by infection control professionals will continue to be valid. As data collected in NHSN shifts increasingly to automated reporting from electronic health records, hospital, and laboratory information systems, the reporting burden should decline and validity should arguably improve both for hospitals and public health agencies (30), although the impact of these automated approaches need to be evaluated. The real challenge for public health practitioners and agencies in the future will not primarily be the data collection and reporting but how public health agencies interpret and act to hold health-care institutions and providers accountable for preventing HAIs. This can be expected to increase the burden on already overstretched public health departments.

MEDICAL PRODUCT SAFETY SURVEILLANCE

A related growing area of federal public health surveillance is medical product safety. Medical products for which public health surveillance is conducted or planned include medications, vaccines, blood, organ, tissues, and medical devices. This type of surveillance is critical for assessing and maintaining safe and high-quality medical products (*see* Chapter 16).

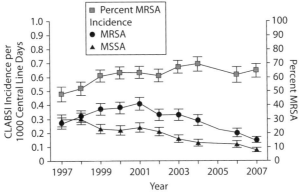

No. of Units   491 514 552 544 520 506 498 478 n/a 488 1039

Figure 15–1 Trends in percent MRSA and incidence of *Staphylococcus aureus* central line-associated bloodstream infections (CLABSI) in intensive care units—National Nosocomial Infections Surveillance System, 1997–2004; National Healthcare Safety Network, 2006–2007 (*20*).

An example of a national safety public health surveillance system is CDC-supported National Electronic Injury Surveillance System–Cooperative Adverse Drug Event Surveillance (NEISS-CADES) project. This system is a collaboration among CDC, the Food and Drug Administration (FDA), and the U.S. Consumer Product Safety Commission. NEISS-CADES provides detailed and nationally representative data on serious adverse drug events (ADEs) from medications used in non-hospital settings. NEISS-CADES produced the first detailed national estimates of ADEs treated in hospital emergency departments, finding that over 700,000 individuals are treated in emergency departments for ADEs each year. NEISS-CADES data have been critical for promoting evidence-based prevention efforts, particularly for older adults and children.

One example of significant public health action supported by surveillance data from NEISS-CADES is cough-and-cold medications. The surveillance data identified high rates of emergency visits for overdoses from these medications among young children (*31*). The FDA and product manufacturers changed recommendations in response to these findings such that the medications should not be used in children younger than 4 years of age. For older adults, NEISS-CADES data found that three commonly used medications (insulin, warfarin, digoxin) caused one-third of emergency department visits related to medications in this age group (*32*). The FDA, HRSA, and non-governmental organizations are now using this information to focus and prioritize medication safety efforts to reduce adverse events from these specific medications.

Using NEISS-CADES date, CDC recently found that antibiotics were 7 of the top 15 medicines implicated in emergency visits for ADEs. CDC has been working to reduce inappropriate use of antibiotics to reduce the emerging threat of antimicrobial resistance. These national data on the risks of harm to individuals is yet another reason to avoid antibiotics when they are not needed (*33*).

Another example of a medical product that is critical for public health is vaccines. CDC monitors the safety of vaccines in collaboration with FDA through the Vaccine Adverse Event Reporting System (VAERS). VAERS is a national reporting system that receives reports on adverse events following immunization and serves as an early warning system to detect problems that may be related to vaccines. Approximately 30,000 VAERS reports are filed annually, with 10% to 15% classified as serious (causing disability, hospitalization, life-threatening illness, or death). All adverse event reports classified as serious are reviewed, with review of available medical records and follow-up at 1 year (*34*).

State and local health agencies often are involved in the investigations of outbreaks related to medical products. Consequently, these national medical product surveillance efforts provide useful information to initiate investigation of outbreaks at a local level, while also providing national data to gauge progress in improving the safety and quality of medical products.

THE WAY FORWARD

Despite the long history of quality measurement and improvement starting with Codman, the disciplines and systems for monitoring the quality of healthcare are still evolving. Concerns about health care quality will only increase as efforts to curb the spiraling costs of health care stimulate anxiety about rationing and other structural impediment to provision of high-quality care. The concepts, development, and implementation of standards and methods for measuring quality of health care are still evolving and will need to incorporate the particular needs and challenges faced by national, state, and local public health agencies, especially for local public health action. Meanwhile, from the other direction, the more traditional public health surveillance systems that operate in the same theater of health-care delivery institutions, such as those for HAI and medical product safety, likewise continue to grow and achieve greater penetration and sophistication, so that these two important enterprises will be sharing content, data, and methods. Measuring quality of health care in the United States has been a priority for many years. It becomes increasingly important as the country reforms how it finances and provides care for its 300 million citizens. Public health surveillance of health care quality will play a key role in the evidence-driven approach needed for effective change.

REFERENCES

1. Donabedian A. The end results of health care: Ernest Codman's contribution to quality assessment and beyond. *Milbank Q* 1989;67:233–267.
2. Neuhauser D. Ernest Amory Codman, M.D. and end results of medical care. *Int J Technol Assess Health Care* 1990;6:307–325.
3. Institute of Medicine. *Medicare: A Strategy for Quality Assurance.* Volume I. K.N. Lohr, ed. Washington, DC: National Academy Press; 1990.

4. Donabedian A. Definition of quality and approaches to its assessment. In: *Explorations in Quality Assessment and Monitoring.* Ann Arbor, MI: Health Administration Press; 1969:178.

5. Donabedian A. *The Criteria and Standards of Quality: Explorations in Quality Assessment and Monitoring.* Ann Arbor, MI: Health Administration Press; 1969.

6. Donabedian A. *Methods and Findings of Quality Assessment and Monitoring: An Illustrated Analysis. Explorations in Quality Assessment and Monitoring.* Ann Arbor, MI: Health Administration Press; 1969.

7. Committee on Quality of Health Care in America. *Crossing the Quality Chasm.* Institute of Medicine; 2001.

8. Institute of Medicine. *Committee on Redesigning Health Insurance Performance Measures, Payment, and Performance Improvement Programs.* Performance Measurement: Accelerating Improvement (Pathways to Quality Health Care Series) National Academies Press; 2006.

9. http://www.qualityforum.org. Accessed August 25, 2009.

10. http://www.cms.hhs.gov. Accessed August 25, 2009.

11. http://www.jointcommission.org. Accessed August 25, 2009.

12. http://www.ncqa.org. Accessed August 25, 2009.

13. Keister LW. Big employers back new drive for comparable quality measures. *Manag Care* 1995;4:20–24.

14. NCQA. Quality At Work: 1998 Annual Report. Washington, DC: National Committee for Quality Assurance; 1999.

15. Rosenthal MB, Landon BE, Normand SLT, *et al.* Employers' use of value-based purchasing strategies. *JAMA* 2007;298:2281–2288.

16. CMS Quality Initiatives—http://www.cms.hhs.gov/QualityInitiativesGenInfo.

17. Medicare "Pay for Performance (P4P) Intiatives. http://www.cms.hhs.gov/apps/media/press/release.asp?Counter=1343. Accessed August 25, 2009.

18. Landon BE, Rosenthal MB, Normand SL, Frank RG, Epstein AM. Quality monitoring and management in commercial health plans. *Am J Manag Care* 2008;14(6):377–386.

19. Edgman-Levitan S, Cleary PD. What information do consumers want and need? *Health Aff (Millwood)* 1996;15:42–56.

20. Cleary PD, Edgman-Levitan S. Health care quality. Incorporating consumer perspectives. *JAMA* 1997;278:1608–1612.

21. Sainfort F, Booske BC. Role of information in consumer selection of health plans. *Health Care Financ Rev* 1996;18:31–54.

22. NCQA State of Healthcare report, Washington, DC: National Committee for Quality Assurance; 2006.

23. Scott RD. The direct medical costs of healthcare-associated infections. Centers for Disease Control and Prevention. 2009. http://www.cdc.gov/ncidod/dhqp/pdf/Scott_CostPaper.pdf. Accessed August 25, 2009.

24. Klevens RM, Edwards JR, Richards CL, *et al.* Estimating healthcare-associated infections and deaths in U.S. hospitals, 2002. *Public Health Rep* 2007;122:160–166.

25. Healthcare-Associated Infections. http://www.hhs.gov/ophs/initiatives/hai. Accessed August 25, 2009.

26. Department of Health and Human Services. "Secretary Sebelius Highlights Two New Reports on Health Care Quality, Says Improving Quality is Key Component of Health Reform". http://www.hhs.gov/news/press/2009pres/05/20090506a.html. Accessed August 25, 2009.

27. Burton DC, Edwards JR, Horan TC, Jernigan JA, Fridkin SK. Methicillin-resistant Staphylococcus aureus central line–associated bloodstream infections in US intensive care units, 1997–2007. *JAMA* 2009;301:727–736.
28. Richards C, Emori TG, Edwards J, Fridkin S, Gaynes R. Characteristics of hospitals and infection control professionals participating in the National Nosocomial Infections Surveillance System-1999. *Am J Infect Cont* 2001;29:400–403.
29. McKibben L, Horan TC, Tokars JI, *et al.* Guidance on public reporting of healthcare-associated infections: recommendations of the healthcare infection control practices advisory committee. *Infection Control Hosp Epidemiol* 2005;26(6):580–587.
30. Tokars JI, Richards C, Andrus M, *et al.* The changing face of surveillance for healthcare-associated infections. *Clin Infect Dis* 2004;39:1347–1352.
31. Schaefer MK, Shehab N, Cohen AL, Budnitz D. Adverse events from cough and cold medications in children. *Pediatrics* 2008;121:783–787.
32. Budnitz D, Shehab N, Kegler S, Richards CL. Medication use leading to emergency department visits for adverse drug events in older adults. *Ann Intern Med* 2007;147:755–765.
33. Shehab N, Patel PR, Srinivasan A, Budnitz D. Emergency Department visits for antibiotic-associated adverse events. *Clin Infect Dis* 2008;47(6):735–743
34. Singleton JA, Lloyd JC, Mootrey GT, Salive M, Chen RT, VAERS Working Group. An overview of the vaccine adverse event reporting system (VAERS) as a surveillance system. *Vaccine* 1999:17;2908–2917.

16

PostMarket Surveillance of Medical Products in the United States

PAUL J. SELIGMAN, THOMAS P. GROSS, M. MILES BRAUN, AND JANET B. ARROWSMITH

INTRODUCTION

Postmarket surveillance is an essential part of medical product development worldwide. Postmarket surveillance is intended to identify unanticipated adverse events (AEs) associated with medical product use, discover interactions not identified before market entry (patient–product, product–product, and product–environment), monitor for unanticipated uses or misuses by prescribers or patients, and identify failures caused by manufacturing, design, labeling, packaging, or maintenance that occur after a medical product is marketed.

Medical products, including pharmaceuticals, medical devices, radiation-emitting electronic products, and biological products, each present unique surveillance challenges based on the uses of the products, the types of premarket evaluations, and their design or development features. The U.S. Food and Drug Administration (FDA) controls market entry of and approves professional labeling for medical products (1–4). Together with product manufacturers, healthcare providers, patients, consumers, and federal, state, and local public health agencies, the FDA monitors marketed medical products for AEs and product problems that occur after market entry. This chapter describes postmarket surveillance practices in the United States and how these practices influence the availability of and labeling for these products.

PREMARKET PRODUCT EVALUATION

Most medical products undergo extensive laboratory and clinical evaluation prior to entry into the U.S. market. Premarket clinical trials for medical products are designed to establish the efficacy of a product and evaluate its safety. Inherent limitations of these trials include their relatively small size and short duration compared to the anticipated market size and duration of use for most medical products. In addition, premarket clinical trials usually exclude patients with significant comorbidities and might not include certain populations such as the elderly, pregnant

women, and children. The inability of clinical trials to study all potential populations and uses for a product and, in the case of medical devices, restriction of clinical trial investigators to the most experienced physician-users generally means that
the product safety profile is incomplete at the time of initial marketing.

Most premarket trials for devices, drugs, and therapeutic biologic products enroll
a total of a few hundred to a few thousand people in studies of varying lengths.
These size constraints make it statistically unlikely to detect rare AEs or ones that
occur following long-term exposure. For example, to reliably detect an event occurring at a rate of one per thousand, a premarket clinical trial would need to expose
3,000 people to an experimental treatment for a sufficient duration to have a 95%
chance of detecting that AE. Given the general size and duration limitations of clinical trials, premarket databases for new medical products are unlikely to reliably
detect AEs or product problems that occur at rates of one per thousand or less.

Vaccines are an exception to these general size limitations because pivotal trials of new vaccines frequently enroll larger numbers of patients; conversely, most
medical devices are not evaluated at all in clinical trials prior to market entry.

GENERAL PRINCIPLES OF POSTMARKET
SURVEILLANCE

Postmarket surveillance is based primarily on observational data. Review and
analysis of AE case reports and device problem reports is an essential component
of postmarket surveillance. Postmarket AEs are untoward clinical outcomes tem-
porally associated with the use of a marketed medical product. AEs might result
from the inherent toxicity of the product, idiosyncratic effects, abuse or misuse,
medical errors, contamination, or product interactions. AEs resulting from errors
in use might be related to packaging problems, name confusion, inadvertent sub-
stitution of one product for another, dose miscalculations, or administration to the
wrong patient or via the wrong route. Medical device problems, which might also
result in AEs, can arise from errors in device assembly or maintenance, inadequate
instructions for use, defective design, or devices that fail to function properly.

Certain AEs and product problem reports must be submitted to the FDA.
Requirements for each product type are discussed below and detailed in
Table 16–1. Important new safety issues might arise from serious and unexpected
AE reports (Table 16–2), serious events that are uncommon in the general population, specific populations at potential risk for AEs, and unanticipated device
failures or problems. These product problems are usually assessed on a product-
by-product basis by manufacturers and the FDA.

SIGNAL DETECTION FOR MEDICAL PRODUCTS

Detection, evaluation, and interpretation of product problem or safety signals are
essential in postmarket safety surveillance (5). A signal is essentially an indication
of a potential safety concern associated with the use of a medical product based on

Table 16–1 Attributes of U.S. Food and Drug Administration Medical Product Problem Reporting Systems, 2009

	AERS (1)	VAERS (2)	MAUDE (3)
Year initiated	1996	1990	1996
Reporting requirements	21CFR314	21CFR600.80	21CFR 803
Coding terminology	MedDRA (4)	MedDRA	NCI (5)
Data mining capabilities	MGPS (6)	PRR(7)&MGPS	under development
Numbers of reports			
Total			
thru 2007	>4 million	>250,000	>2 million
2007 only	>364,000	>31,000	300,000
Reporting time-frames			
Death or serious			
unlabeled	15 days	15 days	User facility: 10 days Manuf/Importer: 30 days
Non-serious and serious, labeled	3 or 12 months	3, 6 or 12 months	
Malfunction			Manuf/Importer: 30 days
Summary (known device events)			3 months
Patient Outcomes (2007)			
Death			2%
Serious	75%	20%	18%
Non-serious	25%	80%	
Malfunction			30%
Summary			50%
Reporter Type (2007)			
Health-care provider	54%	30%	0.5%
Consumer	46%	6%	1%
Sources of Report (2007)			
Direct to the FDA	6%		
Manufacturer	94%	41%	96%
State health officer		24%	
Importer			0.5%
User Facility			2%
Submission method (2007)			
Electronic	65%	under development	10%
Paper	35%	100%	90%
Public access	www.fda.gov/cder NTIS (8)	www.vaers.hhs.gov	www.fda.gov/cdrh

1. Adverse Event Reporting System
2. Vaccine Adverse Event Reporting System
3. Manufacturer and User Facility Device Experience
4. MedDRA: Medical Dictionary for Regulatory Activities
5. NCI: National Cancer Institute
6. MGPS: Multi-item gamma Poisson shrinker
7. PRR: proportional reporting rate
8. NTIS: Technical Information Service (www.ntis.gov)

Table 16–2 Regulatory Definitions of Serious as It Applies to Adverse Drug or Biologic Event Reporting (21 CFR § 314.80, effective April 1, 2008)

A serious adverse drug/biologic event is defined as any event that occurs at any dose and results in one or more of the following:

- Death
- A life-threatening event
- An event resulting in inpatient hospitalization
- An event that prolongs a current hospitalization
- A persistent or significant disability or incapacity
- A congenital anomaly or birth defect
- Any event that, based on appropriate medical judgment, may jeopardize the patient and for which medical or surgical intervention may be required to prevent one of the outcomes listed above

postmarket surveillance and consideration of what is generally known about the product. Signal detection often starts with information on an AE or product problem report form. Generally, a number of factors are considered in identifying a signal. A signal might arise from a report of a previously unknown serious problem, of an event seen rarely in an unexposed population, reports suggesting an increase in the frequency or severity of a known or labeled event, or isolated reports suggesting problems in packaging, maintenance, design, or manufacture. There might be concerns about product name confusion or misuse or unanticipated uses of the product. A program implemented to reduce the risk of an AE or problem might prove to be inadequate. Most signals depend on more than one report, although occasionally a single well-documented report can produce a signal of a new concern.

The ability of postmarket safety surveillance to suggest a relationship between the use of a medical product and an AE depends on the degree to which details and documentation are provided in AE reports. An FDA Guidance describes the elements of good case reporting (6). Manufacturers, distributors, importers, user facilities, and FDA scientists conduct follow-up with reporters to obtain additional data on individual reports; information obtained during follow-up might help clarify the relationship between the problem or event and the product.

Statistically sound analyses of AE and problem reports help detect new signals of AEs and errors. A number of statistical methods to review relative frequencies of events and likelihood analyses are used. The statistical methods and graphical enhancements of data assessments vary depending on the products and reports under evaluation (7–9).

In some circumstances, external data sources are used by manufacturers and regulators to further evaluate a safety signal or assess risks associated with a product or studies are contracted to outside organizations.

CAUSALITY ASSESSMENTS

Table 16–3 lists factors considered in assessing the relationship between exposure to a medical product and an AE. In general, these types of determinations are based on the

Table 16–3 Factors Important in Causality Assessment for Adverse Events Reported in Association with Marketed Medical Products in the United States

- Timing of product administration such that exposure precedes onset of the event
- Abatement or resolution of the event with discontinuation of the suspect product (de-challenge)
- Recurrence or recrudescence of the event with re-exposure to the suspect product (re-challenge)
- Biological plausibility of the event in association with the product
- Confirmatory or supporting laboratory or other objective evidence
- Previous known toxicity of the suspect product

review of a case series. However, a single, well-documented case report might be sufficient to establish a causal relationship between the use of a medical product and an AE. There are no agreed-upon international standards for assessing causality, especially for events that occur commonly in the general population absent exposure to the medical product. In these circumstances epidemiologic studies are used to examine the potential association between and exposure and an AE or product problem (5).

DATA COLLECTION

Manufacturers and importers of medical products and facilities using medical devices (e.g., hospitals and nursing homes) are required to submit AE or problem reports to the FDA. The FDA also receives voluntary reports directly from health-care providers and consumers. Voluntary reports can be submitted to the FDA's MedWatch program by mail, fax, or on a Web-based form at www.fda.gov/medwatch. AE and problem reports submitted to MedWatch are triaged to the appropriate Center (10).

Currently, each FDA Center maintains separate electronic databases for storage, retrieval, and evaluation of AE or product problem reports. Table 16–1 summarizes descriptions of these databases, including the types of reports, reporting requirements, and other aspects of postmarket surveillance. Examples of outside data sources for each center are discussed below.

PUBLIC HEALTH IMPORTANCE OF POSTMARKET SURVEILLANCE

New medical product safety information is communicated to prescribers in updated professional labeling, "Dear Healthcare Provider" letters, safety alerts, and public health notifications. Information is communicated to consumers in Medication Guides and Patient Package Inserts (11–13).

Data from postmarket surveillance are reflected in changes to product packaging, formulation, materials or design, and, on rare occasions, the suspension or withdrawal of a product from the market. Findings from postmarket surveillance activities inform enforcement activities and companies are asked or required to make any of a number of changes to its product or label. In addition, postmarket surveillance data are communicated to the medical–scientific community through peer-reviewed journals, presentations at medical–scientific meetings, and conferences. New safety information is publicly available free of charge from the FDA in safety-related monthly Internet broadcasts or subscription podcasts (*14,15*) and on the MedWatch website (*16*). MedWatch online, a free subscription service, provides information on labeling changes, emerging safety issues, recalls, or other problems associated with regulated products (*16*).

Postmarket safety concerns can result in programs that mitigate or minimize risks associated with a specific product (*17*) or result in an FDA request or requirement that a manufacturer conduct additional epidemiological studies to more fully evaluate a safety concern.

POSTMARKET SURVEILLANCE OF DRUGS

Postmarket safety surveillance for pharmaceuticals, commonly referred to as *pharmacovigilance*, depends on safety signal detection through review and analysis of AE and medical error reports. Automated methods of analyzing AE databases as well as active surveillance systems and hypothesis-driven studies are used to augment a traditional passive surveillance system, the Adverse Event Reporting System (AERS).

The Center for Drug Evaluation and Research (CDER) at the FDA uses the AERS database to store, retrieve, and analyze AE reports. AERS was established in 1996 and contains over 4 million AE reports; about 450,000 reports are submitted annually.[1] AEs are coded using the Medical Dictionary for Regulatory Activities (MedDRA) to facilitate reports retrieval and analysis (*18,19*); previous coding dictionaries and reporting formats limit the usefulness of older data (*20*).

About 95% of AE and error reports are received via product manufacturers, who are required to submit certain reports to the FDA (Table 16–4); the remaining 5% are submitted directly by health-care providers and consumers. Manufacturers obtain new AE information from telephone calls from health-care providers or consumers, marketing staff contacts with providers, the scientific literature, post-approval clinical trials, and other sources.

Statistical tools are used to assist FDA scientists in detecting new signals of AEs and errors in the AERS database. These tools are used to estimate the relative frequency of specific AE–drug combinations as compared to the frequency of the event with all other drugs in the database. There are a number of graphic enhancements of the data and statistical methods, such as Proportional Reporting Rates and Multi-Item Gamma Poisson Shrinker, that are in use or under development (*7–9, 20–23*).

The FDA might require that a manufacturer evaluate a signal detected by a surveillance system. The study might use outside data sources such as health-care

[1] A predecessor computerized database, the Spontaneous Reporting System, initiated in 1967, was phased out in 1996 when AERS came online.

Table 16–4 Key Requirements for Reporting Adverse Drug Experiences for Holders of Approved Drug Applications (21 C.F.R. § 314.80)

- 15-Day "Alert Reports"
    Each adverse drug experience meeting regulatory definitions for both serious and unexpected must be reported to the FDA by the sponsor within 15 calendar days.
    15-day "Alert Report"—follow-up
    Each adverse drug experience reported as a 15-day "Alert Report" must be promptly investigated and any new information must be submitted to the FDA within 15 calendar days of receipt of the new information.

- Periodic Adverse Drug Experience Reports
    Each adverse drug experience classified as *(1)* serious and expected, *(2)* non-serious and unexpected, or *(3)* non-serious and expected must be reported in a periodic report. The reporting interval is quarterly for the first 3 years following U.S. approval and annually thereafter. The periodic report also includes an analysis of the 15-Day "Alert Reports" submitted during the reporting interval.

- Reports from Scientific Literature
    Serious, unexpected adverse drug experiences from scientific or medical journals (case reports or derived from a clinical trial) must be reported as 15-Day "Alert Reports."

- Reports from Postmarketing Studies
    Serious, unexpected adverse drug experiences occurring during a postmarketing study and for which the sponsor concludes that there is a reasonable possibility that the drug caused the adverse drug experience must be reported as a 15-Day "Alert Report."

organizations whose databases link pharmacy records with clinical records. These studies provide rapid estimates of specific event frequencies in exposed and unexposed populations. The FDA might conduct more detailed studies to estimate the frequency of an AE or study risk factors associated with the AE (*24*). There are a variety of other data sources that provide drug AE and medication error information. Among these data sources are the Toxic Exposure Surveillance System (TESS) from the American Association of Poison Control Centers (*25*); MEDMARX, a voluntary system of hospital medication error reports (*26*); medication error reports from the Institute for Safe Medication Practices; and the Drug Abuse Warning Network (DAWN) (*27*). The National Electronic Injury Surveillance System's (NEISS) network of emergency rooms identifies adverse drug events and medication errors requiring emergency room evaluation (*28*).

Registries and monitoring programs established to evaluate or monitor specific drugs, classes of drugs, or specific diseases or as part of risk management plans are also used to characterize signals of potential AEs. Examples include the outcome-specific registry of drug-induced liver injury (DILI) (*29*); drug-specific systems for tracking outcomes in exposed populations such as those for Accutane (*30*), Lotronex (*31*), or Tysabri (*32*); or a population-based registry such as the Organization of Teratology Information Specialists (OTIS) birth defects registry (*33*).

Estimates of exposures (denominators) and physician use or prescribing are available through private databases such as IMS Health (*34*) and Verispan (*35*). Additional data sources under development are discussed in the section "Innovations in Postmarket Surveillance Activities."

POSTMARKET SURVEILLANCE FOR DEVICES

For most medical devices, limited or no clinical data are required before marketing (*36*). Device manufacturers often provide engineering or performance data to the FDA for review prior to marketing, but only the highest risk devices, such as heart valves and defibrillators, undergo evaluation in clinical trials. These trials generally enroll only a few hundred patients and the nature of devices often precludes randomization or blinding.

The Center for Devices and Radiologic Health's (CDRH) electronic reports database, the Manufacturer and User Facility Device Experience (MAUDE) database, was established in 1996. In 2007, MAUDE contained more than 2 million reports (*see* Table 16–1). MAUDE data are updated regularly and are available on the CDRH website with patient or reporter identifiers redacted (*37*). Similarly to AERS, the vast majority of reports in MAUDE are from manufacturers, with a small percentage from user facilities (such as hospitals and nursing homes), voluntary sources, and importers (*38*). Manufacturers and importers are required to submit reports of device-related deaths, serious injuries, and malfunctions to the FDA. User facilities are required to submit reports of device-related deaths and serious injuries to the manufacturer and only deaths to the FDA. Health-care providers and consumers submit reports to MedWatch voluntarily.

In assessing causality, in addition to specific patient characteristics, the following factors are considered: failure potential resulting from design or manufacturing problems; user error potential from improper device assembly or misreading instructions; incorrect clinical use; or inadequate instructions for use. Possible packaging errors, support system failure, adverse environmental factors, maintenance error, adverse device interactions such as electromagnetic interference, or toxic/idiosyncratic reactions are also considered (*39*). Some manufacturers conduct failure analyses on retained or returned products in the event of a reported device problem.

To enhance understanding of clinical safety issues for medical devices, the Medical Product Safety Network (MedSun) was established to provide national medical device surveillance based on a representative subset of user facilities (*13,40*). MedSun currently includes approximately 350 hospitals nationwide. Specialty networks in areas such as laboratory medicine and pediatrics have emerged within MedSun to focus on device-specific issues. A pilot of a human tissue and cell product network is in process.

MedSun publishes monthly newsletters highlighting device reports, FDA actions, and safety initiatives by other agencies; hosts clinical engineering audioconferences; and can conduct rapid initial surveys as well as observational studies for high-profile safety concerns.

To enhance the usefulness of reported data, statistical methods similar to those employed by CDER, are being explored to help detect safety signals in MAUDE. In addition, to better capture exposure and outcome classification, a consistent international nomenclature to identify and define reported device types (e.g., deep brain stimulators) is in development (*41*). An extensive hierarchical vocabulary for adverse device outcomes (e.g., high impedance in pacemakers) also has been developed (*42,43*).

Active surveillance is used for certain high risk devices such as implanted ventricular-assist devices (VADs). In the VAD registry, expected as well as unanticipated device-related AEs are adjudicated by external experts and undergo complete follow-up and reporting by device manufacturers (*44*).

As a condition of marketing approval, manufacturers of the highest risk medical devices are sometimes required to conduct hypothesis-driven postmarket observational studies to augment passive surveillance (*45–47*).

Because of the heterogeneity of medical devices, manufacturers and the FDA typically use an *ad hoc* approach to characterize device risks using external databases. Examples include the use of Blue Cross/Blue Shield claims data to assess the risk of secondary vertebral fractures following vertebroplasty (*48*); incidence and short-term outcomes of primary and revision hip replacement in the United States using national hospital discharge data (*49*); and the prevalence of breast implant rupture using National Cancer Institute breast cancer cohort data (*50*).

To meet FDA mandatory post-approval study requirements, manufacturers often use registries for postmarket device evaluation, such as registries of patients with drug-eluting coronary stents or those with carotid stents. Registries can be used for Center-initiated, applied epidemiologic investigations (*51*), or as means for Department of Health and Human Services agencies to address their respective missions (e.g., National Implantable Cardioverter Defibrillator Registry) (*52*).

Most health-care or administrative claims records do not uniquely identify medical devices; development and use of unique device identifiers that can be incorporated into records and claims data will greatly enhance the usefulness of these datasets in evaluating device performance and safety.

BIOLOGICAL PRODUCT POSTMARKET SURVEILLANCE

Biological products include therapeutics like monoclonal antibodies, vaccines, allergenic extracts and blood, blood components, and blood derivatives as well as human tissue and cell products. Premarket evaluation of most biological therapeutic products is similar to that of pharmaceutical products, whereas vaccines, human tissues, and blood and blood components have unique premarket features.

Premarket studies for new vaccines are generally very large, with individual studies often exceeding 10,000 subjects. Vaccines are intended to prevent disease and most are used in healthy pediatric populations so that even low frequencies of serious AEs are considered unacceptable. For example, in 2005, licensure of a live, attenuated rotavirus vaccine was based on a trial of approximately 70,000 subjects. The trial was powered to exclude a prespecified level of risk of intussusception, a severe AE that led to market withdrawal of the first licensed rotavirus vaccine (*53,54*).

Spontaneous vaccine AE reports are submitted to the Vaccine Adverse Event Reporting System (VAERS), comanaged by the FDA and the Centers for Disease Control and Prevention (CDC), and maintained by a contractor. Follow-up is initiated on all serious vaccine AEs to obtain additional information such as hospital discharge summaries and autopsy reports. These AEs are reviewed to identify signals that often require additional investigation.

Analyses of VAERS data of medical and public health interest, such as alopecia (55) and syncope (56) following vaccination, are published in the peer-reviewed scientific literature. In addition, summaries of the first several years of safety data for newly marketed vaccines are published in the medical literature (57–59), in the CDC's *Morbidity and Mortality Weekly Report* (60,61), and disseminated through the FDA's MedWatch and CBER websites for rapid communication of safety information to health-care providers and the public (62,63).

Every 2 weeks, statistical tools to assess VAERS data for signals of possible vaccine-related safety signals are applied. The two statistical methods currently in use are proportional reporting ratios and the Empirical Bayes Geometric Mean (EBGM). These statistical programs are used to mine the VAERS data for potential associations that could not be detected by individual report review. This process generates new safety signals—for example, photophobia following smallpox vaccination. It also helps assess the strength of known signals or safety concerns. Assessments of the relative effectiveness of data mining[2] methods for VAERS have not demonstrated that one approach is superior to another; there is no gold standard reference for objective evaluation.

The Vaccine Safety Datalink project, managed and principally funded by the CDC, includes data on 5.5 million patients in eight managed care organizations. Started in the early 1990s, it is an ongoing observational monitoring system that is an essential part of U.S. safety monitoring for licensed vaccines. Currently, each health-care organization maintains separate vaccination records, potential AEs, and data on potential confounders. The data include medical claims information and, increasingly, electronic medical records. The Vaccine Safety Datalink has been useful for addressing important safety questions such as the risk of seizures after measles-mumps-rubella vaccine or whole-cell pertussis vaccine. The Vaccine Safety Datalink also permits semi-automated rapid cycle analyses of population-based data for new vaccines. These analyses are performed periodically (e.g., weekly) to assess the safety of new vaccines. Safety signals from rapid cycle analyses generally require additional study. Should a safety concern arise from VAERS or other sources, the Vaccine Safety Datalink can be used to conduct rapid preliminary assessments of vaccine safety concerns using retrospective cohort or other study designs. Examples of such rapid assessments include the first rotavirus vaccine, Rotashield®, which was withdrawn shortly after marketing, and intussusception as well as meningococcal vaccine and Guillain–Barre syndrome (54,61). These preliminary assessments can be of great assistance to public health policy decision makers (64).

For new vaccines, the FDA routinely requires a pharmacovigilance plan according to an internationally standardized format (65). Ideally, these plans are submitted as part of the application for marketing approval, the Biologics License Application (BLA). Studies initiated as part of the pharmacovigilance plan address specific safety concerns or information gaps present at the time of licensure. Another common type of study is a general safety evaluation of a large number of potential vaccine–AE associations. Such required safety studies are often

---

[2] Data mining refers to the use of statistical algorithms to detect unexpected variations in reporting rates for specific AEs for one product as compared to other products in the database.

conducted as observational studies in health maintenance organization (HMO) databases with 25,000 to 50,000 vaccinees.

The Brighton Collaboration is an international organization focused on reaching consensus among volunteer experts on definitions for important AEs following vaccination (66). Such definitions promote better interstudy comparisons of safety data and, potentially, safer vaccines. Examples of finalized case definitions include fever, hypotonic hyporesponsive episode, and intussusception (67).

When a complication of blood collection or transfusion is confirmed to be fatal, FDA regulations require a report be made to the FDA within 7 days after the fatality (68). During the period October 1, 2007 through September 30, 2008 such reports numbered 10 and 72, respectively (69). Regarding the 10 fatalities following collection of blood or blood components, FDA review did not find a causal association between the deaths and collection. With respect to the 72 transfusion recipient fatality reports, FDA concluded that 46 of the deaths were related to the transfusion, 18 were unrelated to the transfusion and in 8 fatalities transfusion was not ruled out as the cause of the fatality.

Tissue establishments are required to report serious adverse reactions involving a communicable disease related to human cell or tissue transplantation (70) to the AERS database. Each AE, including follow-up information, is evaluated by a physician and other health professionals on the FDA's Tissue Safety Team. Non-vaccine biological products, such as plasma derivatives (e.g., factor VIII) and their recombinant analogs, are regulated similarly to drugs, with AE reports submitted to AERS.

As with drugs and devices, registries are also used for biological products. Although there have been no reported cases of congenital syndromes after varicella or rubella vaccine, concerns based on experience with congenital rubella following wild-type infection and with other teratogens have led to registries for pregnancies following live attenuated viral vaccination (71).

INTERNATIONAL COLLABORATIONS

Medical product development and marketing is a global enterprise and has prompted international cooperation and information exchange with other regulatory agencies and public health agencies. The International Conference on Harmonisation of Technical Requirements for Registration of Pharmaceuticals for Human Use or ICH has fostered the development of a number of agreements to implement uniformity in reporting, coding, and terminology (72). The Council for International Organizations of Medical Sciences (CIOMS) has developed a number of consensus documents toward achieving such uniformity (73). The World Health Organization (WHO), including its Global Advisory Committee on Vaccine Safety, and the Pan American Health Organization provide forums for the regular exchange of information regarding postmarket issues. The Uppsala Monitoring Centre in Sweden collects and shares international postmarket reports of drugs that can provide early safety warnings for regulatory agencies worldwide (74). Finally, the Global Harmonization Task Force (75) exchanges information on high-profile device-related adverse events with a number of international regulatory authorities.

INNOVATIONS IN POSTMARKET SURVEILLANCE ACTIVITIES

In 2004, the sudden market withdrawal of a widely prescribed and promoted anti-inflammatory drug, rofecoxib (Vioxx®), focused public attention on the FDA's postmarket drug safety surveillance system. In response, the FDA asked the National Academy of Sciences' Institute of Medicine (IOM) to evaluate the U.S. postmarket safety system. In 2006, IOM released its report, *The Future of Drug Safety: Promoting and Protecting the Health of the Public* (76), providing recommendations for improving pharmaceutical postmarket safety surveillance and identifying additional authorities and resources needed by the FDA. A new law, the Food and Drug Administration Amendments Act (FDAAA), was passed in September 2007, incorporating many of the IOM recommendations (77).

FDAAA and Pharmaceutical Postmarket Surveillance

The FDA has new authority to require postmarket studies and surveillance programs either at the time of approval of a new drug or biologic or when a new safety issue arises following approval, if certain criteria are met. These criteria include the need to further assess a known, serious risk; investigate a new signal of a serious risk; or identify the potential for a possible serious risk. To require additional clinical trials, the FDA must find that its existing capabilities are not sufficient to assess or identify the specific risk and that an observational study alone would not suffice for the proposed risk assessment.

Sponsors must comply with certain reporting requirements, and all trials or studies must be registered in the clinical trials database at the National Institutes of Health (78). The FDA may undertake enforcement actions, including imposition of monetary penalties, if a sponsor fails to comply with the study reporting requirements or fails to complete the required features of a postmarket study.

The law calls for collaborations between public and private organizations to develop a risk identification and analysis system containing safety data. This system is intended to rapidly detect trends, patterns, incidence, and prevalence of drug-induced adverse reactions and ensure that more useful benefit and risk information is available to prescribers and users of pharmaceuticals.

In addition, FDAAA established the Reagan-Udall Foundation, an independent not-for-profit organization, to foster and support collaborative postmarket safety research and to offer fellowship opportunities and advance science and public health practice at the FDA.

Medical Devices

FDAAA includes requirements to strengthen postmarket device surveillance based on the IOM report *Safe Medical Devices for Children* (79). These requirements include annual review of AEs for certain pediatric devices, development of a research agenda to evaluate the short- and long-term safety and effectiveness of pediatric devices, and expansion of the FDA's authority to require manufacturers to conduct postmarket studies when the device is expected to have substantial pediatric use (80).

In addition, FDAAA establishes a system of unique device identifiers and requires quarterly device malfunction reports by manufacturers for lower risk devices.

FUTURE DIRECTIONS AND NEW CHALLENGES

The recent innovations and new directions in postmarket medical product surveillance have arisen primarily to address many of the limitations and weaknesses of the current systems and in response to the expansion of authorities and new requirements of FDAAA. There are four primary areas of ongoing or planned improvements to the postmarket medical product surveillance system. These include: *(1)* improving access to and analysis of the existing large, case report databases; *(2)* expanding the depth and breadth of public and private clinical databases for use in conducting surveillance and studies; *(3)* understanding the scientific basis for AEs and why certain individuals and populations are at increased risk; and *(4)* increasing international cooperation and information sharing.

Improve Analysis of Large Databases of Case Reports

A single, Web-based portal for reporting all problems related to medical products is under development at the FDA, which would require uniform data elements so that AE databases can be combined, permitting uniform analytic approaches *(81)*. Data mining techniques currently in use for specific products hold the potential for real-time signal detection for all products being evaluated. Finally, electronic AE reporting by manufacturers, which is a common pharmaceutical industry practice, might soon become mandatory for both the drug and device industries *(82)*.

Expand the Databases Available for Surveillance and Observational Studies

Increasing use of electronic records by health-care institutions for medical, pharmacy, laboratory, radiology, and administrative information will permit use of these databases as distributed data networks[3] for surveillance and study purposes. Numerous evaluations have demonstrated the usefulness of large, linked databases to investigate surveillance safety signals, to evaluate device performance, to assess compliance with drug monitoring requirements, and to determine compliance with disease-specific treatment guidelines *(83,84)*. These examples offer models for ways to meet statistical, technological, and methodological challenges while addressing privacy, proprietary, and data security concerns. Establishing unique device identifiers will improve the usefulness of these datasets in surveillance of medical devices.

With FDAAA requiring larger datasets, there is interest in the private sector in developing data networks across healthcare institutions. The FDA has established the Sentinel Initiative to identify health-care organizations with the capability and interest in participating in such data networks *(85)*. The goal of these networks is

---

[3] A distributed data network is a systems architecture allowing independent analyses of large separate datasets, which are then integrated to provide an expanded patient population for higher level analyses and studies, while protecting confidential patient information in each of the individual datasets.

to improve postmarket risk assessment for medical products through rapid conduct of relatively inexpensive studies to estimate the potential public health risk of newly identified safety signals with marketed medical products. Challenges include developing data standards and patient privacy protections and resolution of analytic, organizational, governance, and technology issues. Organizational and governance issues include data ownership, data access, and how surveillance priorities are selected, reviewed, and approved.

Understanding the Science of Adverse Events

There have been a number of recent advances in the understanding to the genetic basis of the actions of pharmaceuticals as well as for adverse reactions. The ability to tailor therapies to individuals (e.g., warfarin dosing) and identify potentially at-risk individuals and populations for serious adverse reactions (e.g., carbamazepine) holds great promise for increasingly personalized medicine (86,87). The FDA's Critical Path initiative encourages the development of science to better understand the scientific bases for both the benefits and risks associated with medicines (88).

International Collaboration

With global expansion of medical product development, clinical studies now are conducted on every continent. Standards for the conduct of postmarket surveillance and for sharing AE data have been developed through a number of international agreements. Historically, much of the international cooperation was among agencies and organizations representing the United States, Europe, Japan, Canada, Australia, New Zealand, and Norway. Expanding manufacturing in China and India and rapidly expanding markets for medical products worldwide are changing that dynamic. We anticipate that linked record systems and distributed data networks developed in the United States and Europe will increasingly be piloted by, adapted to, and, where feasible, adopted in other regions, expanding the potential reach and power of medical product surveillance.

Collaborations among the FDA, CDC, manufacturers, distributors, importers, foreign regulatory agencies, prescribers, and consumers are likely to remain the backbone of the postmarket safety surveillance system. These collaborations will be needed to develop data sources and to validate methods of risk identification and analysis by linking clinical, laboratory, pharmacy, and administrative data sets. Refinements and improvements in data reporting standards, data transmission, risk assessment tools, and development of data sources of increasing size and depth will provide continued improvement in medical product risk assessment and risk management.

REFERENCES

1. 21U.S.C.§ 321(g) http://www.fda.gov/opacom/laws/fdcact/fdcact1.htm. Accessed March 31, 2009.
2. 21U.S.C.§ 321(h) http://www.fda.gov/opacom/laws/fdcact/fdcact1.htm. Accessed March 31, 2009.

3. 21 U.S.C.§ 360(hh) http://www.fda.gov/opacom/laws/fdcact/fdcact1.htm. Accessed March 31, 2009.

4. 42 U.S.C. § 262 http://www.fda.gov/opacom/laws/phsvcact/Sec262.htm. Accessed March 31, 2009.

5. Shenfield GM, Le Couteur DG, Rivory LP. Updates in medicine: clinical pharmacology. *Med J Aust* 2002;176:9.

6. Guidance for Industry Good Pharmacovigilance Practices and Pharmacoepidemiologic Assessment at page 13. http://www.fda.gov/cder/guidance/6359OCC.htm. Accessed November 26, 2008.

7. Szarfman A, Machado SG, O'Neill RT. Use of screening algorithms and computer systems to efficiently signal higher-than-expected combinations of drugs and events in the US FDA's spontaneous reports database. *Drug Saf* 2002;25(6):381–392.

8. Szarfman A, Tonning JM, Doraiswamy PM. Pharmacovigilance in the 21st century: new systematic tools for an old problem. *Pharmacotherapy* 2004;24(9):1099–1104.

9. Almenoff J, Tonning JM, Gould AL, *et al*. Perspectives on the use of data mining in pharmaco-vigilance. *Drug Saf* 2005;28(11):981–1007.

10. Kessler DA. Introducing MEDWatch: a new approach to reporting medication and device adverse effects and product problems. *JAMA* 1993;269(21):2765–2768.

11. Guidance: Drug Safety Information-FDA's Communications to the Public. http://www.fda.gov/cder/guidance/7477fnl.htm. March 2007. Accessed March 31,2009.

12. www.fda.gov/cdrh/medicaldevicesafety. Updated March 14, 2009. Accessed March 31, 2009.

13. http://www.fda.gov/cdrh/medsun/about.html. Updated January 14, 2009. Accessed March 31, 2009.

14. http://www.accessdata.fda.gov/scripts/cdrh/cfdocs/psn/index.cfm. Accessed March 31, 2009.

15. http://www.fda.gov/cder/drug/podcast/default.htm. Updated March 10, 2009. Accessed March 31, 2009.

16. http://www.fda.gov/medwatch/elist.htm. Accessed March 31, 2009.

17. Guidance for Industry Development and Use of Risk Minimization Action Plans. http://www.fda.gov/cder/guidance/6358fnl.htm)March 2005. Accessed March 31, 2009.

18. Brown B, Douglas B. Tabulation and analysis of pharmacovigilance data using the medical dictionary for regulatory activities. *Pharmacoepidemiol Drug Saf* 2000;9(6):479–489.

19. Mozzicato P. Standardised MedDRA queries: their role in signal detection. *Drug Saf* 2007;30(7):617–619.

20. Banks D, Woo EJ, Burwen DR, Perucci P, Braun MM, Ball R. Comparing data mining methods on the VAERS database. *Pharmacoepidemiol Drug Saf* 2005;14(9):601–609.

21. Evans SJW, Waller PC, Davis S. Use of proportional reporting ratios (PRRs) for signal generation from spontaneous adverse drug reaction reports. *Pharmacoepidemiol Drug Saf* 2001;10:483–486.

22. DuMouchel W. Bayesian data mining in large frequency tables, with an application to the FDA Spontaneous Reporting System (with discussion). *Am Stat* 1999;53(3):177–190.

23. DuMouchel W, Pregibon D. Empirical Bayes screening for multi-item associations. *Proc KDD 2001*, ACM, NY, 67–76.

24. Graham DJ, Campen D, Hui R, *et al*. Risk of acute myocardial infarction and sudden cardiac death in patients treated with cyclo-oxygenase 2 selective and non-selective non-steroidal anti-inflammatory drugs: nested case-control study. *Lancet* 2005;365(9458):475–481.

25. Watson WA, Litovitz T, Rubin C, *et al.* Toxic Exposure Surveillance System. *MMWR* 9/24/2004;53(suppl);262. www.cdc.gov/mmwr/preview/mmwrhtml/su5301a74.htm. Converted October 4, 2004. Accessed March 31, 2009.

26. MEDMARX Data Report 2006-Drug Names and Medication Errors. www.store. usp.org/OA_HTML/ibeCCtpItmDspRte.jsp?a=b&item=35442. Accessed March 31, 2009.

27. Paulozzi LJ. Opioid analgesic involvement in drug abuse deaths in American metropolitan areas. *Am J Public Health* 2006;96(10):1755–1757.

28. Budnitz DS, Pollock DA, Weidenbach KN, Mendelsohn AB, Schroeder TJ, Annest JL. National surveillance of emergency department visits for outpatient adverse drug events. *JAMA* 2006;296(15):1858–1866.

29. Chalasani N, Fontana RJ, Bonkovsky HL, *et al.* Causes, clinical features, and outcomes from a prospective study of drug-induced liver injury in the United States. *Gastroenterology* 2008;135(6):1924–1934, 1934.e1-4. Epub 2008 Sep 17.

30. Honein MA, Lindstrom JA, Kweder SL. Can we ensure the safe use of known human teratogens?: The iPLEDGE test case. *Drug Saf* 2007;30(1):5–15.

31. Lotronex Tablets (alosetron hydrochloride): Questions and Answers. www.fda. gov/cder/drug/infopage/lotronex/lotronex-qa_0602.htm. Accessed January 3, 2009.

32. TOUCH™ Prescribing Program. www.tysabri.com/tysbProject/tysb.portal/_baseurl/ twoColLayout/SCSRepository/en_US/tysb/home/touch-prescribing/index.xml. Accessed March 31, 2009.

33. http://www.otispregnancy.org/hm/inside.php?id=42. Accessed April 2, 2009.

34. http://www.imshealth.com. Accessed April 1, 2009.

35. http://www.marketresearch.com. Accessed April 1, 2009.

36. Gross TP, Witten CM, Uldriks C. Medical device regulation in the USA. In: Brown SL, Bright RA, Tavris DR, eds. *Medical Device Epidemiology and Surveillance.* West Sussex, England: John Wiley & Sons; 2007:5–19.

37. http://www.fda.gov/cdrh/maude/html. Updated March 6, 2009. Accessed April 2, 2009.

38. http://www.fda.gov/medwatch/safety/3500a.pdf. Accessed April 1, 2009.

39. Medical device problem reporting for the betterment of healthcare. *Health Devices* 1998;27(8):277–292.

40. Food and Drug Administration. Designing a medical device surveillance network. *FDA Report to Congress.* Rockville, MD: U.S. Food and Drug Administration, September 1999.

41. Hefflin BJ, Gross TP, Richardson EA, Coates VH. Medical device nomenclature. In Brown SL, Bright RA, Tavris DR, eds. *Medical Device Epidemiology and Surveillance.* West Sussex, England: John Wiley & Sons; 2007:87–97.

42. National Cancer Institute. Terminology Resources: NCI Enterprise Vocabulary Services (EVS), Dictionaries, FedMed, FDA, CDISC, and NCPDP Terminology. http://www.nci. nih.gov/cancerinfo/terminologyresources/page5. Accessed March 9, 2010 .

43. Food and Drug Administration. Medical Device Event Problem Codes. http://www. fda.gov/cdrh/problemcode Updated April 2, 2009. Accessed March 9, 2010.

44. US Department of Health and Human Services. National Institutes for Health. Interagency Registry for Mechanically Assisted Circulatory Support. http://www. intermacs.org. Accessed April 1, 2009.

45. Food and Drug Administration. Medical Devices—522 Postmarket Surveillance Studies. http://www.fda.gov/MedicalDevices/DeviceRegulationandGuidance/PostmarketRequirements/PostmarketSurveillance/default.htm. Accessed March 9, 2010.

46. Food and Drug Administration. Medical Devices—Post-Approval Studies. http://www. accessdata.fda.gov/scripts/cdrh/cfdocs/cfPMA/pma_pas.cfm. Accessed March 9, 2010.

47. Marinac-Dabic D, Bonhomme M, Lloyo-Berrios N, *et al.* Medical device post-approval studies program: vision, strategies, challenges, and opportunities. FDLI. *Food Drug Law J* 2007;62(3):597–604.

48. Mudano AS, Bian J, Cope JU, *et al.* Vertebroplasty and kyphoplasty are associated with an increased risk of secondary vertebral compression fractures: a population-based cohort study. *Osteoporos Int* 2009;20(5):819–826.

49. Zhan C, Kaczmarek R, Loyo-Berrios N, Sangl J, Bright RA. Incidence and short-term outcomes of primary and revision hip replacement in the United States. *J Bone Joint Surg Am* 2007;89(3):526–533.

50. Brown SL, Pennello G. Replacement surgery and silicone-gel breast implant rupture: self-report by women after mammoplasty. *J Women's Health & Gender-Based Med* 2002;11:255–264.

51. Tavris DR, Dey S, Gallauresi BA, *et al.* Risk of local adverse events following cardiac catheterization by hemostatis device use—Phase II. *J Invas Cardiol* 2005; 17:644–650.

52. National Cardiovascular Data Registry. http://www.accncdr.com/webncdr/ICD/ Default.aspx. Accessed April 1, 2009.

53. Centers for Disease Control and Prevention. Withdrawal of rotavirus vaccine recommendation. *MMWR* 1999;48(43):1007. http://www.cdc.gov/mmwr/preview/ mmwrhtml/mm4843a5.htm. Accessed December 1, 2009.

54. Ruiz-Palacios GM, Perez-Schael I, Velazquez FR, *et al.* Safety and efficacy of an attenuated vaccine against severe rotavirus gastroenteritis. *N Engl J Med* 2006;354:11–22.

55. Wise RP, Kiminyo KP, Salive ME. Hair loss after routine immunizations. *JAMA* 1997;278(14):1176–1178.

56. Braun MM, Patriarca PA, Ellenberg SS. Syncope after immunization. *Arch Pediatr Adolesc Med* 1997;151(3):255–259.

57. Izurieta HS, Haber P, Wise RP, *et al.* Adverse events reported following live, cold-adapted, intranasal influenza vaccine. *JAMA* 2005;294(21):2720–2725. Erratum in: *JAMA* 2005;294(24):3092.

58. Wise RP, Iskander J, Pratt RD, *et al.* Postlicensure safety surveillance for 7-valent pneumococcal conjugate vaccine. *JAMA* 2004;292(14):1702–1710.

59. Braun MM, Mootrey GT, Salive ME, Chen RT, Ellenberg SS. Infant immunization with acellular pertussis vaccines in the United States: assessment of the first two years' data from the Vaccine Adverse Event Reporting System (VAERS). *Pediatrics* 2000;106(4):E51.

60. Belongia E, Izurieta H, Braun MM, *et al.* Postmarketing Monitoring of Intussusception After RotaTeq™ Vaccination—United States, February 1, 2006–February 15, 2007. *MMWR* 2007;56:218–222.

61. Woo J, Ball R, Braun M, *et al.* Update: Guillain-Barre Syndrome Among Recipients of Menactra® Meningococcal Conjugate Vaccine—United States June 2005–September 2006. *MMWR* 2006;55(41):1120–1124.

62. Food and Drug Administration. Vaccines, Bloods and Biologics. http://www.fda.gov/ cber. Accessed April 1, 2009.

63. Food and Drug Administration. MedWatch: The FDA Safety Information and Adverse Event Reporting Program. http://www.fda.gov/medwatch. Updated April 1, 2009. Accessed April 1, 2009.

64. Braun MM. Toward better vaccine safety data and safer vaccination. *Pediatrics* 2008;121:625–626.

65. Food and Drug Administration. Guidance for Industry: E2E Pharmacovigiliance Planning. http://www.fda.gov/downloads/Drugs/GuidanceComplianceRegulatory Information/Guidances/ucm073107.pdf. Accessed March 8, 2010.

66. The Brighton Collaboration—Setting Standards in Vaccine Safety. http://www. brightoncollaboration.org/internet/en/index.html. Accessed April 1, 2009.

67. http://www.brightoncollaboration.org/internet/en/index/html.definition_guidelines. html. Accessed April 1, 2009.

68. 21 C.F.R. § 606.170.

69. Fatalities Reported to FDA Following Blood Collection and Transfusion. Annual Summary for Fiscal Year 2008. http://www.fda.gov/downloads/BiologicsBlood Vaccines/SafetyAvailability/BloodSafety/UCM113904.pdf. Accessed March 10, 2010.

70. 21 C.F.R. § 1271.

71. Chang S, Ball R, Braun MM. Elective termination of pregnancy after vaccination reported to the Vaccine Adverse Event Reporting System (VAERS): 1990–2006. *Vaccine* 2008;26(19):2428–2432.

72. International Conference on Harmonisation of Technical Requirements for Registration of Pharmaceuticals for Human Use (ICH). http://www.ich.org. Accessed April 1, 2009.

73. Council for International Organizations of Medical Sciences. http://www.cioms.ch/. Updated January 26, 2009. Accessed April 1, 2009.

74. Uppsala Monitoring Centre. http://www.who-umc.org/. Accessed April 1, 2009.

75. Global Harmonization Task Force. http://www.ghtf.org. Updated March 19, 2009. Accessed April 1, 2009.

76. Institute of Medicine of the National Academies. http://www.iom.edu/?id=37339. Updated March 19, 2009. Accessed April 1, 2009.

77. Psaty BM, Korn D. Congress responds to the IOM drug safety report–in full. *JAMA* 2007;298(18):2185–2187.

78. National Institutes of Health—Clinical Trials. http://www.clinicaltrials.gov. Accessed April 1, 2009.

79. Institute of Medicine of the National Academies. Safe Medical Devices for Children. http://www.iom.edu/CMS/3740/18614/28277.aspx. Updated March 18, 2009. Accessed April 1, 2009.

80. Food and Drug Administration. Regulatory Information. 21 U.S.C. 360c §522. http:// www.fda.gov/opacom/laws/fdcact/fdcact5a2.htm#sec522. Accessed April 1, 2009.

81. http://www.fda.gov/cdrh/postmarket/mdpi.html. Updated March 4, 2009. Accessed April 1, 2009.

82. Safety Reporting Requirements for Human Drug and Biological Products; 68 FR 12405–12497, March 14, 2003, proposed rule.

83. Lazarou J, Pomeranz BH, Corey PN. Incidence of adverse drug reactions in hospitalized patients: a meta-analysis of prospective studies. *JAMA* 1998;279(15):1200–1205.

84. Gurwitz JH, Field TS, Harrold LR, et al. Incidence and preventability of adverse drug events among older persons in the ambulatory setting *JAMA* 2003;289:1107–1116.

85. Food and Drug Administration. Sentinel Initiative. http://www.fda.gov/Safety/ FDAsSentinelInitiative/default.htm. Accessed March 8, 2010.

86. Food and Drug Administration. Drug Safety Newsletter. http://www.fda.gov/Drugs/ DrugSafety/DrugSafetyNewsletter/ucm119991.htm. Accessed March 8, 2010.

87. Food and Drug Administration. Drug Safety Newsletter. http://www.fda.gov/Drugs/ DrugSafety/DrugSafetyNewsletter/ucm109173.htm Accessed March 8, 2010.

88. Food and Drug Administration. Critical Path Initiative. http://www.fda.gov/oc/initia-tives/criticalpath/. Accessed March 8, 2010.

17

Surveillance in Low-Resource Settings

Challenges and Opportunities in the Current Context of Global Health

MICHAEL E. ST. LOUIS, HENRY WALKE, HELEN PERRY, PETER NSUBUGA, MARK E. WHITE, AND SCOTT DOWELL

The fundamental principles and practice of public health surveillance for global health and in low-resource countries do not differ from industrialized countries. However, a number of contextual factors are substantially different in low-resource settings (LRS). The interplay of national and international structures and norms is greater (*1–3*). The need to do more with less—while pervasive in public health—is thrown into sharper relief when the burden of disease is great and the financial and human resources are few (*4,5*). In addition, the strategy for strengthening surveillance is more complicated, and the sustainability of surveillance is more precarious when there is a heavy influence of external (international) partners, who might be influenced by a wide and frequently changing array of global perspectives about health priorities, and whose assistance might end or be delivered with unpredictable timing (*6,7*). This chapter offers some strategies for managing efforts to conduct surveillance and to improve surveillance systems in LRS in the current context of global health.

PUBLIC HEALTH SURVEILLANCE IN THE CURRENT ENVIRONMENT OF GLOBAL HEALTH

In the first decade of the 21st century there have been dramatic increases in the awareness of global health and resources allocated to it (*7–9*). Over the same period, public health surveillance has become a topic that commands attention and resources from a much broader community of partners (*10–12*). The threats of biologic terrorism after the 2001 anthrax attacks in the United States, the economic impact of severe acute respiratory syndrome (SARS) in 2003, the threat of a severe human influenza pandemic emerging from persistent avian epidemics of the H5N1 influenza virus, and the sudden emergence of novel 2009 Influenza A H1N1 of swine origin to a global pandemic in 2009 have put public health surveillance high not only on the global health agenda but also on national security agendas (*13,14*). Reflecting this heightened focus, the World Health Report of 2007 focused on global health security and emphasized the corresponding need to strengthen public health surveillance across the globe (*15*).

This increased attention and resources, along with advances in technology, would ideally catalyze rapid advances in global public health surveillance. However, despite the welcome additional resources, the proliferation of new partners with whom to transact support for surveillance and the disparate ways in which resources are sometimes made available to low-income countries can create new challenges (*2,3*). The majority of increases in global health spending in the past decade have come for highly targeted, disease-specific efforts, at times displacing investments in the more general, cross-cutting, health systems components, such as surveillance systems (*6,7*). Moreover, the increased alignment of public health surveillance with national and international security agendas might represent a threat as well as an opportunity, bringing greater resources to poor countries but potentially introducing considerations and approaches other than the best public health practices (*14,16*). It will be important to ensure that increased resources for surveillance around the world in coming years leads to improved surveillance that results not only in enhanced health security for industrialized nations but also improved health of people in the poorest countries (*14,17*).

International Partners and Networks for Surveillance

An increasingly complex array of organizations, partnerships, and global and regional networks now operate in global health (*1,18*), and many or most have some impact in the domain of surveillance. The World Health Organization (WHO) continues to provide overall global leadership on public health surveillance, but its shrinking proportionate share of global health funding and the sheer number of new organizations operating in the sphere challenge its ability to provide that needed leadership (*7,19*). In addition, other United Nations agencies and the World Bank and other international development banks have a history of supporting disease prevention programs in LRS (*7*), and these official multilateral agencies now increasingly underwrite surveillance initiatives. Most notable, however, are the many private or quasi-private global health organizations founded only since approximately 2000, including such preeminent global health organizations as the Global Alliance for Vaccines and Immunizations (GAVI); the Global Fund for AIDS, TB, and Malaria (GFATM); the Bill and Melinda Gates Foundation; and Google.org (*18*). Each of these has become a major supporter and influence on leaders in global health, including surveillance. In 2007 alone, the Gates Foundation and Google.org launched initiatives specifically for global health information and surveillance totaling more than $170 million (*20,21*), an unprecedented private sector investment in health information and surveillance. The Rockefeller Foundation has been a strong supporter of regional surveillance initiatives such as for emerging diseases in the Mekong River Delta

Basin. The more than 100 Global Health Partnerships (GHPs) founded in the past decades often include a surveillance component for their diseases of special interest. In an interesting and important variation on this theme, the Health Metrics Network (HMN) was the first GHP to target a cross-cutting health system issue (i.e., health information systems, including surveillance). Each of these organizations can be a source of technical and/or financial support for improved public health surveillance.

In addition to individual organizations, there are a growing number of networks operating to support, coordinate, and harmonize surveillance (Table 17–1; ref. *22*). Such networks, and others, can be among the most important and useful sources of information, technical assistance, mentoring, and tools to surveillance programs in LRS. For example, the INDEPTH Network (*see* http://www.indepth-network.net/) is a membership organization of Demographic Surveillance Systems (DSS) that represents a valuable source of data to provide estimates of vital events and to characterize selected diseases or outcomes, such as the major causes of and risk factors for childhood mortality in a country (*23,24*). Data from DSS have been used to document the burden of disease and the distribution of health interventions among the very poor (*25*) and to help document, for example, the impact of the demographic transition (to chronic diseases) in the setting of high HIV-related mortality (*26*). Globally, the International Emerging Infections Program (IEIP), a core component of the U.S. Center for Disease Control (CDC) Global Disease Detection (GDD) Program, implements similar high-quality, laboratory-based infectious public health surveillance at the population level in local areas, providing important, pathogen-specific estimates of incidence and burden of disease (*27*). However, despite—or, to some degree, because of—this plethora of new resources and potential partners, understaffed and underequipped Ministries of Health, and surveillance units in poor countries are often challenged by the "transaction costs" of interacting with many different partners and networks, each dealing with a specific aspect of surveillance (*6*). Assistance can be fragmented, and the proliferation of international partners with different programs, schedules, funding streams, and monitoring requirements greatly increases the complexity of managing the total enterprise of surveillance in many LRS (*28*). In addition, receiving resources or participating in specific networks might require the purchase or use of certain equipment or adoption of systems that complicate or contribute to fragmenting the broader surveillance and health protection enterprise in the countries. Importantly, the acceptance of external funding often obligates government personnel time and opportunity cost from the national health system, expenditures that also must be considered when accepting external offers of assistance (*29*).

To optimize the opportunities of the coming decade, the community of global surveillance practitioners needs to adopt the spirit and norms of the 2005 Paris Declaration of Aid Effectiveness (*30*), promoting country ownership of programs; use of country systems; and development of and adherence to consensus global standards that put improved performance much more within reach of poor countries (*31*). Early donor efforts in this regard show that this is far from a trivial undertaking either technically or sociologically, even for the best-intentioned

Table 17–1 Examples[1] of Types of Global Networks that Support Surveillance in Specific Subject Matter Areas

Network and contact URL	Description	Coverage, 2008
World Health Organization IHR (www.who.int/ihr)	IHR Focal Points in Geneva, six Regions, and all countries effectively establish a global network for detection and response to public health emergencies	All WHO Member States
Global Influenza Surveillance Network (GISN) http://www.who.int/csr/disease/influenza/influenzanetwork/en/	Surveillance for circulating human influenza illness and viruses	All Regions > 80 countries
Global Polio Surveillance Network http://www.polioeradication.org/casecount.asp	Surveillance for acute flaccid paralysis (AFP) and maintenance of appropriate laboratory testing of AFP cases	Global, but focused especially on the remaining polio-endemic countries
Global Outbreak Alert and Response Network (GOARN) http://www.who.int/csr/outbreaknetwork/en/	Secretariat at WHO maintains global vigilance for outbreaks and coordinates a network of trained responders to assist with outbreak investigation and control	Global scope includes more than 80 partner institutions across all WHO regions
Training Programs in Epidemiology and Public Health Interventions Network (TEPHINET) http://www.tephinet.org/	Supports field epidemiology training programs (FETP) globally. Extensive informal networks led to reporting of and response to outbreaks of Ebola, SARS, and other diseases	Currently has member organizations in more than 30 countries
International Food Safety Authorities Network (INFOSAN) (http://www.who.int/foodsafety/fs_management/infosan/en)	Network of national food safety authorities, developed and managed by WHO in collaboration with the Food and Agriculture Organization of the United Nations (FAO)	Currently 177 national food safety authorities participate
Global Foodborne Infections Network (GFN) (formerly Global Salm-Surv Network) (http://www.who.int/salmsurv/en)	Promotes integrated, laboratory-based surveillance and fosters intersectoral collaboration among human health, veterinary, and food-related disciplines through training courses and activities around the world	Training courses provided in all WHO regions
Global Disease Detection Program (US CDC) (http://www.cdc.gov/cogh/gdd)	Network of CDC-supported programs in emerging infectious diseases, supplements WHO's IHR and GOARN networks	GDD Centers in 6 countries on 5 continents, plus collaborations in multiple other countries

(continued)

Table 17–1 (*continued*)

Network and contact URL	Description	Coverage, 2008
Global Emerging Infections Surveillance System (US DOD) http://www.geis.fhp.osd.mil/aboutGEIS.asp	Network of U.S. Department of Defense research and preventive health units that can assist with surveillance efforts in their regions in both military and civilian populations	Two U.S.-based facilities and five research programs outside of the United States
Health Metrics Network (HMN) http://www.who.int/healthmetrics/en/	Global Health Public-Private Partnership working to strengthen health information systems to promote better health and better accountability	Supports activities in more than 70 countries globally
INDEPTH Network http://www.indepth-network.org/	International organization for the demographic evaluation of populations and their health in developing countries through Demographic Surveillance Sites (DSS)	Currently 35 DSS in 18 countries are monitoring population vital events and particular diseases or conditions
Integrated Disease Surveillance and Response (IDSR) http://www.who.int/csr/labepidemiology/projects/diseasesurv/en or http://www.cdc.gov/idsr/	A strategy supported by WHO AFRO for integrated surveillance of outbreak-prone diseases and other major public health conditions	WHO Africa, Region
Asia Pacific Strategy for Emerging Diseases (APSED) http://www.wpro.who.int/NR/rdonlyres/FCEEBB9D-21BB-4A16-8530-756F99EFDB67/0/asia_pacific.pdf	A strategy for surveillance for emerging diseases in the WHO WPRO and SEARO regions	WHO Asia and SE Asia Regions
Global Tobacco Surveillance Systems https://www.who.int/tobacco/surveillance/en/	The GTSS includes the collection of data through four surveys: the Global Youth Tobacco Survey (GYTS) for youth; the Global School Personnel Survey (GSPS); and the Global Health Professions Students Survey (GHPSS) for adults	GTSS surveys have been conducted in more than 130 countries in all WHO Regions
ChemiNet http://www.who.int/environmental_health_emergencies/ChemiNet3.pdf	A Global public health chemical incident alert, surveillance, and response network	Global network of institutions, agencies, laboratories, WHO Collaborating Centers, poison centers, etc.

[1] Table is not a complete enumeration of surveillance support activities and networks, but includes only selected examples to demonstrate the types of resources potentially available.

international organizations (*32*), but it remains an essential part of the a code of good behavior for all international organizations and individuals operating in the field of public health surveillance (*30,33*).

Policy Regarding Public Health Surveillance in Global Health

The overriding policy development of the past several decades relevant to public health surveillance is the 2005 revision of the International Health Regulations (IHRs) (*34,35*). The new IHR sharply broadens the range of infectious diseases and other public health events of international concern (PHEICs) from just three diseases listed in prior revision of the IHR to a much broader set of known and emerging diseases as well as non-infectious hazards; shifts the focus from control at borders to detection and control at the source; and, most importantly, requires countries to document capacity for detection, verification, and response to PHEICs within their borders. This last provision established a new requirement for surveillance capacity and performance that will need to be both developed and measured for accountability. Unfortunately, this new requirement for global surveillance has not yet been matched by resources dedicated to assisting LRS to meet the standard—a classic "unfunded mandate." Nonetheless, the IHR 2005 sets a new bar for surveillance system performance that will stimulate surveillance authorities in poor countries and their national and international partners to strengthen surveillance programs in every country substantially by 2012, when the IHR requires achievement of the new global surveillance capacity standards (*36*).

Advances in Technology

Technological advances could empower global surveillance and, in particular, surveillance in LRS. The information and communication technology (ICT) revolution continues, including: power-sparing computers tolerant of harsh environmental conditions; expansion of the Internet and its users; and vastly expanded penetration of cellular networks to cover the majority of even the poorest populations (*37*). The last factor allows voice calling for emergencies and text message reporting of human and animal diseases. Many health surveys in LRS are now being implemented on handheld computing devices with global positioning system (GPS) capacity, resulting in improved accuracy, sampling, supervision, and timeliness of analysis and reporting (*38,39*). Laboratory testing technology is also advancing, with more assays being implemented in simpler formats usable in environments with weak infrastructure (*40,41*). Further innovation in biotechnology and initiatives such as the Grand Challenges in Global Health (*42*) promise to continue to spin off new laboratory tools to support surveillance in areas that have lacked laboratory capacity in the past. These technology advances create tremendous opportunities for improving surveillance, but sustained pressure toward identification of best global practices, harmonization, and standardization will be needed in all these areas. Active dissemination of emerging best practices will need to be championed by organizations such as WHO and the HMN, so that the poorest countries will not each independently need to assess and experiment with how to incorporate each of these innovations into their national surveillance programs. Most importantly, surveillance systems are made fundamentally of humans, and new technologies need to be introduced in ways that enhance the function of the people who fill diverse roles in surveillance systems. It is critical not to foresee that computers or other types of automation will eliminate the need for adequate human capacity in the form of vigilant clinical, laboratory, and public health surveillance officers who are well-trained for their roles. Instead, new technology should be envisioned to support those workers to do their jobs better and more efficiently.

Low-Resource Settings

The remainder of this chapter addresses the special situation of surveillance in LRS, in the light of the growing global interest, resources, opportunities, and expectations for surveillance. Several recent reviews have provided excellent updates on the broad field of public health surveillance in low resources (43) and for specific diseases (44). The pressure for global reporting of disease threats in poor countries needs to be met by thoughtful, appropriate design of the next generation of surveillance systems, recognizing that one is building not in a vacuum but on a complex, diverse set of ongoing systems that differ from country to country.

GENERAL CONSIDERATIONS FOR SURVEILLANCE IN LOW-RESOURCE SETTINGS

Value of Surveillance

Regardless of setting, surveillance is the basic tool of public health that informs public health action. Without the ongoing collection and analysis of health data to inform public health decision making, essential health policy decisions in poor countries are made on the basis of information or advice from elsewhere. Too often, decisions are not made at all. Surveillance can be expensive or inexpensive, and in countries with very few health resources, it is particularly important to ensure that the human and financial resources expended on surveillance are commensurate with the burden and importance of the public health problem being addressed.

In spite of these considerations, examples abound of the value of public health surveillance for informing decision making in LRS. Smallpox and other disease eradication campaigns demonstrated how high-quality surveillance could be conducted in LRS to achieve public health goals (45). Funded globally, the smallpox eradication campaign, like the current polio and guinea worm eradication efforts, delivered enormous value in terms of savings in mortality, morbidity, and vaccine expenditures for each year after the success of the campaigns. Polio eradication requires intensive nationwide surveillance to identify all cases of acute flaccid paralysis, coupled with an effective laboratory network capable of obtaining and transporting stool specimens, culturing polio viruses, and accurately differentiating wild-type polio from vaccine-derived strains. The presence of wild-type polio viruses, the characterization of any viruses obtained, and the geographic distribution of cases and persons with asymptomatic viral shedding are all critical pieces of information informing substantial decisions about the public health response, such as instituting mass vaccination campaigns or enhancements of routine infant immunization, the type of vaccine to use, and the geographic extent of the response (*46*).

More complex and costly public health decisions, such as whether to invest limited resources in a national commitment to provide a new vaccine to all children in the population, often require more detailed surveillance information useful for measuring disease burden and monitoring the burden over time. The impact of such diseases might differ substantially among regions and countries (*47*) so that surveillance findings are needed to guide long-term commitments of resources.

Emerging infectious diseases have the potential to cause widespread public concern or panic, leading to economic as well as health losses. The outbreak of SARS in 2003 resulted in more than 8,000 confirmed cases worldwide, with almost 800 deaths, and economic losses estimated at more than $30 billion (*48*). Avian influenza is a top concern of wealthy countries because of the potential for a global pandemic, as well as the impact of widespread poultry outbreaks on human health and the considerable impact on the poultry industry and individual farmers (*49*). High-quality surveillance, such as in Thailand and Egypt, can minimize the economic and public health impact by containment of poultry outbreaks and earlier identification and treatment of human disease (*50,51*). It is plausible that current efforts to identify, treat, and interrupt transmission of H5N1 strains rapidly in settings where human infections have occurred has already contributed to reducing risk or at least setting back the clock for evolution toward viruses that are more transmissible among humans.

TYPES OF SURVEILLANCE

Structured and Unstructured Surveillance

The most fundamental and relevant distinction in types of global health surveillance is between systems that capture and use *structured* versus *unstructured* data (Fig. 17–1). Most traditional types of public health surveillance involve a structured approach to gain information on a defined number of specific diseases or conditions of high priority to public health, typically reflected by a structured process involving explicit case definitions and precise reporting procedures from throughout the health system. This is also frequently called *routine surveillance, indicator-based surveillance, surveillance for notifiable conditions*, and a number of other terms that reflect the specific intent to bring specific types of illness or specific scenarios under a systematic, structured system of surveillance that involves disseminating explicit case definitions and reporting requirements

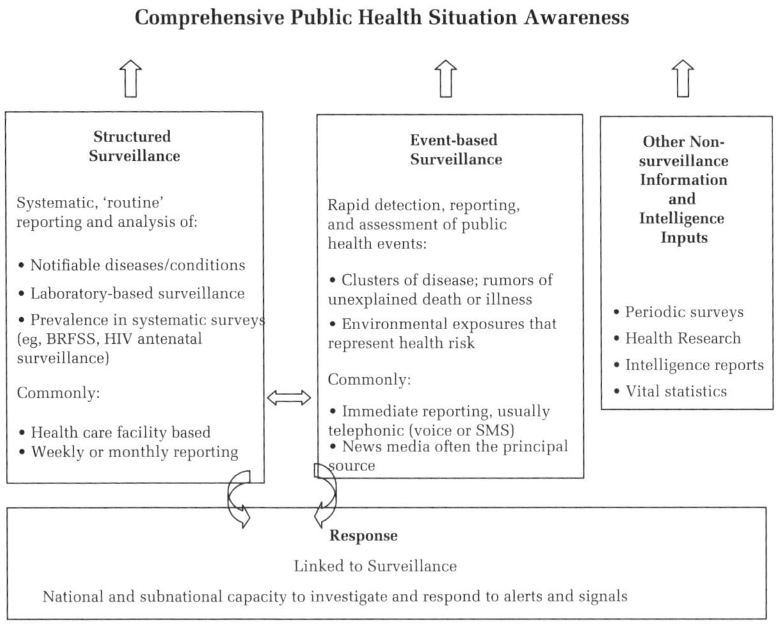

Comprehensive Public Health Situation Awareness

Figure 17–1 Comprehensive Public Health Situation Awareness. Two Main Categories of Public Health Surveillance Systems—Structured Surveillance and Event-based (Unstructured) Surveillance—and their linkage to each other and to Response Capabilities, along with other inputs contributing to overall Comprehensive Public Health Situation Awareness. Adapted from WHO WPRO, A Guide to Establishing Event-Based Surveillance, 2008.

throughout the jurisdiction. Classical, structured surveillance is represented well by the WHO Standards for Surveillance issued in 1999 (*52*).

More recently, new systems specifically attuned to emerging diseases (for which there can be no explicit case definition, unanticipated events, and rumors) have been developed to detect information about potential health threats in novel and unstructured ways (*12,53,54*). GPHIN, based on "Web-crawler" technology that searches continuously for certain key words in mass media, blogs, and all types of Internet-based information has revolutionized outbreak detection in the world for WHO and now yields the first signal for more than 70% of important outbreaks (*49,53,55*). The general process of active and passive search for unstructured signals and reports suggesting emerging outbreaks has been termed *event-based surveillance* (*56*). The optimal relationship between structured and unstructured (or event-based) surveillance has been articulated well in the formulation of an "Epidemic Intelligence" framework at the European Centers for Disease Control, although the term *indicator-based surveillance* is awkward and frequently a source of confusion (*57*). As a term, *Epidemic Intelligence* suffices to characterize the situation regarding disease epidemics but fails to capture important non-infectious health risks (such as extreme weather, climate change, or occupational health risks). This new requirement for a broader, integrated, more real-time synthesis of diverse types of structured and unstructured data has recently been defined somewhat awkwardly as *Biosurveillance* in the United States (*see* Chapter 14), but that term does not extend to include either health status associated with chronic diseases nor the monitoring of risk factors representing intermediate and longer-term threats to the population. Other terms have been offered for this highest-level comprehension of the health status of the population, the associated threats to health, and the opportunities for health protection and improvement, including: *Health Situation Awareness*, *Health Status Monitoring*, *Health Intelligence*, and others. However, a true consensus term for this concept has not yet emerged. Nonetheless, this capacity for high-level comprehension of population health status and risks, including at least the fusion of diverse surveillance systems plus other information feeds, will be increasingly expected by policy makers in LRS as well. In most settings, it is fair to say that the fusion of different streams of surveillance information with incorporation of other diverse types of nonsurveillance information has not yet been brought together seamlessly to provide the type of comprehensive, real-time, comprehensive health situation awareness that policymakers increasingly demand (*see* Fig. 17–1).

Choice of Surveillance Approaches in Low-Resource Settings

There is no single best approach to public health surveillance any more than there is a single protocol for conducting medical research. Different approaches are appropriate and efficient to address different information needs. The more specifically the question to be addressed can be articulated, the more appropriate the surveillance design can be for informing the public health decision. In reality, choosing a surveillance approach always involves compromises or trade-offs between desirable attributes—for example, between timeliness and representativeness or between sensitivity and specificity (*58–60*). Cost is also an important consideration in choosing a surveillance approach. In addition to direct costs such as the printing of reporting forms or computer programming and hardware, it is important to consider the value of the time health workers spend on entering information and the potential political costs to national governments of reporting diseases where stigma might reduce vital income exports or damage tourism. Failure to consider all the costs of a system may contribute to system failure (*61*).

Table 17–2 lists principal types of or approaches to both structured and event-based surveillance employed in LRS, along with relative advantages and disadvantages for each, as well as other types of health information collection that are *not* surveillance activities according to the definition used in this book (*see* Chapter 20) but that are closely tied to core surveillance efforts in LRS and that are commonly considered by stakeholders in those settings to be components of "surveillance." Some of these categories are logical subcategories of others (e.g., population-based surveillance in a limited jurisdiction is really a specific type of sentinel surveillance), but they have grown sufficiently distinct and important in the current environment of global health and particularly in LRS that it is worth identifying them separately. For a country that wishes to get a comprehensive view of its current surveillance activities, it can be useful to develop a table with

Table 17-2 Principal Types of Surveillance Systems and Closely-Aligned Health Information Sources in Low-Resource Settings

Type of surveillance system	Explanation and examples	Particular strength	Particular drawback or cost
1. Notifiable public health surveillance from all facilities and providers	Most comprehensive or "passive" surveillance systems for outbreak-prone diseases and uncommon but important conditions. Typically managed by a unit of the MOH charged with surveillance and outbreak response (which usually is distinct from the unit responsible for the National Health Information System).	The only system that yields baseline data on key conditions across the entire public health jurisdiction down to local levels. Also—along with event-based surveillance—the only system that potentially provides a continually updated epidemic intelligence over the entire jurisdiction under surveillance.	Because of comprehensive scope of coverage, both data quality and timeliness of detection might lag, often severely. Also, data are almost always "thinner" (limited data collected for each case) than in more intensive surveillance approaches, such as in sentinel surveillance.
2. Surveillance data from disease control programs	AIDS, HIV prevalence, TB, malaria, polio and other vaccine-preventable diseases, and other disease reporting established as a component of a disease control program. Often managed through a monitoring and evaluation unit integrated into the disease control program, but outside the surveillance and outbreak response unit.	Generally, high-quality data reported with timeliness appropriate for the disease in question (e.g., daily/weekly for polio eradication, annually for HIV/AIDS). Information constitutes an essential input for managing these high-priority public health programs.	Compartmentalization of surveillance efforts might be associated with redundant, parallel building of components (data entry fields, databases, schemes for transmission of reports, etc.) while also creating barriers to sharing of data (e.g., linked HIV and TB registries) and sharing of surveillance resources.
3. Sentinel surveillance	The implementation of surveillance not comprehensively across all territory and population for which a public health authority has jurisdiction, but only in an explicit subset of the territory or its facilities. Surveillance for antimicrobial resistance in *N. gonorrheae* in the United States at 26 clinics across the United States is an example, as are many efforts to assess the potential impact of introducing new vaccines through sentinel surveillance. The Global Influenza Surveillance Network (GISN) operates globally through sentinel surveillance sites.	Particularly important and useful in the systematic and more detailed investigation of a subset of cases to assess trends in characteristics that could not be universally evaluated, such as intensive laboratory investigation of pathogens.	Sentinel surveillance does not yield early warning of outbreaks other than coincidentally in a very small sample of the total population and does not engage the public health community in most of the country (a strength as well as a weakness). Sentinel surveillance often borders on and might need to be treated as research.

(continued)

Table 17–2 (continued)

Type of surveillance system	Explanation and examples	Particular strength	Particular drawback or cost
4. Active, population-based surveillance in limited areas	A subset (but an important and growing subset) of sentinel surveillance involves actively trying to ascertain all of a set of selected events in a defined geographic region, usually while vigilantly tracking the population denominator (births, deaths, in- and out-migration, etc.) The Active Bacterial Core program in the U.S. and INDEPTH Demographic Surveillance Sites (DSS) in low-resource settings are examples.	Near universal ascertainment of events under active surveillance allow accurate determination of burden of disease, attributes of an infectious pathogen and its health consequences, vital events (in countries without other ongoing vital events data), and other health events and outcomes.	The area under surveillance does not necessarily reflect the country as a whole and might well differ from the Hawthorne Effect (intensified observation changes things) and because of the intervention trials often carried out in DSS and other such settings.
5. Syndromic surveillance	This term is used in two very different ways: (1) traditionally, it refers to case definitions that do not depend only on laboratory results, but depend only on a clinical syndrome (e.g., acute watery diarrhea); (2) recently, it is used to electronic systems that attempt to gain situation awareness of rapidly emerging clusters of disease by automated aggregation and analysis of electronic signals from different sources.	Syndromic surveillance has high sensitivity. When a syndrome is important, highly characteristic, and present in all or most patients (e.g., smallpox), highly effective syndromic surveillance can result.	Syndromic surveillance, except for very specific syndromes such as acute flaccid paralysis (AFP) or hemorrhagic fever, tends to generate large amounts of data and signals. Truly important signals are at risk to get lost in a "needle in the haystack" effect.
6. Ongoing, periodic surveys for public health monitoring and action	Surveillance surveys may be conducted on a stable, ongoing basis (i.e., annually or more frequently), to guide public health interventions. Examples include BRFSS in the U.S.; HIV sentinel surveillance in antenatal clinics as practiced in most sub-Saharan African countries; and global surveillance for tobacco use in youth.	Prevalence data potentially quickly available at relatively low cost (relevant especially for highly prevalent conditions rather than rare conditions). Trend data quickly available at relatively low cost.	Local data is not available except where sampling occurs. Absolute magnitude of condition often is not determined (depends on statistical nature of sampling).

| 7. Population-based surveys | Not a surveillance system per se, but a critical source of high quality population health data that in most low resource settings are critical to calibrating surveillance findings. Examples include the USAID-supported Demographic Health Surveys (DHS) and the UNICEF-supported Multiple Indicator Cluster Surveys (MICS). An extreme example outside the health sector but critical to the public health information grid is the population census. | Yields statistically valid estimates of health outcomes and population denominators at a point in time. Surveillance systems almost never do so, unless highly resource-intensive and generally restricted to a modest-sized population that can be effectively covered. | High cost, low frequency of replication (often 5–10 years), and—for sample surveys—lack of estimates at subnational and local levels. Inability to estimate relatively rare outcomes (such as maternal mortality). |
| 8. Event-based surveillance | The organized and rapid capture of unstructured information about events that are a potential risk to public health. This includes both events involving occurrence of disease in humans and events that reflect a risk for potential exposure of humans (such as disease in animals or environmental contamination events). | The rapid detection of and response to events that fall outside of the predefined conditions that are the objects of structured surveillance. | Potential for large number of false-positive alerts that consume valuable resources and attention. One might miss the critical needle in the haystack because of noise. |

categories such as in Table 17–2 and to use it to list by category the diverse, specific public health surveillance systems operating in the country. This will often turn into a long and heterogeneous list, with entries in all or most of the categories. Each surveillance system could have a diverse geographic coverage and might have its own sponsorship, technical, and financial support from different international partners. Such an inventory can be used to identify for redundancies, gaps, and inefficiencies, as well as to identify strengths on which to build.

Surveillance systems such as those underlying disease elimination or eradication efforts often have an especially complex relationship to other surveillance systems. They often have substantially more resources than other surveillance programs while, by definition, pursuing a decreasing burden of visible disease (*62,63*). This can be addressed by integrating surveillance and control efforts together where there is a natural fit, as is done in WHO's Regional Office for Africa Integrated Public health surveillance and Response networks (*see* below), which was developed in large part on the infrastructure of established polio eradication surveillance systems (*64,65*). Surveillance systems for eradication of guinea worm and onchocerciasis have helped contribute to pragmatic delivery of other basic surveillance and to health situation awareness in the most remote and challenging situations in the world.

COORDINATION, HARMONIZATION, AND INTEGRATION OF SURVEILLANCE SYSTEMS IN LOW-RESOURCE SETTINGS

The terms *coordination*, *harmonization*, and *integration* have often been used in overlapping ways with regard to efforts to improve the efficiency and effectiveness of surveillance in LRS. We use the term *coordination* to refer to efforts to maintain mutual awareness of activities and promote efficiencies, while not changing the actual processes of any of involved surveillance systems. It is the "lightest" of approaches. A main purpose for coordination is the sharing of resources for common tasks (*2*). A good example was the coordination in Rwanda of efforts to develop a laboratory network to support HIV/AIDS testing, on the one hand, with the government's intent to establish a national laboratory system for communicable diseases surveillance that collects, transports, safely handles, sorts, and processes specimens for infectious diseases beyond HIV, including bacterial pathogens. Funds were leveraged to common purpose, so that not only were the HIV/AIDS laboratory objectives achieved but sharing of common resources, training, and requirements enhanced the overall laboratory capacity for the country (*66*).

Harmonization is the attempt to require that different surveillance programs each independently adhere to the same norms, rules, and processes (such as data standards, standardized data dictionaries, data interfaces, and software development standards), resulting in convergence to eventual interoperability of those systems (see Chapter 5 for discussion of interoperability of surveillance information systems). Harmonization in this sense reduces the complexity of dealing with different systems on the part of health-care and surveillance workers and promotes the ability to link data across surveillance systems. Furthermore, it helps to establish the basis for truly integrated systems of surveillance and health information when the technical infrastructure in an area sufficiently matures. Examples of harmonization of surveillance practices include the publication of Standards for Surveillance by WHO (52) and a Technical Framework for Strengthening Health Information Systems by HMN (67). Globally, emerging frameworks and standards such as Health Level Seven (HL7), International Classification of Diseases (ICD), and others point to an upcoming era when health and surveillance data can be transmitted rapidly, efficiently, and reliably anywhere in the world telecommunications. Harmonized and interoperable surveillance systems can remain functionally and operationally independent, and do not need to be recast as an integrated package of activities and modules.

True "integration" of systems is the most ambitious of these three concepts, involving development of a seamless or common set of processes shared by all. Since the mid-1990s, WHO has been promoting what it calls an integrated approach to public health surveillance (68). This integrated approach seeks to improve overall national communicable public health surveillance by streamlining resources and coordinating surveillance functions at all levels of the health system. Integration attempts to provide countries with a framework to produce systems that are effective, efficient, and sustainable and to organize all public health surveillance activities into a common public service (69).

Special opportunities for integration occur when a system is newly designed and implemented. For example, the Integrated Disease Surveillance and Response (IDSR) strategy was developed by the WHO Regional Office for Africa (AFRO) in 1998 (70). In IDSR, integration focused on organizing a system around surveillance functions rather than individual disease-specific requirements. In this approach, the functions of surveillance (detection, reporting, analysis, interpretation, response, feedback, and evaluation) are linked to each level of the health system and incorporate the supporting structures of laboratory services, communication, training, and supervision (71). A powerful example of the potential utility of applying a standardized logical approach across different surveillance activities can be seen in the application of the concept of "thresholds for action" to different types of public health surveillance data in the WHO AFRO IDSR framework and approach (Table 17–3).

At the current time, the concept of harmonization as defined above, which focuses on making incremental but tangible progress toward standards-based interoperable systems, probably offers the most broadly feasible approach for large-scale strengthening of national systems of surveillance (6). To the extent the international standards can be articulated and defined for public health surveillance, all countries will benefit—especially the poorest countries—because they should be drawn upward in global efforts to make health-related data systems more interoperable and efficient. This might also help toward leapfrogging in surveillance over a generation of infrastructure, like that which has been largely achieved in sub-Saharan Africa with the widespread adoption of cellular telephone systems without having passed through a phase of copper wire telephony. Sustained leadership in championing, developing, and promoting consensus standards for public health surveillance will be needed on the part of WHO, HMN, and other leadership organizations in global health.

Table 17–3 Examples of Action Thresholds and Response Actions Linked to Public Health Surveillance Efforts in Low Resource Settings

Disease or Condition	Surveillance Objective	Action Threshold	Response Action
Example of an epidemic-prone disease			
Cholera	Detect and respond promptly and appropriately to cases and outbreaks of watery diarrhea	A single suspected case of cholera	• Report case-based information immediately. • Manage and treat the cause according to national guidelines. • Enhance strict hand-washing and patient isolation procedures. • Obtain stool specimen from five patients within 5 days of onset of acute watery diarrhea and before antibiotic treatment is started. • Conduct case-based investigation to identify similar causes not previously reported.
Example of a disease targeted for eradication or elimination			
Poliomyelitis (acute flaccid paralysis; AFP)	Identify all cases of paralytic poliomyelitis	One suspected case if AFP	• Report suspected case immediately. • Conduct case-based investigation. • Obtain 2 or more stool specimens within 14 days of onset of paralysis for viral isolation. • Respond according to national polio program guidelines.
Example of a disease that is endemic			
Malaria	Monitor impact of program interventions	When coverage of program intervention is at moderate or high levels, any lack of decline for in-patient deaths in children less than age 5 years.	• Review the effectiveness of the program interventions (e.g., resistance to insecticide in the bed net, anti-malarial drug resistance). • Evaluate the quality of the data. • Review data for any surveillance biases (e.g., increase or decrease in number of patients resulting from a change in drug availability).

(continued)

Table 17–3 (*continued*)

Disease or Condition	Surveillance Objective	Action Threshold	Response Action
Example of surveillance for a risk factor			
Tobacco use	Monitor prevalence of use	Rise in prevalence by age group	• Review regulations regarding tobacco sales to minors • Raise taxes • Ban or restrict advertising
Example of event-based surveillance			
H5N1 disease outbreaks in poulty	Detect any introduction or presence of the virus	Any presence of H5N1 in domestic poultry	• Implement culling of affected flocks, more intensive surveillance for surrounding flocks, etc. • Initiate active surveillance for human disease among cullers, nearby populations, health-care workers, etc. • Attempt to assure access to effective antiviral agents at nearby hospitals.
Release of a dangerous chemical	Immediate awareness of potential chemical event	Any release of a dangerous chemical or of chemical with uncertain safety profile	• Surveillance among first responders and nearby populations • Deployment of specific remedies and general emergency supplies

AN ENABLING ENVIRONMENT FOR PUBLIC HEALTH SURVEILLANCE

There are many potential obstacles that can derail public health surveillance in LRS. A critical, high-level consideration in any setting is to work systematically toward establishing an environment that enables the various forms of surveillance to flourish. Outside of technical requirements, such as defined protocols for collection and analysis of data, important issues to consider are the legal, administrative, and financial structures that support surveillance; basic public health laboratory capacity; the existence of a trained public health workforce; and, of course, political commitment and leadership (*22,72*).

Public law infrastructure establishes the powers and duties of the government in promoting the population's health (*73*). Countries have diverse governance systems and a varying array of legal frameworks and procedures under which public health surveillance operates. National, state, and local governmental authorities have different legal responsibilities and capacities for surveillance and response. Whether the governmental structure is a more or less centralized system, absence of a public health legal framework breeds conflict between different levels of government or, worse, leads to inaction resulting from inadequate clarity of legal responsibilities.

In LRS, governmental and administrative structures as well as technical strategies are needed that support diverse surveillance activities simultaneously and use scarce human and financial resources efficiently. As described earlier, the impact of donor-driven priorities or international concerns in a country often results in multiple, vertical, disease-specific surveillance programs using separate information systems, personnel, vehicles, and office space at every administrative level of the country. In Pakistan, for example, the acute flaccid paralysis surveillance system, the Lady Health Worker information system, and the Health Management Information System report to separate programs in different agencies in the government (74). Integration of similar surveillance functions across multiple diseases can plausibly lead to greater efficiency but only if resources are maintained and technical leadership for surveillance and health awareness is recognized as a major governmental responsibility. Instead, such integration is frequently adopted mainly as a cost-cutting measure rather than in a drive for higher levels of function and most often results in substantial loss of functionality across the formerly "vertical" but at least functioning systems. Integration truly directed at strengthening surveillance could be enhanced by creating surveillance units at every administrative level, staffed by trained personnel, who can perform coordinated surveillance and response. Public health surveillance and health information systems in general require important financial commitments. These investments could be offset in the future by savings from improvements in the efficiency in the health-care system (31), but virtually every effort at integration of surveillance systems that starts without explicit and attentive high-level commitment to meet the real information requirements of priority public health programs ends in failure and need to bring back the dedicated or vertical surveillance programs.

The organizational structure should also facilitate communication among health-related agencies within the government, including, for example, those responsible for vital statistics, food and drug administration, and medical research. National public health agencies such as CDC, the Finnish National Public Health Institute (KTL), and the United Kingdom's Health Protection Agency (HPA) are examples where countries have grouped essential public health capacities under one organizational structure (75).

The existence of solid, basic public health laboratory capacity, matched to country priority diseases, is vital for public health surveillance. The laboratory is not only a good source of surveillance data, but health workers are also more likely to complete reporting and specimen submission requirements if they know they will receive a timely laboratory result. Without a functional public health laboratory, surveillance is essentially limited to syndromes or symptoms and in emergencies; countries are left dependent on a regional reference laboratory or the private or academic community. Improving the quality of laboratory testing in resource-constrained countries requires a systematic approach (76). Hiring personnel and purchasing equipment are important, but attention should also be directed to the quality of laboratory systems, including such issues as developing uniform formats for documents and records, process control, facilities and safety, and training. Promoting the establishment of laboratory networks, which include all administrative levels of the country, can also facilitate standardization and sharing of procedures and protocols. In the Jordan Ministry of Health at the national level, the public health laboratorians frequently join the weekly surveillance meeting, a practice that can result in vital information sharing and team building across expertise domains.

Public health surveillance requires an adequately staffed and trained workforce to function well. A basic surveillance workforce includes heath workers as the front line of surveillance, epidemiologists, public health laboratorians, and, increasingly, informatics specialists. Health workers need training in detection and reporting mechanisms. Surveillance is typically a low priority for health-care providers with heavy patient loads, but ancillary health staff can be trained. Trained epidemiologists, who can aggregate, analyze, and synthesize surveillance data; identify aberrations; and generate informative reports, are an essential part of the workforce. Basic descriptive analysis is needed for the peripheral levels of a public health system, but more sophisticated skills such as the ability to create thresholds for action, conduct surveillance evaluations, and analyze regional data sets are needed for the provincial and federal levels. Functioning public health laboratory systems require trained laboratory scientists who excel in their basic disciplines but who also appreciate the special requirements of surveillance and outbreak response. Even in LRS, or perhaps *especially* in LRS in the 21st Century, informatics specialists are also needed (*see* Chapter 5). Informaticians should be able to help translate information generation, flow, and processing for public health surveillance into the most robust and efficient design and architecture for the local ICT infrastructure and the human capacity context.

An especially good source of epidemiologists to lead surveillance and response systems are the field epidemiology training programs (FETPs) (77). In these programs, MOH staff are engaged in a 2-year, competency-based, in-service training that includes surveillance, outbreak response, and public health program management (78). Graduates of these programs have taken leadership roles for surveillance in federal or provincial health departments (79). Recruiting and retaining such personnel within the ministry of health will depend on creation of the appropriate epidemiologist and surveillance career paths, competitive salaries, and administrative units in which to use their skills.

Political commitment and leadership is essential to create an enabling environment for surveillance. A culture of evidence-based decision making can be fostered through training "tomorrow's leaders" in public health, either through applied epidemiology programs such as FETPs or interdisciplinary in-service training programs for policymakers and program managers such as Data for Decision Making (DDM) (80). A key attribute of these programs is mentoring of participants while they apply their newly acquired skills. Ultimately, political commitment is best obtained when decision makers facing a policy issue can easily access and utilize information from public health surveillance systems.

OPPORTUNITIES IN COMING YEARS, AND THE ATTENDANT NEED FOR EVIDENCE-BASED APPROACHES TO STRENGTHENING SURVEILLANCE

Two major global consensus goal frameworks involving health were negotiated by nearly all nations near the start of the new millenium: the IHR 2005, as discussed previously, and the Millenium Development Goals (MDGs) (81). Each of these frameworks lay out ambitious goals to be reached in all countries by 2012 through 2016 for the IHR, and by 2015 for the MDGs, and, to a large degree, define the overarching goal structure for global health in the early 21st century. Strengthened surveillance is the essence of the IHR, and it is a critical requirement for monitoring progress in the three of the eight MGDs that directly relate to health. In addition, beyond the health security goals of the IHR and the health promotion goals of MDGs, the highest additional priority in global health is arguably the need to address the emerging global health crises precipitated by climate change; once again, strengthened and appropriately sensitized surveillance has been consistently identified one of the most fundamental requirement (82–84).

Because of these multiple goals for which surveillance is either the main or an essential element, we are confident that industrialized countries and global health stakeholders will continue to invest more in surveillance in LRS in coming years. Low-resource countries have an opportunity to use the high global focus on biosecurity to help build a strong infrastructure and a capacity for surveillance in a comprehensive fashion that addresses the diverse health needs of their own citizens, while simultaneously reducing pandemic and other threats to all nations. Such win–win solutions need to be identified in case studies and disseminated as models.

More generally, the global scientific community collectively needs to strengthen the evidence for what works to improve surveillance. Many organizations are now working in this domain, and a new level of scientific rigor needs to be brought to an area that has often been more of an art or a craft than a science in the past. The principles of critical appraisal and systematic review of evidence need to be applied to strengthening public health surveillance as they have been applied to health care services in the past (85,86). To do less is to miss a great opportunity for building one essential health system element—surveillance—in the decade that sees the countdown to both the MDGs and IHR core capacities.

REFERENCES

1. Fidler DP. Germs, governance, and global public health in the wake of SARS. *J Clin Invest* 2004;113(6):799–804.
2. Calain P. From the field side of the binoculars: a different view on global public health surveillance. *Health Policy Plan* 2007;22(1):13–20.
3. Sridhar D, Batniji R. Misfinancing global health: a case for transparency in disbursements and decision making. *Lancet* 2008;372(9644):1185–1191.
4. Narasimhan V, Brown H, Pablos-Mendez A, *et al.* Responding to the global human resources crisis. *Lancet* 2004;363(9419):1469–1472.
5. Garrett L. The challenge of global health. *Foreign Aff* 2007;86(1):14.

6. Samb B, Evans T, Dybul M, *et al*. An assessment of interactions between global health initiatives and country health systems. *Lancet* 2009;373(9681):2137–2169.

7. Ravishankar N. Financing of global health: tracking development assistance for health from 1990 to 2007. *Lancet* 2009;373(9681):2113–2124.

8. Fauci AS. The expanding global health agenda: a welcome development. *Nat Med* 2009;13(10):1169–1171.

9. Schieber GJ, Gottret P, Fleisher LK, Leive AA. Financing global health: mission unaccomplished. *Health Aff (Millwood)* 2007;26(4):921–934.

10. *Brilliant L. 2006. Help stop the next pandemic.* http://www.ted.com/index.php/talks/larry_brilliant_wants_to_stop_pandemics.html. Accessed January 10, 2009.

11. Heymann DL, Rodier G. Global surveillance, national surveillance, and SARS. *Emerg Infect Dis* 2004;10(2):173–175.

12. Morse SS. Global infectious disease surveillance and health intelligence. *Health Aff (Millwood)* 2007;26(4):1069–1077.

13. Cecchine G, Moore M. Infectious disease and national security-strategic information needs. *Rand Corporation Techinal Report* 2006.

14. Calain P. Exploring the international arena of global public health surveillance. *Health Policy Plan* 2007;22(1):2–12.

15. World Health Organization, Heymann DL, Prentice T, Reinders LT. *The World Health Report 2007. A Safer Future: Global Public Health Security in the 21st Century.* Geneva: World Health Organization; 2007.

16. Katz R, Singer DA. Health and security in foreign policy. *Bull World Health Organ* 2007;85(3):233–234.

17. Beaglehole R, Bonita R. Challenges for public health in the global context—prevention and surveillance. *Scand J Public Health* 2001;29(2):81–83.

18. Cohen J. Global health. Public-private partnerships proliferate. *Science* 2006;311(5758):167.

19. McDougall CW, Upshur RE, Wilson K. Emerging norms for the control of emerging epidemics. *Bull World Health Organ* 2008;86(8):643–645.

20. Murray CJ, Frenk J, Evans T. The Global Campaign for the Health MDGs: challenges, opportunities, and the imperative of shared learning. *Lancet* 2007;370(9592):1018–1020.

21. Google.org Battles Bugs & Viruses 2008. http://www.google.com/intl/en/press/pressrel/20081021_googleorg.html. Accessed March 3, 2010.

22. Hitchcock P, Chamberlain A, Van Wagoner M, Inglesby TV, O'Toole T. Challenges to global surveillance and response to infectious disease outbreaks of international importance. *Biosecur Bioterror* 2007;5(3):206–227.

23. Lindblade KA, Hamel MJ, Feikin DR, *et al*. Mortality of sick children after outpatient treatment at first-level health facilities in rural western Kenya. *Trop Med Int Health* 2007;12(10):1258–1268.

24. Sankoh O, Ngom P, Clark S, De Savigny D. Levels and Patterns of Mortality at INDEPTH Demographic Surveillance Systems. In: Jamison D, ed. *Disease and Mortality in Sub-Saharan Africa*. World Bank; 2006.

25. Victora CG, Huicho L, Amaral JJ, *et al*. Are health interventions implemented where they are most needed? District uptake of the integrated management of childhood illness strategy in Brazil, Peru and the United Republic of Tanzania. *Bull World Health Organ* 2006;84(10):792–801.

26. Tollman SM, Kahn K, Sartorius B, Collinson MA, Clark SJ, Garenne ML. Implications of mortality transition for primary health care in rural South Africa: a population-based surveillance study. *Lancet* 2008;372(9642):893–901.

27. Katz MA, Tharmaphornpilas P, Chantra S, et al. Who gets hospitalized for influenza pneumonia in Thailand? Implications for vaccine policy. *Vaccine* 2007;25(19):3827–3833.

28. Manning R, Organisation for economic co-operation and development. *Efforts and Policies of the Members of the Development Assistance Committee: Development Co-Operation Report 2007.* Paris: Organisation for Economic Co-operation and Development; 2008.

29. Biesma RG, Brugha R, Harmer A, Walsh A, Spicer N, Walt G. The effects of global health initiatives on country health systems: a review of the evidence from HIV/AIDS control. *Health Policy Plan* 2009;24(4):239–252.

30. OECD. 2005; *Paris Declaration on Aid Effectiveness: Ownership, Harmonization, Alignment, Results, and Mutual Accountability.* Paris http://www.oecd.org/dataoecd/11/41/34428351.pdf. Accessed June 27, 2009.

31. Stansfield S. Structuring information and incentives to improve health. *Bull World Health Organ* 2005;83(8):562.

32. Naimoli JF. Global health partnerships in practice: taking stock of the GAVI Alliance's new investment in health systems strengthening. *Int J Health Plann Manage* 2009;24(1):3–25.

33. Pfeiffer J, Johnson W, Fort M, et al. Strengthening health systems in poor countries: a code of conduct for nongovernmental organizations. *Am J Public Health* 2008;98(12):2134–2140.

34. World Health Organization. *International Health Regulations (2005), 2nd ed.* World Health Organization 2008.

35. World Health Organization. Resolution WHA58.3. Revision of the International Health Regulations. In Fifty-eight World Health Assembly. 2005.

36. Rodier G. New rules on international public health security. *Bull World Health Organ.* 2007;85(6):428–430.

37. Reidpath DD, Allotey P. Opening up public health: a strategy of information and communication technology to support population health. *Lancet* 2009;373(9668):1050–1051.

38. Vanden Eng JL, Wolkon A, Frolov AS, et al. Use of handheld computers with global positioning systems for probability sampling and data entry in household surveys. *Am J Trop Med Hyg* 2007;77(2):393–399.

39. Yu P, de Courten M, Pan E, Galea G, Pryor J. The development and evaluation of a PDA-based method for public health surveillance data collection in developing countries. *Int J Med Inform* 2009;78(8):532–542.

40. Urdea M, Penny LA, Olmsted SS, et al. Requirements for high impact diagnostics in the developing world. *Nature* 2006;444 (Suppl 1):73–79.

41. Houpt ER, Guerrant RL. Technology in global health: the need for essential diagnostics. *Lancet* 2008;372(9642):873–874.

42. Cohen J. Public health. Gates Foundation picks winners in Grand Challenges in Global Health. *Science* 2005;309(5731):33–35.

43. Nsubuga P, White ME, Thacker SB, et al. Public health surveillance: a tool for targeting and monitoring intervention. In: Jamison D, ed. *Disease Control Priorities in Developing Countries,* 2nd ed. New York: Oxford University Press; 2006.

44. M'ikanatha NM, Lynfield R, Van Beneden CA, de Valk H. *Infectious Disease Surveillance.* Malden, MA: Blackwell Publishing. 2008.

45. Thompson RC. The eradication of infectious diseases. *Parasitol Today* 1998;14(11):469.

46. Centers for Disease Control and Prevention. Laboratory surveillance for wild and vaccine-derived polioviruses. *MMWR* 2007;56:965–969

47. Ochiai RL, Acosta CJ, Danovaro—Holiday MC, *et al*. A study of typhoid fever in five Asian countries: disease burden and implications for controls. *Bull World Health Organ* 2008;86(4):260–268.

48. Lee J, McKibbin WJ. Globalization and disease: the case of SARS. *Asian Economic Papers* 2004;3:113–131.

49. Heymann DL. SARS and emerging infectious diseases: a challenge to place global solidarity above national sovereignty. *Ann Acad Med Singapore* 2006;35(5):350–353.

50. Meleigy M. Egypt battles with avian influenza. *Lancet* 2007;370(9587):553–554.

51. Olsen SJ, Ungchusak K, Birmingham M, Bresee J, Dowell SF, Chunsuttiwat S. Surveillance for avian influenza in human beings in Thailand. *Lancet Infect Dis* 2006;6(12):757–758.

52. World Health Organization. *WHO Recommended Surveillance Standards*, 2nd ed. World Health Organization; 1999.

53. Grein TW, Kamara KB, Rodier G, *et al*. Rumors of disease in the global village: outbreak verification. *Emerg Infect Dis* 2000;6(2):97–102.

54. Heymann DL, Rodier GR. Hot spots in a wired world: WHO surveillance of emerging and re-emerging infectious diseases. *Lancet Infect Dis* 2001;1(5):345–353.

55. Brownstein JS, Freifeld CC, Madoff LC. Digital disease detection—harnessing the Web for public health surveillance. *N Engl J Med* 2009;360(21):2153–2155, 2157.

56. World Health Organization. Regional Office for the Western Pacific. A Guide to establishing event-based surveillance. 2008; http://www.wpro.who.int/NR/rdonlyres/92E766DB-DF19-4F4F-90FD-C80597C0F34F/0/eventbasedsurv.pdf. Accessed March 11, 2010.

57. Paquet C, Coulombier D, Kaiser R, Ciotti M. Epidemic Intellligence: a New Framework for Strengthening Disease Surveillance in Europe. *Eurosurveillance* 2006;11(12).

58. Buehler JW, Hopkins RS, Overhage JM, Sosin DM, Tong V. Framework for evaluating public health surveillance systems for early detection of outbreaks: recommendations from the CDC Working Group. *MMWR Recomm Rep* 2004;53(RR-5):1–11.

59. Doroshenko A, Cooper D, Smith G, *et al*. Evaluation of syndromic surveillance based on National Health Service direct derived data—England and Wales. *MMWR Morb Mortal Wkly Rep* 2005;54 Suppl:117–122.

60. Murray CJ, Frenk J. Health metrics and evaluation: strengthening the science. *Lancet* 2008;371(9619):1191–1199.

61. Cash RA, Narasimhan V. Impediments to global surveillance of infectious diseases: consequences of open reporting in a global economy. *Bull World Health Organ* 2000;78(11):1358–1367.

62. Taylor CE, Cutts F, Taylor ME. Ethical dilemmas in current planning for polio eradication. *Am J Public Health* 1997;87(6):922–925.

63. Taylor CE, Taylor ME, Cutts F. Ethical dilemmas in polio eradication. *Am J Public Health* 1998;88(7):1125.

64. Perry HN, McDonnell SM, Alemu W, *et al*. Planning an integrated disease surveillance and response system: a matrix of skills and activities. *BMC Med* 2007;5:24.

65. White M, Herrera DJG, Lim-Quizon MC. Joined-up public-health initiatives. *Lancet* 2006;367(9519):1301–1302.

66. World Health Organization. A. Documentation of the laboratory networking in implementation of integrated disease surveillance and response in Rwanda. *Unpublished report* 2006.

67. Health *Metrics Network. Framework and Standards for Country Health Information Systems,* 2nd ed. Geneva: Health Metrics Network 2008.

68. World Health Organization. An integrated approach to communicable disease surveillance. *Wly Epidemiol Rec* 2000;75:1–8.
69. White M, McDonnell S. Public health surveillance in low- and middle-income countries. In: *Principles and Practice of Public Health Surveillance,* 2nd ed. 2000:287–315.
70. World Health Organization. Regional Office for Africa: Integrated Disease Surveillance and Response: A Regional Strategy for Communicable Diseases, 1999–2003. 1999.
71. World Health Organization, Regional Office for Africa, Division of Communicable Disease Prevention and Control. Guide for the Use of Core Integrated Disease Surveillance and Response Indicators in the African Region. 2005 (June).
72. Baker MG, Fidler DP. Global public health surveillance under new international health regulations. *Emerg Infect Dis* 2006;12(7):1058–1065.
73. Gostin LO. Public health law in a new century: part I: law as a tool to advance the community's health. *JAMA* 2000;283(21):2837–2841.
74. Pakistan's Public Health Surveillance System: A Call to Action. *Working Paper: World Bank.* August 15, 2005.
75. Koplan JP, Dusenbury C, Jousilahti P, Puska P. The role of national public health institutes in health infrastructure development. *BMJ* 2007;335(7625):834–835.
76. Martin R, Hearn TL, Ridderhof JC, Demby A. Implementation of a quality systems approach for laboratory practice in resource-constrained countries. *AIDS* 2005;19 (Suppl 2):S59–S65.
77. Nsubuga P, White M, Fontaine R, Simone P. Training programmes for field epidemiology. *Lancet* 2008;371(9613):630–631.
78. White ME, McDonnell SM, Werker DH, Cardenas VM, Thacker SB. Partnerships in international applied epidemiology training and service, 1975-2001. *Am J Epidemiol* 2001;154(11):993–999.
79. Jones DS, Tshimanga M, Woelk G, *et al.* Increasing leadership capacity for HIV/AIDS programmes by strengthening public health epidemiology and management training in Zimbabwe. *Hum Resour Health* 2009;7(69): doi10.1186/1478-4491-7-69.
80. Pappaioanou M, Malison M, Wilkins K, *et al.* Strengthening capacity in developing countries for evidence-based public health: the data for decision-making project. *Soc Sci Med* 2003;57(10):1925–1937.
81. United Nations. *The Millenium Development Goals Report.* New York: United Nations; 2008.
82. Frumkin H, Hess J, Luber G, Malilay J, McGeehin M. Climate change: the public health response. *Am J Public Health* 2008;98(3):435–445.
83. St Louis ME, Hess JJ. Climate change: impacts on and implications for global health. *Am J Prev Med* 2008;35(5):527–538.
84. Costello A, Abbas M, Allen A, *et al.* Managing the health effects of climate change: Lancet and University College London Institute for Global Health Commission. *Lancet* 2009;373(9676):1693–1733.
85. Bjorndal A. Improving social policy and practice: knowledge matters. *Lancet* 2009;373(9678):1829–1831.
86. Chalmers I, Glasziou P. Avoidable waste in the production and reporting of research evidence. *Lancet* 2009;374(9683):86–89.

18

State and Local Public Health Surveillance in the United States

GUTHRIE S. BIRKHEAD AND
CHRISTOPHER M. MAYLAHN

Public health surveillance as discussed in this book was first defined by Alexander Langmuir in the 1960s (*1*). He expanded the traditional concept of surveillance in public health from the monitoring of persons who were exposed to contagious diseases to permit early detection of illness, to the monitoring of health and disease in whole populations to guide population-based public health measures. Langmuir defined the meaning of public health surveillance as the "continued watchfulness over the distribution and trends of incidence [of disease] through the systematic collection, consolidation and evaluation" of public health data with "the regular dissemination of the basic data and interpretations to all who have contributed and to all others who need to know." He added, "The concept, however, does not encompass direct responsibility for control activities. These traditionally have been and still remain with the state and local health authorities" (*1*).

Langmuir's definition and its accompanying caveat highlight a key feature of public health surveillance at the state and local level that differs from surveillance at the national level in the United States, which is the close link between surveillance and disease control activities. The legal authority for both disease control and public health surveillance often resides at the state or local level. The impetus for these legal requirements is the need to prevent and control specific health problems at the community level—functions that traditionally have been carried out by state and local public health agencies because of their knowledge of and proximity to the population. The link between surveillance and community action is critical and is the primary justification for surveillance activities and public health reporting requirements locally. Using data to monitor trends or to suggest research hypotheses, although an important purpose of surveillance data, is not usually the primary aim of surveillance at the state and local level. Surveillance is synonymous with control to many state and local public health professionals, policymakers, legislators, and members of the public. Therefore, both the historical definition of surveillance—reporting linked directly to control—and Langmuir's broader definition apply at the state and local level.

The Institute of Medicine recommends that every health department regularly and systematically collect, assemble, analyze, and make available information about the health of the community, including statistics on health status, community health needs, and epidemiologic and other studies of health problems (2). They noted that "state and local public health authorities engage in a variety of activities, including monitoring the burden of injury and disease in the population through surveillance systems; identifying individuals and groups that have conditions of public health importance with testing, reporting, and partner notification; providing a broad array of prevention services such as counseling and education; and helping assure access to high-quality health care services for poor and vulnerable populations" (p.102). A 2001 survey of public health agencies confirmed that community assessment, epidemiology and surveillance were commonly performed by the majority of the nation's local health departments (3).

In this chapter, we discuss the history and features that characterize public health surveillance at the state and local level. We also describe some new developments in surveillance strategies and briefly mention the challenges faced by public health surveillance practitioners in carrying out this core public health function.

HISTORY OF STATE AND FEDERAL COLLABORATION ON SURVEILLANCE

The partnership between states and the federal government in the United States to conduct public health surveillance began in the late 1800s. States voluntarily submitted data from communicable disease reports to the federal government starting in 1878 when Congress authorized the Marine Hospital Service to collect such information. The first national summary of notifiable diseases was published in 1912. The uniformity of these national surveillance efforts was improved by the development in 1913 of a model state statute for reporting of 53 diseases, first to state health departments and then forwarded to the Surgeon General. This model law divided conditions of interest into infectious, occupational, and venereal diseases, as well as injuries. The underlying principle for selection of reportable conditions was the ability or need to undertake public health measures, often for affected individuals and their direct contacts.

An important milestone in the state/federal collaboration around public health surveillance came in 1950 with a national meeting of a group of state and territorial epidemiologists, convened through the efforts of Alexander Langmuir at the Communicable Disease Center (now Centers for Disease Control and Prevention, or CDC) (4). This group established the Conference (now Council) of State and Territorial Epidemiologists (CSTE). CSTE was designated by the Association of State and Territorial Health Officials to have shared responsibility with CDC for determining those diseases recommended for states to list in their reporting requirements and to submit reports voluntarily, without identifying information, to CDC. This was named the National Notifiable Disease Surveillance System (NNDSS) (5,6).

CSTE has continued to provide a forum to discuss surveillance issues for epidemiologists working in state, territorial, and local health departments and in the federal government. CSTE has designated state-based epidemiologists as surveillance "consultants" to provide expertise in content areas such as infectious diseases and environmental health to CDC and other federal, state, and international agencies. In addition to CSTE, professional organizations representing state surveillance interests have worked collaboratively with the federal government to coordinate surveillance efforts within and across the topical areas. Examples include the National Association for Public Health Statistics and Information Systems in the area of vital registration; the National Association of Central Tumor Registrars regarding cancer registries; the National Association of Chronic Disease Directors on issues related to chronic diseases; and the State and Territorial Injury Program Directors Association on intentional and unintentional injuries.

CSTE and CDC have collaborated to develop the scientific basis of public health surveillance. Case definitions for reportable communicable diseases, which are necessary for the uniform classification of disease cases, were first published in 1990 (7) and updated periodically (8). Following the 1994 National Surveillance Conference, the methods of conducting surveillance were specified for new diseases being added to the NNDSS (9). Chronic disease indicators and case definitions were established in 1998 (10) and subsequently updated (11,12). CSTE provided input into the development of guidelines for the evaluation of surveillance systems (13), an important step to assure that surveillance systems are well designed and appropriately monitored to meet the goals set for them. A framework for evaluating public health surveillance systems for early detection of disease outbreaks has also been developed (14).

CSTE and CDC have established a set of standards for electronic collection and dissemination of surveillance data in the Public Health Information Network (PHIN) (15,16) and the National Electronic Disease Surveillance System (NEDSS) (17). These standards help ensure comparability of data from different data sources and over time. The rapid growth of electronic health information systems has underscored the need for interoperability between systems to facilitate the monitoring of the health of communities, permit analysis of trends and detection of emerging public health problems, and set public health policy.

FEATURES OF STATE AND LOCAL PUBLIC HEALTH SURVEILLANCE

The Legal Basis for Many Surveillance Systems Resides at the State and Local Level

Surveillance activities at the state and local level are usually based on specific state and local public health laws or regulations. These legal provisions often require physicians, other health-care providers, laboratories, and hospitals to report, by name, persons with diseases of public health importance to the health department. Reporting requirements are placed either in statute, requiring legislative action to amend, or in rule or regulation, which health departments and boards of health amend through administrative procedures. State laws are the basis for most surveillance activities, but large cities and counties within states may establish additional reporting requirements. States often share surveillance data with CDC and other federal agencies on a voluntary basis or as a condition of receiving federal funds, but surveillance data with personal identifying information collected under state and local legal authority are almost never sent to CDC or other federal agencies.

Surveillance and control activities are authorized in state statutes as part of the "police powers" of states (18). These provisions balance the needs of society to protect the public health and realize benefits for society that individuals acting alone could not, with the right of privacy of individuals (19,20). This tension between the needs to protect the public's health and individual privacy—as illustrated by the controversy about reporting the name of persons with HIV infection in the late 1990s (21)—is an ongoing challenge.

Most states have laws requiring reporting of some or all communicable diseases, vital events, cancer, environmental and occupational conditions, and injuries. In general, health-care providers are required to provide information about persons with reportable conditions to the health department for surveillance purposes, but the individual citizens are not required to give information about themselves. State and local public health authorities have legal authority to isolate individuals infected with same highly contagious diseases detected by a surveillance system, as well as to isolate individuals infected with some highly contagious diseases detected by a surveillance system as well as to quarantine persons who have been exposed to such individuals for the presumed incubation period. The severe acute respiratory syndrome (SARS) epidemic in 2003 provides a recent example where this was done (22).

The Purposes of Surveillance at the State and Local Level are Closely Linked to Public Health Action

The primary purposes of surveillance at the state and local level are to trigger disease control activities and to plan, implement, and evaluate health promotion and disease prevention programs. It is primarily at the state and local level that society can "expeditiously implement interventions to prevent disease" (23). Surveillance might involve identifying persons with diseases that require public health follow-up (e.g., to prevent transmission to others). The information can also be used to identify populations at high risk or that have experienced health disparities in order to target public health programs.

The close link between surveillance and disease prevention/control activities undertaken by state and local health departments can be illustrated at four levels:

Surveillance Helps Assure Accurate Diagnosis and Treatment

One specific purpose for surveillance at the state and local level is to assure the accurate diagnosis and appropriate treatment of an individual with a disease or condition of public health importance. For example, botulism is a rare disease often linked to contaminated food. Suspicion of the diagnosis of botulism is based on symptoms and medical history (*24*). Because it is rare, clinicians might need assistance in making the diagnosis and accessing specific treatment (botulinum antitoxin). Reporting of suspect cases to the health department has several purposes. Public health workers have the expertise to advise physicians in making a diagnosis. State public health laboratories perform laboratory diagnostic tests for botulism that commonly are not done in clinical laboratories. Antitoxin, which is available in limited supplies, is stored at federal quarantine stations and released to physicians only after a request from a state health official. Public health workers play a similar role in assuring the correct diagnosis and treatment of sexually transmitted diseases (*25*) and tuberculosis (*26*).

Surveillance Enables Appropriate Public Health Management of Persons Exposed to Disease

Identifying contacts of communicable disease cases and assuring that prevention or prophylactic measures are applied is a second purpose of surveillance. One example is identifying people who have been in contact with a case of meningococcal meningitis in a household or daycare setting for the purpose of administering antibiotic prophylaxis (*27*). Such follow-up must happen very quickly following the report of a case to prevent other people from being infected or to prevent contacts who are incubating disease from becoming ill, making the timeliness of surveillance reporting important. Similar efforts occur following the report of cases of sexually transmitted diseases such as syphilis or gonorrhea, often referred to as "partner notification." Information about recent sexual partners is solicited on a voluntary basis from reported cases. Partners are notified of their exposure and encouraged to undergo testing and prophylaxis to prevent disease (*25*). Rapid reporting can result in the treatment of partners during the incubation period of disease before they become infectious, thus breaking the chain of transmission. These partner notification activities might also identify the sources of infection for index cases and allow them to receive treatment.

Surveillance Identifies Disease Outbreaks

Identifying and removing the source of disease transmission in an outbreak is a third purpose of surveillance. In the botulism example discussed above, local health officials undertake an investigation of confirmed or suspected botulism cases to determine source of the infection. This often involves collecting food samples and having them analyzed at the public health laboratory. Surveillance reporting can thus lead to a recall of contaminated food items and can also alert other practitioners to be on the lookout for more cases. In the non-communicable disease area, surveillance can lead to the identification of clusters of injuries, such as farm injuries related to new farming equipment or farming practices and alerting the farming community to be careful and avoid risks (*28*), or an unusual pattern of teen suicide attempts, prompting a community response to prevent further attempts and potential fatalities (*29,30*). Methods for early disease detection surveillance systems, such as the space–time permutation scan statistic (*31*) that relies on local data, are an important tool for state and local health departments to use in identifying disease outbreaks.

Surveillance Guides Population-Based Public Health
Prevention Programs

Monitoring the health status and disease trends in the community and then determining the need for and effectiveness of public health programs is a fourth purpose of surveillance. Surveillance programs monitor disease outcomes and can measure determinants and risk factors for communicable and non-communicable diseases. Because many health problems result from a combination of unfavorable environmental and social conditions, interpersonal factors, and adverse behavioral patterns, information about these determinants is key in designing effective intervention strategies. The use of various surveillance systems, including disease reporting, health behavior surveillance, disease registries, and administrative data can be helpful for this purpose. These can include health status measures, population characteristics, access to and utilization of care, or community and environmental attributes linked to health and disease.

The need to link action to outcome has led to an increasing emphasis on measuring indicators that are causally related to health status but are not health outcomes themselves. These are called proximal indicators (*32*). As discussed in Chapter 13, these may also be regarded as proximal determinants, because they are linked to other changes, often in a theoretical construct, to health outcomes. For example, programs to reduce smoking prevalence often seek to change attitudes and beliefs about tobacco use, limit exposure to tobacco advertising, increase social support for non-smoking, and alter norms about tobacco use and environmental tobacco smoke, all of which might be the focus of surveillance. As these change, it is reasonable to expect that smoking prevalence and the associated health consequences will decline (*33,34*).

Data about disease patterns and epidemics can reveal variations in sociodemographic, geographic, behavioral, and clinical characteristics that are useful in targeting efforts. Local data can also assist public health practitioners to make informed, evidenced-based decisions that lead to more effective prevention and control interventions. Some state health departments have developed Web-based data query systems (*35*) to give practitioners and the public access to community health data. At the local level, geographic information systems (GIS) can facilitate targeting and evaluation.

The Methods of Surveillance at the State and Local Level are Linked to the Purposes

Methods for conducting surveillance can vary by purpose and governmental level. Table 18–1 provides an example of how surveillance purposes and methods for meningococcal invasive disease might differ at the local, state, and national level. Meningococcal invasive disease is a rare but severe and rapidly progressive contagious disease resulting in overwhelming meningitis or bloodstream infection and death in 8% to 15% of cases despite antibiotic therapy. At the local level, immediate disease control activities are the primary purpose of

Table 18–1 Purposes, Desired Attributes and Methods of Public Health Surveillance at the Local, State, and National Public Health Governmental Levels for Meningococcal Invasive Disease

Purposes	*Surveillance Attributes*	*Methods*
Local Health Department Level		
Assure proper diagnosis and treatment of cases	Timeliness Sensitivity	Case reporting by clinicians and emergency departments
Initiate prophylaxis of contacts	Completeness of detection	Laboratory reporting of clinical isolates to detect clinical cases
State Health Department Level		
Monitor and assure appropriate local surveillance and control	Completeness of reporting	Collect data from local health department
	Positive predictive value of reports	State public health laboratory confirmation of diagnosis
Detect inter-county clusters		
Assess impact of vaccination programs		Review hospital discharge and mortality data for unreported cases
Obtain resources and institute regulatory action to control disease		Assess vaccine usage and coverage
National Level		
Monitor nationwide trends	Complete demographic and risk factor data	Collect data from state health department
Characterize epidemiology and vaccine efficacy for disease	Positive predictive value	Conduct special studies and surveys
Detect inter-state outbreaks	Comparability	
Obtain resources	Flexibility	

surveillance for meningococcal disease. For example, it is recommended that close contacts of meningococcal disease cases must be observed closely for early symptoms of disease and should receive antibiotic prophylaxis as soon as possible, but usually within 24 to 48 hours after confirmation of the index case (*27*). With these purposes in mind, local surveillance is based on reporting of clinically supected cases by physicians and emergency departments (EDs) even before laboratory confirmation has been obtained. The desired attributes of such reporting are timeliness and sensitivity—that is, all possible cases should be reported. False-positive reports are tolerated because of the potential seriousness of the disease outcome.

In some states, such as those where there are local health departments, direct disease control measures are not a state health department responsibility. In this example, the purposes of state-level surveillance are to monitor and assure that appropriate local surveillance is occurring, to assess epidemiologic features of the disease across the state, and to measure the success of immunization programs to prevent meningococcal disease. Important attributes of states' surveillance activities are complete reporting and assuring that all cases are confirmed as meningococcal disease. Appropriate methods for surveillance at the state level include review of case data submitted by local health departments, review of laboratory reports, and assessment of vaccination coverage.

Characterizing the epidemiology of meningococcal invasive disease, rather than direct provision of disease control activites in the community, is the primary goal at the national level. Because this disease is so rare, it is only at the national level where sufficient numbers of cases to study the epidemiology and risk factors for meningococcal disease, and the efficacy of vaccines to prevent meningococcal disease, can be examined. Therefore, the methods of surveillance employed at the national level include aggregating local and state data (*see* descriptions below for NNDSS and BRFSS) and conducting surveys of nationally representative samples. This latter method usually cannot be used to generate estimates for each state or locality.

Surveillance, Public Health Practice, and Research at the State and Local Level

The previous section highlighted disease prevention and control functions as key purposes of surveillance at the state and local level. Developing hypotheses and conducting research are of secondary importance at these levels and are usually not sufficient to justify population-based public health surveillance activities, especially those that involve mandated reporting.

State and local public health surveillance is not viewed as a research activity (*36*). Unlike research, which often is not mandated in state regulations, public health surveillance activities such as disease reporting are mandated by state law. Public health surveillance practiced at the state and local level does not meet the federal definition of research because its purposes are not to contribute to generalizable knowledge but rather to undertake prevention and control steps among ill or at-risk persons or in specific communities. These purposes are usually made explicit in laws and regulations authorizing surveillance.

In recent years, there has been discussion among federal, state, and local public health professionals about whether surveillance constitutes research in some cases (*37*). Research is defined in the federal code of regulations as a "systematic investigation … designed to develop or contribute to generalizable knowledge" (*38*). Activities that meet this definition are required to undergo 45 CFR part 46 review and considerations by an institutional review board (IRB).

The fact that surveillance is not research does not lessen the need to maintain individual confidentiality. Model legislation has been developed that outlines specific principles to protect individual privacy and confidentiality during collection, storage, use, and dissemination of public health data (*39*). Surveillance data collected at the state or local level to control a specific disease are sometimes used subsequently for research purposes. In these cases, IRB review is necessary.

SURVEILLANCE SYSTEMS OF IMPORTANCE AT THE STATE AND LOCAL LEVEL

The following section describes surveillance systems that play important roles in most state and local public health jurisdictions in the United States. In addition, use of data collected for other purposes for surveillance is described.

Reportable Disease Surveillance

Example: Communicable Disease Surveillance

Reporting cases of communicable diseases from health-care providers to health departments was one of the earliest forms of surveillance. States develop legal reporting requirements using as a guide the list of communicable diseases recommended as part of the NNDSS (*40*) as well as local public health priorities. Most case definitions require laboratory test results to confirm a surveillance report but also contain a clinical case definition to enable providers to report cases without or in advance of laboratory confirmation. All states require reporting of selected notifiable diseases by health-care providers (Fig. 18–1). Hospitals often require infection control practitioners to fulfill the reporting function for attending physicians. In recent years, laboratories have become an increasingly important source for reporting of diagnostic test results. In most states, clinical laboratories are also required to report individuals with reportable diseases. Increasingly, states are collecting laboratory data on these diseases in electronic form (*41*). Electronic reporting increases the completeness and timeliness of reporting (*42*). State statutes authorizing reporting generally provide for protection of this confidential information, but the specificity of these protections varies (*43*). Information that identifies an individual patient is not sent to CDC.

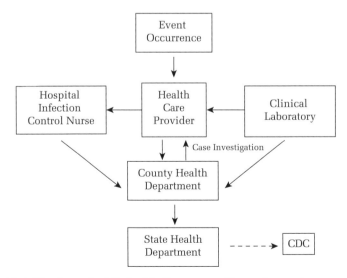

Figure 18–1 The flow of public health disease surveillance data at the state and local level.

Completeness and timeliness are key attributes of communicable disease surveillance. Completeness is enhanced by relying on laboratory reporting because there are relatively few laboratories to interact with to ensure complete reporting, and many have electronic systems that enable automated reporting of positive test results. Effective laboratory reporting requires that physicians order appropriate laboratory tests so that specific diagnoses can be made. For example, reportable diarrheal diseases might be missed if stool cultures are not ordered and patients receive symptomatic treatment only. Concerns have been expressed that cost-cutting measures in medicine will result in under-diagnosis and under-reporting of conditions of public health interest (*44*). Capitation in managed care, for example, could create situations where diagnostic testing in cases of diarrheal or respiratory illness is not ordered to save costs, resulting in no specific reportable diagnosis being made.

Disease Registry Surveillance

Example: Cancer Surveillance

Statutory reporting of individuals with specific diseases or conditions to a disease registry is employed for surveillance of chronic diseases. For example cancer registries are like disease notification systems, except that individual records are maintained open, to accept more information over time, rather than closed after the acute illness is resolved, and longitudinal data are collected on individuals. This enables surveillance of disease at different stages: prior to diagnosis (risk factors for illness, efficacy of screening and prevention programs), treatment (health-care access, treatment success), and mortality (combination of prevention, screening, and treatment efficacy).

Cancer registries are an example of this kind of surveillance and have been established in all states. The methods used for cancer registration have been well-documented (*45,46*). Cancer registries obtain information about people diagnosed with cancer using reports from physicians and diagnostic laboratories. Depending on resources available, the information might include not only basic demographic data on the individual and type of tumor but also encompass detailed data on the anatomic site of the tumor, the stage at diagnosis, the cell type of the cancer, and treatment and follow-up clinical information. Death certificates are matched periodically to registries to enable calculation of cancer-specific mortality rates. When a person is diagnosed with more than one type of cancer, information is obtained for each separate tumor in a case report. Most registries include reports of all malignant cancers.

In most state-based cancer registries, reporting of cancer cases is required in state law. All information reported to cancer registries is considered confidential, with strict procedures in place to protect the privacy of cancer patients and to limit the release of information to outside investigators. Research studies involving data with patient identifiers must obtain IRB approval. Furthermore, release of individual-level data for small geographic areas is restricted, and when there is a low number of cases in a small area, the exact number of cases is not revealed.

If sufficient resources are expended, cancer registry data can be of high quality, relatively complete, and representative of a state's population. Some registries, especially in states that lack the resources to maintain them, are not timely in releasing information and might be incomplete. Some state cancer registries do not have the resources to track clinical outcomes in reported cases other than mortality.

Sentinel Surveillance

Example: Influenza Surveillance

Sentinel surveillance systems obtain surveillance reports from a limited number of sites that are more or less representative of the population. Such systems require fewer resources than case-based reporting systems and can provide higher quality information, often enriched with more intensive laboratory testing than would be feasible or needed on a total population sample. This approach is used to obtain an estimate of disease activity for common diseases in populations, such as viral influenza. Despite influenza's public health importance and preventability, individual cases of influenza are not generally reportable in most states because the large number of cases would overwhelm the communicable disease surveillance system and because public health action is usually not taken in response to each case. In addition, the clinical definition of influenza is not specific and laboratory confirmation is not often sought.

Sentinel physicians or clinics are a selected group who agree to report cases of influenza-like respiratory illness and could obtain nasopharyngeal swabs for viral diagnosis from some ill patients. Reports of aggregate data are usually submitted by sentinel sites to the state or local health department each week. Sentinal surveillance for influenza is helpful to determine the level of disease activity in the population and to inform clinicians and the public about which strains of influenza are circulating and whether they are resistent to antiviral agents. This permits antiviral prophylaxis and treatment of persons at risk for complications. Vaccine efficacy in each influenza season can be determined by investigation of selected outbreaks.

States often conduct other types of sentinel surveillance for influenza such as monitoring rates of absenteeism in selected occupational settings or schools. Some states receive pneumonia and influenza mortality reports from the vital registrars in cities participating in the national 121 Cities Mortality Reporting System (47). Data from all these sources, combined with reports of influenza outbreaks, allow state communicable disease epidemiologists to report to CDC on a weekly basis the level of influenza activity in their states.

Periodic Population Surveys

Example: Behavioral Risk Factors Surveillance System

Periodic surveillance commonly is used to estimate the proportion of people engaging in a particular health risk or health protection behavior (e.g., smoking, high-fat food consumption, or immunized with pneumococcal vaccine). Sometimes, population-based behavioral surveillance is conducted to obtain information about an emerging or priority issue as was the case in the early years of the HIV epidemic. The Behavioral Risk Factors Surveillance System (BRFSS), an example of this kind of surveillance, is the primary source of state-based information on risk behaviors and health-related conditions among adults (*48*). States select a random sample of adults for a telephone interview that includes questions about their knowledge, attitudes, behaviors, and risk factors associated with the leading causes of disease and mortality. Every state uses similar methods for selecting respondents and the same core questions to facilitate comparisons. After appropriate weighting, the selection process results in a representative sample for each state so that statistical inferences can be made from the information collected (*see* Chapter 12 for more discussion of the BRFSS).

BRFSS data can be combined with other data at the state and local surveillance systems to characterize patterns of risk, disease, and their determinants across a state or in local communities. An example is the public health surveillance of cancer. Relevant risk factors and behaviors from BRFSS can be combined with reports of cancer incidence from cancer registries. GIS can assist in the epidemiologic investigation of potential cancer clusters and can facilitate a linkage with other data systems—for example, those containing environmantal exposure data. These combined data can help guide local cancer screening and treatment programs targeting high-risk or underserved communities.

Syndromic Surveillance

Example: Surveillance of Diseases Capable of Mass Transmission

Syndromic surveillance is the name given to the review of medical information on signs and symptoms of disease before a specific diagnosis is made. Since the events of September 11, 2001 and the subsequent anthrax attacks, there is a greater interest in collecting and analyzing such data as an early warning system for mass intentional attacks with biological agents (*49*). Many states have developed pilot syndromic surveillance systems as part of the activities carried out with federal preparedness funding. The usefulness of sydromic surveillance for this purpose is unknown, partly because such attacks are rare. Such systems could be useful for detecting naturally occurring epidemics, such as annual influenza. CDC has proposed a national Biosense project where syndromic data are received and reviewed simultaneously at the state and federal level (*50*). In 2007 CDC was charged with developing, in collaboration with state and local surveillance partners, the national strategy for biosurveillance, which is outlined briefly in Chapter 14.

State level syndromic surveillance systems have typically involved collection of chief complaint or provisional diagnostic data from EDs and collection of pharmacy claims data for drugs used to treat diseases of interest. ED data are not collected uniformly, coded, or put in electronic form. Early syndromic surveillance systems had to develop methods to get ED chief complaint data from the ED log into an electronic form. Because there are no standard chief complaint or provisional diagnosis nomenclatures, computer programs to group words or phrases indicative of different clinical syndromes (e.g., "fever" and "cough" for infectious respiratory illness) had to be developed and customized to each ED's specific circumstances. These data are then collected daily and analyzed for "signals," unusual clusterings of illness that might be indicative of an outbreak. Other types of data used for syndromic surveillance include, but are not limited to, review of pharmacy claims for prescription and non-prescription drugs of interest, and chief complaint data from ambulance runs. Syndromic surveillance systems typically have not had special legal authorization, although care needs to be taken that state and federal confidentiality laws are not violated in the establishment of such systems (51).

To date, most published reports have not found a high positive predictive value for disease signals arising from syndromic surveillance systems, and the experience of many health departments is that such signals rarely indicate a true common source outbreak (52). In fact, such systems might be more useful to provide assurance that a large outbreak is *not* occuring. Because the utility of syndromic surveillance is uncertain, it is appropriate to share the monthly or annual experience about syndromic surveillance clusters with health department leadership so decisions about the prioritization or resources devoted to this activity can be made (53,54). Because state and local governments are the primary responders to a possible syndromic cluster, many state and local surveillance practitioners have not been supportive of federalizing these systems because they believe that if such systems are indeed worthwhile, they should be a local or state responsibility (55).

Information Systems Useful for Surveillance

Information systems containing data collected for other purposes that exist in states and local communities might be useful for public health surveillance.

Vital Registration

Example: Infant Mortality Surveillance

All states and most major cities require the registration of live births and deaths (usually including fetal deaths) among their residents. The reporting forms used are based on the national standard certificate (or standard data set when used in electronic reporting). Electronic registration of the birth and death certificate is becoming common, which minimizes the burden, accelerates the calculation of birth and death rates, and facilitates the linkage of the two events. Although the main purpose for collecting vital events is the legal registration of vital status, states use the data on births and deaths to track population health, monitor the leading causes of death, make population projections, forecast disease trends, and plan needed health services.

Infant mortality is a widely used measure of population health. The calculation of infant mortality rates requires knowing the number of live births and deaths up to age 1 year, using the standard birth and death certificates. Information about infant deaths can be used in combination with perinatal surveillance data to ascertain mortality patterns, risk factors, and impact of public health initiatives. Variations exist in quality of cause of death information, but systematic analysis of such data is critical to improve quality, as well as to draw insights for how to promote the health of the population. (56,57)

Administrative Data on Health

Example: Asthma Surveillance

The most common administrative data systems used for public health surveillance at state and local levels are hospital discharge data, ED utilization, health insurance and Medicaid billing data, managed care encounter data, pharmacy information systems, and the claims data maintained by the federal Center for Medicare and Medicaid Services for Medicare recipients. These systems are not designed for public health surveillance, although their use can supplement information for a number of surveillance systems. Their primary function is reimbursement, monitoring health-care costs, and assessing general patterns of care. The accuracy and completeness of diagnostic information is uncertain. In addition, people often have multiple encounters with the health-care system so the lack of unique identifiers in administrative data systems makes it difficult to eliminate duplicate counts or follow the longitudinal course of individual patients. However, alternative approaches using case reporting by medical providers would pose a burden on the public health system, thus making administrative systems a more feasible approach for disease-specific surveillance. In the future, universal electronic medical records systems could enable surveillance in all medical settings (*see* below). The advantages of such systems are their relative availability in electronic form, defined population coverage, and low cost for secondary uses like surveillance.

Asthma is an example of a disease where hospital and ED data are used for surveillance purposes. Asthma-related hospitalization data can be used to identify geographic areas or population subgroups experiencing disparities. Because asthma hospitalizations are an AHRQ-defined ambulatory care sensitive condition (*58,59*), this information can also be used to inform prevention programs, based both in community and clinical settings.

THE FUTURE OF STATE AND LOCAL PUBLIC HEALTH SURVEILLANCE

Surveillance strategies employed at the state and local level will likely be shaped by three key forces discussed elsewhere in this book—maintaining a well-trained surveillance workforce, taking advantage of the electronic data revolution, and integrating surveillance activities both within and between public health programs and community and health-care settings.

State and local health departments can serve as incubators for new surveillance methods or applying old surveillance methods in new ways. A recent example has been the extension of traditional laboratory reporting for communicable diseases, to new areas of chronic disease such as diabetes. Diabetics are recommended to have periodic laboratory testing to detect glycosylated hemoglobin (hemoglobin A1c) as a measure of the adequacy of the success of their medical treatment. At least one local health department—in New York City—has undertaken a pilot program to require reporting from laboratories of hemoglobin A1c levels with the eventual plan to use the data to assist clinicians and patients who have poor performance on this indicator (*60*). Innovative new surveillance approaches can raise a number of issues. In this case, resources to track individual providers and patients, as well as the feasiblilty of using lab data in this way, might need further study. Concerns about confidentiality raise the question about whether informed consent is necessary when obtaining data from individuals. The "intrusion" by public health into the domains of individual privacy and the practice of medicine is problematic to some, because diabetes poses no communicable disease risk to the wider population. This initiative points to the complicated relations between public health surveillance, privacy claims, and the duty of public health to protect vulnerable populations (*61*).

State and local public health surveillance practitioners have been involved actively in discussions of the future course of national public health surveillance. The PHIN standards form the basis for a "virtual" national public heath surveillance system. It is important to maintain surveillance as a collaborative process among national, state, terriotorial, tribal and local public health systems. The electronic revolution in health care might finally bear fruit to provide high-quality, timely data to determine public health priorities and guide public health programs. Public health surveillance at state and local levels will continue to expand beyond infectious diseases. Surveillance needs to be visible as a supra-categorical, core public health function. Collaboration and integration across surveillance domains needs to be encouraged for efficiency and access to new data sources. Surveillance practitioners should foster improved data quality through coordinated evaluation, training, and development of new surveillance methods. Expanding and improving public health surveillance efforts require engaging national, state, and local public health partners and leveraging the strengths at each level to be successful.

REFERENCES

1. Langmuir AD. The surveillance of communicable diseases of national importance. *N Engl J Med* 1963;268:182–192.
2. Committee on Assuring the Health of the Public in the 21st Century, Board on Health Promotion and Disease Prevention, Institute of Medicine of the National Academies. *The Future of the Public's Health in the 21st Century.* Washington, DC: The National Academies Press; 2002.
3. Beitsch LM, Brooks RG, Grigg M, Menachemi N. Structure and functions of state public health agencies. *Am J Public Health* 2006;96(1):167–172.
4. Koplan JP, Thacker SB. Fifty years of epidemiology at the centers for disease control and prevention: significant and consequential. *Am J Epidemiol* 2001; 154(11):982–984.
5. Koo D, Wetterhall SF. History and current status of the National Notifiable Diseases Surveillance System. *J Public Health Manag Pract* 1996;2:4–10.
6. Centers for Disease Control and Prevention. National Notifiable Disease Surveillance System. http://www.cdc.gov/ncphi/disss/nndss/nndsshis.htm.
7. Wharton M, Chorba TL, Vogt RL, Morse DL, Buehler JW. Case definitions for public health surveillance. *MMWR Recomm Rep* 1990;39(RR-13):1–43.

8. Centers for Disease Control and Prevention. Case definitions for infectious conditions under public healths surveillance. http://www.cdc.gov/ncphi/disss/nndss/casedef/.

9. Meriwether R A. Blueprint for a national public health surveillance system for the 21st century. *J Public Health Manag Pract* 1996;2(4):16–23.

10. Lengerich EJ. Indicators for chronic disease surveillance: consensus of CSTE, ASTCDPD, and CDC. Atlanta, GA: Council of State and Territorial Epidemiologists, 1999 Nov.

11. Centers for Disease Control and Prevention, Council of State and Territorial Epidemiologists, and Association of State and Territorial Chronic Disease Program Directors. Indicators for chronic disease surveillance. *MMWR Recomm Rep* 2004;53(RR11):1–6.

12. Pelletier AR, Siegel PZ, Baptiste MS, Maylahn C. Revisions to chronic disease surveillance indicators, United States, 2004. *Prev Chronic Dis* 2005;2(3):A15. Published online June 15, 2005.

13. Guidelines Working Group. Updated guidelines for evaluating public health surveillance systems. *MMWR Recomm Rep* 2001;50(RR-13):1–35.

14. Buehler JW, Hopkins RS, Overhage JM, Sosis DM, Tong V. Framework for evaluating public health surveillance systems for early detection of outbreaks: recommendations from the CDC Working Group. *MMWR Recomm Rep* 2004;53(RR-05):1–11.

15. Centers for Disease Control and Prevention. Public Health Information Network standards, specifications, and functions. Atlanta, GA: US Department of Health and Human Services, CDC, 2003. http://www.cdc.gov/phin.

16. Broome CV, Loonsk J. Public Health Information Network—improving early detection by using a standards-based approach to connecting public health and clinical medicine. *MMWR* 2004;53 (Suppl):199–202.

17. The National Electronic Disease Surveillance System Working Group. National Electronic Disease Surveillance System (NEDSS): a standards-based approach to connect public health and clinical medicine. *J Public Health Manag Pract* 2001;7(6):43–50.

18. Gostin LO. Public health law: a review. *Curr Issues Publ Health* 1996;2:205–214.

19. Gostin LO, Lazzarini Z, Neslund VS, Osterholm MT. The public health information infrastructure. *JAMA* 1996;275:1921–1927.

20. Gostin LO. Health care information and the protection of personal privacy: ethical and legal considerations. *Ann Int Med* 1997;127:683–690.

21. Gostin LO, Ward JW, Baker AC. National HIV case reporting for the United States—a defining moment in the history of the epidemic. *N Engl J Med* 1997;337:1162–1167.

22. Speakman J, Gonzalez F, Perez MT. Quarantine in severe acute respiratory syndrome (SARS) and other emerging infectious diseases. *J Law Med Ethics* 2008;31(s4):63–64.

23. Istre GR. Disease surveillance at the state and local levels. In: Halperin W, Baker EL, eds. *Public Health Surveillance*. New York: Van Nostrand Reinhold; 1992.

24. Heymann DL, ed. *Control of Communicable Disease Manual*, 19th ed. *American Public Health Association*, Washington, DC: 2008.

25. Centers for Disease Control and Prevention, Workowski KA, Berman SM. Sexually transmitted diseases treatment guidelines, 2006. *MMWR Recomm Rep* 2006;55(RR-11):1–94.

26. Kaye K, Frieden TR. Tuberculosis control: the relevance of classic principles in an era of acquired immunity deficiency syndrome and multidrug resistance. *Epidemiol Rev* 1996;18(1):52–63.

27. Centers for Disease Control and Prevention. Control and prevention of meningo-coccal disease and control and prevention of serogroup C meningococcal disease: Evaluation and management of suspected outbreaks. Recommendations of the Advisory Committee on Immunization Practices. *MMWR* 2005;54(RR-07):1–21.

28. Centers for Disease Control and Prevention. Injuries associated with self-unloading forage wagons–New York, 1991–1994. *MMWR* 1995;44(32):595–597, 603.

29. Birkhead GS, Galvin VG, Meehan PJ, O'Carroll PW, Mercy JA. The emergency department in surveillance of attempted suicide: findings and methodologic considerations. *Public Health Rep* 1993;108:323–331.

30. Centers for Disease Control and Prevention. Fatal and nonfatal suicide attempts among adolescents—Oregon, 1988–1993. *MMWR* 1995;44(16):312–315, 321–323.

31. Kulldorff M, Heffernan R, Hartman J, Assunção R, Mostashari F. A space-time permutation scan statistic for disease outbreak detection. *PLoS Med* 2005;2(3):e59. Epub 2005 Feb 15.

32. Navarro AM, Voetsch KP, Liburd LC, Giles HW, Collins JL. Charting the future of community health promotion: recommendations from the National Expert Panel on Community Health Promotion. Prev Chronic Dis [serial online] 2007 Jul [Date cited]. http://www.cdc.gov/pcd/issues/2007/jul/07_0013.htm.

33. Best Practices of Comprehensive Tobacco Control Programs. Atlanta, Ga: U.S. Department of Health and Human Services, Centers for Disease Control and Prevention, National Center for Chronic Disease Prevention and Health Promotion, Office on Smoking and Health; 1999.

34. Reducing Tobacco Use: A Report of the Surgeon General. Atlanta, Ga: U.S. Department of Health and Human Services, Centers for Disease Control and Prevention, National Center for Chronic Disease Prevention and Health Promotion, Office on Smoking and Health; 2000.

35. Friedman DJ, Parrish RG. Characteristics, desired functionalities, and data-sets of state web-based data query systems. *J Public Health Manag Pract* 2006;12(2):119–129.

36. Snider DE, Stroup DF. Defining research when it comes to public health. *Public Health Rep* 1997;112:29–32.

37. Mariner WK. Public confidence in public health research ethics. *Public Health Rep* 1997;112:33–36.

38. Code of Federal Regulations, Title 42, Volume 1, Parts 1 to 399. Revised October 1, 2006. [From the U.S. Government Printing Office via GPO Access].

39. Hodge JG, Gostin LO, Gebbie K, Erickson DL. Transforming public health law: The Turning Point Model State Public Health Act. *J Law Med Ethics* 2006;34(1):77–84. Published Online.

40. Centers for Disease Control and Prevention. Summary of notifiable diseases, United States, *MMWR.* 2008;55:1–94. http://www.cdc.gov/mmwr/summary.html. Accessed May 18, 2009.

41. Smith PF, Birkhead GS. Electronic clinical laboratory reporting for public health surveillance. In: Nkuchia M. M'ikanatha, R Lynfield, Van Beneden CA, de Valk H, eds. *Infectious Disease Surveillance*. Blackwell Publishing; 2007:341–350.

42. Overhage JM, Grannis S, McDonald CJ. A comparison of the completeness and timeliness of automated electronic laboratory reporting and spontaneous reporting of notifiable conditions. *Am J Public Health* 2008;98:344–350.

43. Gostin LO, Hodge JG, Valdiserri RO. Informational privacy and the public's health: the Model State Public Health Privacy Act. *Am J Public Health* 2001;91:1388–1392.

44. Azaroff LS, Lax MB, Levenstein C, Wegman DH. Wounding the messenger: the new economy makes occupational health indicators too good to be true. *Internat J Health Services* 2004;34(2):271–303.

45. Monk E, Smart C, eds. *Central Cancer Registries: Design, Management and Use.* Harwood Academic Publishers; 1994.

46. Jenson OM, Parkin DM, MacLennan R, Muir CS, Skeet R, eds. *Cancer Registration: Principles and Methods.* IARC Scientific Publications, Number 95. Lyons, France, 1991.

47. Baron RC, Dicker RC, Bussell KE, Herndon JL. Assessing trends in mortality in 121 U.S. cities, 1970–79, from all causes and from pneumonia and influenza. *Public Health Rep* 1988;103:120–128.

48. Mokdad AH. The behavioral risk factors surveillance system: past, present, and future. *Ann Rev Public Health* 2009;30:43–54. First published online as a Review in Advance on January 19, 2009.

49. Buehler JW. Review of the 2003 National Syndromic Surveillance Conference–lessons learned and questions to be answered. *MMWR* 2004;53(Suppl):18–22.

50. Bradley CA, Rolka H, Walker D, Loonsk J. Biosense: implementation of a national early event detection and situational awareness system. *MMWR* 2005;54(Suppl):11–19.

51. Drociuk D, Gibson J, Hodge J. Health information privacy and syndromic surveillance. *MMWR* 2004;53(Suppl):221–225.

52. Mostashari F, Hartman J. Syndromic surveillance: a local perspective. *J Urban Health* 2003;80(Suppl 1);1099–3460.

53. Steiner-Sichel L, Heffernan R, Layton M, Weiss D. Field investigations of emergency department syndromic surveillance. Signals—New York City. *MMWR* 2004;53(Suppl):184–189.

54. Terry W, Ostrowsky B, Huang A. Should we be worried? Investigation of signals generated by an electronic syndromic suveillance system—Westchester County, New York. *MMWR* 2004;53(Suppl):190–195.

55. Mostashari F, Hartman J. Syndromic surveillance: a local perspective. *J Urban Health* 2003;80(2):11–17.

56. Murray CJL, Kulkarni SC, Michaud C, *et al.* Eight Americas: investigating mortality disparities across races, counties, and race-counties in the United States. *PLoS Med* 2006;3(9):e260. doi:10.1371/journal.pmed.0030260.

57. Ezzati M, Friedman AB, Kulkarni SC, Murray CJ. The reversal of fortunes: trends in county mortality and cross-county mortality disparities in the United States. *PLoS Med* 2008;5(4):e66.

58. AHRQ quality indicators. *Guide to Prevention Quality Indicators: Hospital Admission for Ambulatory Care Sensitive Conditions.* Rockville, MD, Agency for Healthcare Research and Quality (AHRQ); 2007:59 (AHRQ Pub; no 02-R0203).

59. AHRQ quality indicators. *Prevention Quality Indicators: Technical Specifications [version3.2].* Rockville, MD: Agency for Healthcare Research and Quality (AHRQ); 2008:22.

60. Goldman J, Kinnear S, Chung J, Rothman DJ. New York City's initiatives on diabetes and HIV/AIDS: implications for patient care, public health and medical professionalism. *Am J Publ Health* 2008;98(5):807–812.

61. Fairchild AL, Alkon A. Back to the future? Diabetes, HIV, and the boundaries of public health. *J Health Politics Policy Law* 2007;32(4):561–593.

19

Public Health Workforce Needs for Surveillance

DENISE KOO AND HERMAN TOLENTINO

Earlier chapters of this book described the expanding scope of public health surveillance. As the mission of public health has expanded, so too has the science and applications of public health surveillance. And as the critical monitoring function of surveillance is applied to an increasing range of areas, workforce needs have grown accordingly. This chapter provides a brief description of the evolution of surveillance data skill areas, some of the critical disciplines needed to conduct surveillance in the era of technology and (where they have already been defined) competencies needed by the existing workforce in public health, particularly in the arena of data management, analysis, and interpretation. We emphasize particularly the crucial need for a relatively new discipline of public health—the informatician. A definition of public health informatics and competencies for public health informaticians are described. The chapter concludes with ideas for how to take a more strategic approach to recruiting new persons into the workforce and developing and retaining the existing public health workforce needed for the new world of public health surveillance.

BACKGROUND

Clearly, recognition of the relevance of surveillance as a domain of epidemiology in public health practice is increasing, as described in great detail in this book. Surveillance is foundational for all areas of public health, providing critical information regarding the baseline condition of the public health system for a given disease or injury. In fact, surveillance is applied, as described in Chapter 14, to preparedness for even the possibility of a problem, one in which no seasonal baseline exists (e.g., terrorism). This application of the surveillance function to situation awareness and as an early warning system is consistent with the expansion to surveillance for events earlier in the causal chain, not just disease, injury or death but also potential indicators, exposures, behaviors, and hazards.

Expansion of content included in surveillance has occurred simultaneously with an increased expectation of information availability, attributable largely to explosive growth in use of computers and information technology. Advances in technology facilitate instantaneous availability of data in electronic format, thereby putting pressure on public health officials to know it all in real time despite unremitting increases in the number and variety of data sources. Cognizant of the opportunities provided by these advances in information technology, public health officials hope to collect the majority of these data through electronic capture or transfer of existing data (especially data within the healthcare system) and not through the labor-intensive, manual data-collection methods that remain common practice. However, as described in Chapter 5, connectivity is not automatic nor is interoperability and useful information exchange. Public health officials should create information exchange agreements, agree to use certain data standards, clean the data, and evaluate the reliability, validity, and meaning of these data—for example, whether they represent the diseases of interest and whether statistical aberrations signal that a true increase might be occurring.

GENERAL WORKFORCE NEEDS

Although electronic data systems that monitor for health threats increasingly are becoming automated, human expertise is—and will always be—critical to recognizing potential cases of disease, diagnosing disease, reporting data, interpreting data, and communicating findings to all stakeholders. This human capacity is particularly key in developing countries where workforce gaps are particularly acute and where penetrance of training in advanced technology is minimal. For this reason, the health workforce—particularly the public health workforce—is fundamental to sustaining and enhancing surveillance capacity.

Surveillance data come from a variety of sources. Most often, clinicians recognize disease threats or poisoning from chemicals or other toxins, request laboratory confirmation, and report these findings to state and local health departments. In addition, clinicians also provide data related to adverse events following immunization or even medical errors. Surveillance data also come from such nonclinical sources as police reports, injury compensation records, and environmental monitoring systems. After collecting the data, public health workers should synthesize, analyze, interpret, investigate, and act on the findings. Professionals from diverse disciplines—working in a nation's health system and at all levels of government and geographic jurisdictions—provide a range of skills necessary for the components of a national or international surveillance system to work effectively to protect the health of the public. The astute clinician remains a critical link—particularly in infectious disease or other forms of biosurveillance—but other personnel have become increasingly critical. Infection-control professionals, pharmacists, law enforcement officials, coroners, and medical examiners are often the first to recognize events that require prompt interventions of public health personnel.

In light of the importance of each of these professionals to the effectiveness of the national or international surveillance system, workforce initiatives are needed to ensure that the right talent is in the right job at the right time. Efforts should focus on enhancing skills and availability of not only the public health workers who bind the surveillance system together but also the diverse disciplines that contribute vital information and expertise. For example, teaching clinicians to recognize cases and report them early and accurately will also improve a nation's ability to respond rapidly.

WORKFORCE DEVELOPMENT FRAMEWORK

One key to improving the global surveillance system will be the establishment of a systematic framework for continuous learning and training to ensure that current and future workers are prepared to meet the challenges ahead. Such a system would identify the disciplines and professional roles and competencies necessary for surveillance, target these disciplines for recruitment, and offer training and career development paths to increase competencies identified for both those in primary roles (e.g., epidemiologists, informaticians, environmental health specialists, and laboratorians) and those in supporting roles (e.g., physicians, nurses, and public health managers).

The foundation for such a system would be a workforce surveillance system similar to the foundational role of surveillance in public health (*see* Fig. 19–1). Surveillance of the workforce would enumerate and describe the public health workforce and support forecasting of workforce needs (*see* Fig. 19–2). Just as we define cases of illness for surveillance, we would need to define the key disciplines to monitor, their roles in surveillance, and the competencies required for each. This monitoring of the workforce would lead to identification of gaps in the workforce, which should lead to research into the underlying basis for such gaps ("risk factor identification," Fig. 19–2), and priority setting among the gaps. The "intervention evaluation" step would involve careful assessment of methods for addressing the gaps, whether targeted recruitment efforts, competency-based training of existing workforce, or incentives for new or existing workforce. The implementation step involves running programs for workforce recruitment, development, retention, and evaluating their impact through formative and summative evaluation, as well as ongoing surveillance and monitoring.

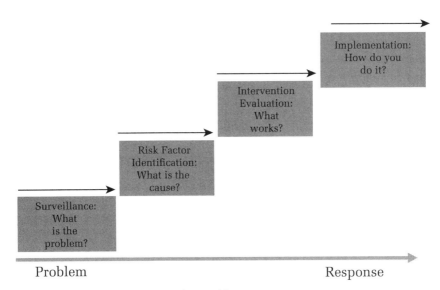

Figure 19–1 Public health approach to problems.

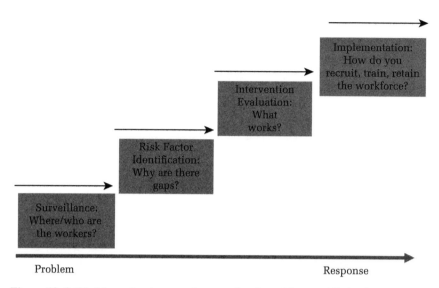

Figure 19–2 Workforce development framework, adapted from public health approach.

CRITICAL COMPETENCIES, WITH EXAMPLES FROM TWO DISCIPLINES

Challenges posed by data and information overload necessitate evolution of the field of public health surveillance, particularly in the arena of connectivity and scientific interpretation of data. We list connectivity first because public health officials should link with many different partners to integrate data from myriad sources for public health surveillance. Many of these partners exist within the field of public health but beyond traditional boundaries for detailed data sharing and collection (e.g., in other countries, as referenced in Chapter 17). Other data-sharing partnerships also being strengthened include those within the health-care system, as with pharmacy and emergency department data. Newer partnerships include those outside the traditional realms of public health and the larger health system (e.g., homeland security, defense, and law enforcement). For many of these, public health has had relationships and recognized the possible uses of those data, but in the past it was difficult to access the data and we often did not maintain the partnerships to the degree necessary to share data for public health surveillance purposes. Technological advances have largely removed the physical access barrier, if not the policy and organizational ones.

For example, in the United States, certain state and local health departments have begun to participate in regional health information exchange collaborations, potentially expanding the types and sources of data public health practitioners can evaluate and use for decision making. A regional health information organization (RHIO) is a geographically defined group of organizations with a business stake in improving the quality, safety, and efficiency of health-care delivery and that have agreed to share resources to facilitate standards-based access to and retrieval of health information. Public health participation in such RHIOs provides an important influence on the development of these building blocks for a future national network of health information. Examples of state and local health departments participating in regional health information exchanges include Tennessee and West Virginia, with Carespark RHIO; Marion County Health Department, with the Indiana Health Information Exchange; Eastern Washington State, with Inland Northwest Health Services; and New York City Department of Health with multiple RHIOs and the NY eHealth Collaborative.

When public health practitioners need to establish electronic connectivity to gain access to new data sources, they require additional informatics-related competencies, for example, even to understand what new terminology like *health information exchange* means and to leverage health information exchange activities that might be taking place in their localities. Even after collaborative relationships and connectivity are established and data are shared (in a technically accessible and acceptable fashion, with appropriate security), the problem of interpretation remains. Evaluating data can be challenging, as they are often collected for different purposes or use similar terms with different definitions. Data collected outside the health realm might not have the meaning we understand in the public health world. Even data collected within the public health realm in countries with fewer resources might use different definitions for cases (or contain less information to confirm a case). And data collected within the health-care setting by clinicians across the country might not signify what we assume (especially data collected for such administrative purposes as for billing) (*1*). These are scientific concerns relevant to the methodology of surveillance. In fact, we should prioritize and focus by evaluating which surveillance data sources and methods provide the most accurate picture of disease or illness or how some might be used together to provide the big picture (*2,3*).

> *"Where is the wisdom we have lost in knowledge? Where is the knowledge we have lost in information?"*
>
> —*T.S. Eliot*

Data management and informatics constitute critical workforce competencies—particularly for epidemiologists and statisticians, whose disciplines and identities revolve around data and information. Informatics, or information science, is the study of information and how it is organized, stored, retrieved, presented, and used. Public health informatics has been defined as the systematic application of information and computer science and information technology to public health research, practice, and learning (*4*). Given the information explosion, this is a critical competency area for the quantitative and data-oriented public health disciplines.

Epidemiologists, especially those working in state and local health departments, are expected increasingly to manage information systems or make choices regarding information technology tools, often without adequate training in informatics. Communication barriers exist between information technologists and epidemiologists as often is the case between two distinct disciplines. Information systems supporting public health surveillance must be designed based on public health program needs, as defined by epidemiologists, program managers, and others. Increasingly, the role of translator between epidemiologists and others and the information technology team is filled by public health informaticians, a relatively new discipline within public health. The public health informatician is dually trained both in public health and in informatics; skilled informaticians fill this vital translational role and recognize the potential role of technology in transforming public health practice. In the following paragraphs, we describe general categories of informatics competencies for public health professionals and, subsequently, the more specific competency requirements for public health epidemiologists and informaticians. Competencies are the knowledge, skills, and abilities demonstrated by organization or system members that are critical to the effective and efficient function of the organization or system (5). The information, described below, is based on two recent national competency development efforts in the United States. The workforce needs for public health surveillance are not limited to epidemiologists and informaticians, but similar efforts to define specific competencies for other public health workforce disciplines critical to surveillance have not yet arisen.

Core Informatics Competencies for All Public Health Professionals

During 2001 through 2002, a working group of public health informaticians and educators drafted a consensus set of public health informatics competencies for the general public health professional (6). These informatics competencies were designed to complement the more general set of *Core Competencies for Public Health Professionals*, developed by the Council on Linkages Between Academia and Public Health Practice. The working group defined three classes of informatics competencies—those related to (a) use of information *per se* for public health practice; (b) use of information technology to increase one's individual effectiveness as a public health professional; and (c) management of information technology projects to improve effectiveness of the public health enterprise (e.g., the state or local health department). For each competency, expertise levels are suggested for three professional workforce segments—front-line staff (including administrative staff); senior-level technical staff (including epidemiologists); and supervisory and management staff. These general informatics competencies provided a useful starting point for defining competencies for all public health professionals in this critical field.

Competencies for Applied Epidemiologists

During 2004 through 2006, the U.S. Centers for Disease Control and Prevention (CDC) and the Council of State and Territorial Epidemiologists (CSTE) convened an expert panel to define *Competencies for Applied Epidemiologists in Governmental Public Health Agencies* (applied epidemiology competencies [AECs]) to improve the practice of epidemiology within the public health system (7,8). The document, developed collaboratively with extensive input from local, state, and federal public health agencies as well as academia, defines the discipline of applied epidemiology and describes expected competencies for different tiers of practicing epidemiologists working in governmental public health agencies. During the process, the group paid special attention to the definition of competencies for epidemiologists in the arenas of public health surveillance and informatics, forming a special subgroup of epidemiologists and informaticians to describe the competencies needed.

AECs contained an entire competency statement related to "conducting surveillance activities," which included 5 subcompetencies and 30 sub-subcompetencies (Table 19–1). Certain subcompetencies included in this document probably would not have appeared had the standard been developed one to two decades ago; these subcompetencies related substantially to the interface of epidemiology with information systems. These subcompetencies defined the need for epidemiologists to be cognizant of and use data standards, to participate actively in information system design, and to define requirements for information systems that serve epidemiologic purposes. One competency related to linking of relational databases and then subsetting them into data sets for analysis, something now facilitated by technology. Public health surveillance and informatics-related competencies also appear under other competencies, such as using new or existing information systems, the data management competency, and the competency related to using principles of informatics in data collection, processing, and analysis. The latter included competencies to "combine data and information from multiple sources to create new information to support public health decision-making" and to "participate in development of data models to ensure representation of epidemiologic needs in associated databases and information systems." The European CDC has followed this model in defining core competencies for public health epidemiologists working in the European Union (9).

Competencies for Public Health Informaticians

Because public health surveillance, at its core, concerns data and information for action, and because in this technological era of information explosion, knowledge management is key, the relatively new discipline of public health informatics has become increasingly crucial. Unfortunately, this discipline is often confused with being "just information technology."

In 2005 through 2007, CDC initiated a collaboration, through the Association of Schools of Public Health, with the University of Washington School of Public Health to define competencies for public health informaticians. This effort involved local, state, and federal public health partners as well as academia. The workgroup defined public health informatics in accordance with the definition cited earlier in this chapter and defined a public health informatician as a "public health professional who works in practice, research, or academia and whose primary work function is to use informatics to improve the health of populations" (10). Perhaps because of the relative newness of this field, this workgroup defined competencies for only two tiers of public health informaticians—the public health informatician and the senior public health informatician. Although the workgroup accepted that public health informaticians needed to be competent in the eight domains defined for all public health professionals by the Council on Linkages between Academic and Public Health Practice (11), this group initially determined that informatics—especially for the informatician— warranted its own new domain of competencies. (The group intended to but

Table 19–1 Surveillance Competencies for Applied Epidemiologists, United States, 2008

Tier 1: Entry-Level or Basic Epidemiologist	Tier 2: Mid-Level Epidemiologist	Tier 3a: Senior-Level Epidemiologist: Supervisor or Manager	Tier 3b: Senior Scientist/Subject Area Expert
B. Conduct surveillance activities	**B. Conduct surveillance activities**	**B. Oversee surveillance activities**	**B. Organize surveillance**
1. N/A	1. Design surveillance for the particular public health concern being considered.	1. Approve surveillance for the particular public health concern being considered.	1. Evaluate validity of conducting surveillance for the particular public health concern being considered.
a. N/A	a. Identify types of surveillance methods for specific public health problems.	a. Examine potential surveillance methods for specific public health problems.	a. Examine types of surveillance methods for specific public health problems.
b. N/A	b. Identify information systems to support surveillance systems.	b. Approve information systems to support surveillance systems.	b. Recommend information systems to support surveillance systems.
c. N/A	c. Recommend types of surveillance systems for specific public health problems.	c. Decide on types of surveillance systems for specific public health problems.	c. Determine type of surveillance systems for specific public health problems.
d. N/A	d. N/A	d. Review anticipated costs and benefits of initiating a new surveillance system.	d. N/A
e. N/A	e. Identify additional burden to public health system and reporting entity anticipated to result from the proposed surveillance system.	e. Decide whether to impose the additional burden to public health system and reporting entity that is anticipated to result from the proposed surveillance system.	e. Evaluate additional burden to public health system and reporting entity anticipated to result from the proposed surveillance system.
2. Identify surveillance data needs.	2. Identify surveillance data needs.	2. Decide on surveillance data needs.	2. Evaluate surveillance data needs.

a. Create case definitions based on person, place, and time.	a. Create case definitions based on person, place, and time.	a. Verify case definitions based on person, place, and time.	a. Evaluate case definitions based on person, place, and time.
b. N/A	b. Describe sources, quality, and limitations of surveillance data.	b. Decide on sources of surveillance data.	b. Evaluate sources, quality, and limitations of surveillance data.
c. N/A	c. Define data elements to be collected or reported.	c. N/A	c. Assess adequacy of data elements to be collected or reported.
d. N/A	d. Identify mechanisms to transfer data from source to public health agency.	d. Decide on mechanisms to transfer data from source to public health agency.	d. Assess mechanisms to transfer data from source to public health agency.
e. N/A	e. Define timeliness required for data collection.	e. Decide on acceptable timeliness for data collection and frequency for reporting.	e. Evaluate timeliness requirements for data collection.
f. N/A	f. Determine frequency of reporting.	f. N/A	f. Assess frequency of reporting.
g. Recognize potential uses of data to inform surveillance systems.	g. Describe potential uses of data to inform surveillance-system design.	g. Decide on surveillance system design.	g. Create surveillance system design on the basis of potential uses of data.
h. N/A	h. Define the functional requirements of the supporting information system.	h. Approve functional requirements of the supporting information system.	h. Assess functional requirements of the information system.
3. Implement new or revise existing surveillance systems.	3. Implement new or revise existing surveillance systems.	3. Supervise or manage implementation of new or revision of existing surveillance systems.	3. Implement new or revise existing surveillance systems.

(continued)

Table 19–1 (continued)

Tier 1: Entry-Level or Basic Epidemiologist	Tier 2: Mid-Level Epidemiologist	Tier 3a: Senior-Level Epidemiologist: Supervisor or Manager	Tier 3b: Senior Scientist/Subject Area Expert
a. Define objectives and uses of surveillance system.	a. Define objectives and uses of surveillance system.	a. Approve objectives and uses of surveillance system.	a. Develop guidelines for objectives and uses of surveillance systems.
b. Test data collection, data storage, and analytical methods, as directed.	b. Test data-collection, data-storage, and analytical methods.	b. Validate data collection, data storage, and analytical methods.	b. Validate data collection, data storage, and analytical methods.
c. Assist in creating working surveillance system.	c. Create working surveillance system.	c. N/A	c. Create working surveillance system.
d. Collect data for verification of defined surveillance-system parameters (e.g., timeliness, frequency).	d. Verify that data collection occurs according to the defined surveillance-system parameters (e.g., timeliness, frequency).	d. Verify that data collection occurs according to the defined surveillance system parameters (e.g., timeliness, frequency).	d. Assess performance of data collection systems against defined surveillance system parameters (e.g., timeliness, frequency).
e. Classify potential cases according to whether they meet the case definition.	e. Ensure correct classification of cases according to the case definition.	e. N/A	e. N/A
f. Interview persons experiencing illness to solicit necessary information.	f. Interview persons experiencing illness to solicit necessary information.	f. N/A	f. N/A
g. Assist in monitoring data quality.	g. Monitor data quality.	g. Ensure that data quality is monitored.	g. Monitor data quality.
h. Maintain working relationships with reporting entities.	h. Create working relationships with reporting entities.	h. Ensure working relationships with reporting entities.	h. Create working relationships with reporting entities.
i. Provide feedback to reporting entities and other organizations or persons who need information regarding the data or system.	i. Provide feedback to reporting entities and other organizations or persons who need information regarding the data or system.	i. Ensure provision of feedback to reporting entities and other organizations or persons who need information regarding the data or system.	i. Synthesize information concerning surveillance system for communicating to reporting entities and other organizations or persons who need information regarding the data or system.

Column 1	Column 2	Column 3	Column 4
4. Report key findings from the surveillance system.	4. Identify key findings from the surveillance system.	4. Synthesize key findings from the surveillance system and other pertinent information for use by decision makers.	4. Synthesize key findings from the surveillance system and other pertinent information for use by decision makers.
a. Provide system's results to senior epidemiologists.	a. Examine system's results in the context of current scientific knowledge.	a. Interpret system's results in the context of current scientific knowledge and other available information.	a. Interpret system's results in the context of current scientific knowledge.
b. Recognize implications to public health programs.	b. Identify implications to public health programs.	b. Examine implications to public health programs.	b. Examine implications to public health programs.
c. Assist in developing conclusions from the surveillance data.	c. Develop conclusions from the surveillance data.	c. Determine relative priority of each conclusion from the surveillance data before making recommendations to decision makers.	c. Determine relative priority of each conclusion from the surveillance data before making recommendations to decision makers.
d. Communicate results to senior staff.	d. Communicate results to agency managers and to reporters of surveillance data (*see* Communication Competencies).	d. Communicate synthesized information to decision makers and the public.	d. Communicate synthesized information to decision makers and the public.
5. Support evaluation of surveillance systems.	5. Conduct evaluation of surveillance systems.	5. Ensure evaluation of surveillance systems.	5. Design and conduct evaluation of surveillance systems.

(*continued*)

Table 19-1 (*continued*)

Tier 1: Entry-Level or Basic Epidemiologist	Tier 2: Mid-Level Epidemiologist	Tier 3a: Senior-Level Epidemiologist: Supervisor or Manager	Tier 3b: Senior Scientist/Subject Area Expert
a. Collect data necessary for evaluation of surveillance systems by using national guidance and methods.* b. Assist in preparing recommendations for modifications to surveillance systems on the basis of evaluation. c. N/A d. Assist in implementing changes to surveillance system on the basis of results of evaluation.	a. Evaluate surveillance systems by using national guidance and methods.* b. Propose recommendations for modifications to surveillance systems on the basis of evaluation. c. N/A d. Implement changes to surveillance system on the basis of results of evaluation.	a. Ensure evaluation of surveillance systems by using national guidance and methods.* b. Appraise recommendations for modifications to surveillance systems on the basis of evaluation. c. Decide whether to modify surveillance systems on the basis of recommendations. d. Ensure that changes to surveillance system are implemented on the basis of results of evaluation.	a. Evaluate surveillance systems by using national guidance and methods.* b. Develop or review recommendations for modifications to surveillance systems on the basis of evaluation. c. Decide whether to modify surveillance systems on the basis of recommendations. d. Ensure that changes to surveillance system are implemented on the basis of results of evaluation.

See Centers for Disease Control and Prevention (US). Updated guidelines for evaluating public health surveillance systems; recommendations from the Guidelines Working Group. *MMWR Recomm Rep* 2001;50(RR-13):1–35.

Source: CDC/CSTE Competencies for Applied Epidemiologists in Governmental Public Health Agencies.

did not have the resources to revisit this decision at the end.) They defined 13 competencies for public health informaticians in a ninth domain (Table 19–2), with subcompetencies and sub-subcompetencies for most of these. These competencies comprised strategic direction for public health informatics; knowledge management; leveraging use of standards; meeting the knowledge, information, and information systems needs of users; operation of information technology projects; communications; information systems evaluation; research in public health informatics; interoperability with systems, including those outside public health; confidentiality, security, and integrity of data and systems; and workforce development.

WORKFORCE DEVELOPMENT STRATEGIES

Simply defining the competencies—the knowledge, skills, and abilities—is insufficient for development of competent practitioners. These competencies should be used by practitioners to assess their current skills, create career development plans, and plan their own training. Employers should use these to create career ladders for employees, develop position descriptions and job qualifications, develop training plans for employees, and assess the capacity of their organization. CDC and CSTE have assembled a toolkit for AECs to facilitate their use. The toolkit, available from CDC and CSTE websites (6), includes the competencies themselves but also includes self-assessment tools, sample position descriptions, and a slide set to disseminate the competencies further. We encourage educators to design programs that meet the continuing education needs of the current workforce in public health agencies and incorporate critical elements of practice into their programs that develop new public health workers.

The Association of Schools of Public Health evaluated AECs and mapped them to several curricula in schools of public health. Their committee concluded that certain competencies can only be acquired through experiential learning and practica (12). Just as physicians are not ready to practice medicine until they complete a medical residency, public health professionals must learn how to apply these principles on the job, preferably under the tutelage of an experienced mentor. It is critical for public health professionals to learn the basic knowledge needed to practice in their fields, but they also need to learn how to apply the abstract principles and knowledge to the reality of government practice, community rules, and policies. CDC and its partners manage public health "residencies" that provide a systematic opportunity for exposure to this kind of subjective knowledge, especially through CDC's Epidemic Intelligence Service (EIS) and Public Health Informatics Fellowship Programs.

Learning on the Job: the Epidemic Intelligence Service

Since 1951, CDC has managed EIS (13), a 2-year training and service program with a focus on applied epidemiology (14,15). The EIS program emphasizes the public health practice of epidemiology and plays a critical role in developing practitioners

Table 19–2 High-Level Competencies for Public Health Informaticians, United States, 2009

Public Health Informatician	Senior Public Health Informatician
1. Supports development of strategic direction for public health informatics within the enterprise.	1. Leads creation of strategic direction for public health informatics.
2. Participates in development of knowledge-management tools for the enterprise.	2. Leads knowledge management for the enterprise.
3. Uses standards.	3. Ensures utilization of standards.
4. Ensures that knowledge, information, and data needs of project or program users and stakeholders are met.	4. Ensures that knowledge, information, and data needs of users and stakeholders are met.
5. Supports information system development, procurement, and implementation that meet public health program needs.	5. Ensures that information system development, procurement, and implementation meet public health program needs.
6a. Manages information technology (IT) operations related to project or program (for public health agencies with internal IT operations).	6a. Ensures IT operations are managed to effectively support public health programs (for public health agencies with internal IT operations).
6b. Monitors IT operations managed by external organizations.	6b. Ensures adequacy of IT operations managed by external organizations.
7. Communicates with cross-disciplinary leaders and team members.	7. Communicates with elected officials, policy-makers, agency staff, and the public.
8. Evaluates information systems and applications.	8. Ensures evaluation of information systems and applications.
9. Participates in applied public health informatics research for new insights and innovative solutions to health problems.	9. Conducts applied public health informatics research for new insights and innovative solutions to health problems.
	10. Ensures that public health information systems are interoperable with other relevant information systems.
	11. Uses informatics to integrate clinical health, environmental risk, and population health.
	12. Develops solutions that ensure confidentiality, security, and integrity while maximizing availability of information for public health.
	13. Contributes to progress in the field of public health informatics.

10. Contributes to development of public health information systems that are interoperable with other relevant information systems.
11. Supports use of informatics to integrate clinical health, environmental risk, and population health.
12. Implements solutions that ensure confidentiality, security, and integrity while maximizing availability of information for public health.
13. Conducts education and training in public health informatics.

Source: Karras BT, Davies J, Koo D, and the Working Group on Competencies for Public Health Informaticians. *Competencies for Public Health Informaticians.* Seattle, WA: US Department of Health and Human Services, Centers for Disease Control and Prevention and the University of Washington's Center for Public Health Informatics; 2009.

experienced in the most current methods of public health surveillance, an area not often included in academic training. In addition to learning about surveillance, EIS officers learn how to evaluate and contribute to actual surveillance systems, and through their training and work, they disseminate new surveillance methods across the country. Since 1951, more than 3,000 professionals have served in EIS, including physicians, veterinarians, nurses, dentists, engineers, and persons with doctoral degrees in multiple health-related fields (e.g., epidemiology, anthropology, sociology, and microbiology). A majority of EIS graduates remain employed in public health after completing the program. EIS serves as an international model for training public health practitioners of epidemiology, with more than 30 programs around the world patterned after it (*16*).

Learning on the Job: the Public Health Informatics Fellowship Program

Recognizing the potential transformational role of informatics in public health, in 1996 CDC initiated a program modeled after EIS, the Public Health Informatics Fellowship Program (PHIFP), a 2-year training and service program with a focus on applied informatics (*17*). PHIFP emphasizes the public health practice of informatics, and although small, the program fills a critical gap in the public health workforce. Since 1996, approximately 70 professionals have trained and served in PHIFP, including physicians, computer and information scientists, librarians, nurses, engineers, and other master's and doctoral-degree holders (e.g., epidemiology, anthropology, and sociology). A majority of PHIFP graduates remain employed in public health after completing the program. Other countries and organizations (e.g., Vietnam, China, Pakistan, and the European CDC) have expressed strong interest in developing new fellowship programs modeled after this one.

CHALLENGES IN DEVELOPING WORKFORCE FOR PUBLIC HEALTH SURVEILLANCE

Several challenges face those in the workforce arena. As mentioned earlier, only a few systems of surveillance for the public health workforce exist, some of which are inadequate; therefore, baseline and ongoing information concerning the numbers of workers in the needed fields is limited. The science of workforce development and taking a systematic, rigorous approach to developing the workforce, is relatively new in public health. The U.S. CDC only formed an Office of Workforce and Career Development in 2004. There are few standards and certification processes for the public health workforce, and clinical partners such as physicians often do not learn about their role in the public health surveillance system (as it is not yet a required component of medical education). And because the health impact of workforce development is indirect, or long-term, and no specific, compelling disease is attached to this critical component of the infrastructure, obtaining funding for this area is challenging. As in the business world, when funding is tight, workforce development is often the first program cut.

Additionally, given the rapidly evolving nature of modern surveillance approaches with links to public health informatics, fewer experts or established scientific principles are available. Where experts are available, whether epidemiologists or informaticians, they often have limited experience with teaching it, and too few case examples are available to illustrate the principles. Epidemiologists sometimes resist using data standards, citing lack of responsiveness to their program needs, and too few are able to analyze data distributed in relational databases (rather than simple flat files). Yet, as noted earlier, these are critical competencies for epidemiologists practicing in this electronic era.

FUTURE DIRECTIONS

The increasing emphasis on reuse of data already captured for other purposes (e.g., National Health Information Network [*18*] and NEDSS, biosurveillance) and the increasing connectivity between electronic health records and public health surveillance systems present exciting new opportunities for public health. These developments also highlight challenges and gaps in the science and methods of surveillance and the training needs of the health workforce. Data management and informatics comprise especially critical workforce competencies among existing disciplines of public health, particularly for epidemiologists and others whose disciplines and identities revolve around data and information. The efforts to define competencies for applied epidemiologists and public health informaticians are a critical first step toward closing these workforce gaps. CDC, state and local health departments, and academic institutions should use these competencies as targets for their workforce development programs, in partnership with other relevant stakeholders in public health (e.g., nonprofit partners with interest in workforce development, the Public Health Informatics Institute, the Public Health Data Standards Consortium, the American Public Health Association, and the American Medical Informatics Association in the United States). These competencies can drive development of projects linking public health information systems with clinical, environmental, and other related systems and contribute to development of the existing public health workforce.

However, effective development of a sustainable surveillance workforce requires more than training; systematic activities directed at recruitment and retention of professionals also are needed. Serious public health workforce shortages exist in disciplines that perform surveillance functions, and these limit the current capacity and plans for enhancement in the United States. States and communities nationwide report needing more public health nurses, epidemiologists, laboratory workers, informaticians, and environmental health experts, and the Association of Schools of Public Health estimates that 250,000 more public health workers will be needed by 2020 simply to maintain current capacity (*19–23*). We need specific, targeted programs such as EIS and PHIFP, as well as educational programs targeted at current public health workers. We also need system-wide or policy-level solutions, such as addressing gaps such as the lack of a job series at the federal level for recruiting informaticians or a lack of understanding of the complexity of the science of epidemiology or informatics and, thus, noncompetitive salaries. Toward this end, Utah and Minnesota have already taken steps to incorporate the informatician class into their human resource departments' job classification schemes.

Just as we strive to be rigorous in our science and practice of public health, so too should we apply systematic, rigorous processes to ensure a prepared, diverse, and sustainable workforce.

REFERENCES

1. Birnbaum HG, Cremieux PY, Greenberg PE, Jacques LeLorier J, Ostrander J, Venditti L. Outpatient diagnostic errors: unrecognized hyperglycemia. *Eff Clin Pract*2002;5:11–16.
2. Centers for Disease Control and Prevention. Syndromic surveillance: reports from a national conference, 2003. *MMWR* 2004:53(Suppl).
3. Koo D. Leveraging syndromic surveillance. *J Public Health Manag Pract* 2005;11:181–183.
4. Yasnoff WA, O'Carroll PW, Koo D, Linkins RW, Kilbourne E. Public health informatics: Improving and transforming public health in the information age. *J Public Health Manag Pract* 2000; 6: 67–75.
5. Nelson JC, Essien JDK, Loudermilk R, Cohen D. *The Public Health Competency Handbook: Optimizing Individual and Organization Performance for the Public's Health*. Atlanta, GA: Center for Public Health Practice of the Rollins School of Public Health; 2002.
6. O'Carroll PW, Public Health Informatics Competencies Working Group. Informatics competencies for public health professionals. Northwest Center for Public Health Practice Web site. http://nwcphp.org/docs/phi/comps/phic_web.pdf. Published August 2002. Accessed April 28, 2009.
7. Competencies for Applied Epidemiologists in Governmental Public Health Agencies. U.S. Centers for Disease Control and Prevention and Council of State and Territorial Epidemiologists Web sites. http://www.cdc.gov/AppliedEpiCompetencies and http://www.cste.org/competencies.asp. Published November 2008. Accessed April 28, 2009.
8. Birkhead GS, Davies J, Lemmings J, Miner K, Koo D. Developing competencies for applied epidemiology: From process to product. *Public Health Rep* 2008;123 (Suppl 1):67–118.
9. Core competencies for public health epidemiologists working in the area of communicable disease surveillance and response, in the European Union. European Center for Disease Prevention and Control Web site. http://ecdc.europa.eu/en/files/pdf/Publications/Core_comp.pdf. Published Stockholm, Sweden; January 2008. Accessed April 28, 2009.
10. Centers for Disease Control and Prevention and University of Washington's Center for Public Health Informatics. Competencies for Public Health Informaticians.U.S. Centers for Disease Control and Prevention and University of Washington Center for Public Health Informatics Web sites: http://www.cdc.gov/informaticscompetencies and http://www.cphi.washington.edu/resources/competencies.html. Published September 2009. Accessed December 27, 2009.

11. Core Competencies for Public Health Professionals. Council on Linkages between Academia and Public Health Practice. Public Health Foundation Web site. http://www.phf.org/link/corecompetencies.htm. Accessed April 28, 2009.

12. Applied Epidemiology Competencies Curriculum and Practicum Project Task Force Report. Association of Schools of Public Health Web site. http://www.asph.org/document.cfm?page=600. Accessed April 28, 2009.

13. Epidemic Intelligence Service. U.S. Centers for Disease Control and Prevention Web site. http://www.cdc.gov/eis. Accessed April 28, 2009.

14. Langmuir AD, Andrews JM. Biological warfare defense. 2. The Epidemic Intelligence Service of the Communicable Disease Center. *Am J Public Health.* 1952;42:235–238.

15. Thacker SB, Dannenberg AL, Hamilton DH. The Epidemic Intelligence Service of the Centers for Disease Control and Prevention: 50 years of training and service in applied epidemiology. *Am J Epidemiol.* 2001;154:985–992.

16. White M, McDonnell SM, Werker D, Cardenas V, Thacker SB. The applied epidemiology and service network in the year 2000. *Am J Epidemiol.* 2001;154:993–999.

17. Public Health Informatics Fellowship Program Web site. http://www.cdc.gov/PHIFP. Accessed April 28, 2009.

18. National Health Information Network. U.S. Department of Health and Human Services Web site. http://healthit.hhs.gov/portal/server.pt?open=512&objID=1142&parentname=CommunityPage&parentid=2&mode=2&in_hi_userid=10741&cached=true. Accessed April 28, 2009.

19. More than 250,000 Additional Public Health Workers Needed by 2020 to Avert Public Health Crisis (Press Release). Association of Schools of Public Health Web site. http://www.asph.org/userfiles/finalasphworkforcerelease.pdf. Released February 27, 2008; Washington, DC. Accessed April 28, 2009.

20. 2007 State public health workforce survey results. Association of State and Territorial Health Officials Web site. http://www.astho.org/pubs/WorkforceReport.pdf. Published Arlington, VA; 2008. Accessed April 28, 2009.

21. 2004 State public health employee worker shortage report: A Civil Service recruitment and retention crisis. Association of State and Territorial Health Officials Web site. http://www.astho.org/pubs/Workforce-Survey-Report-2.pdf. Accessed April 28, 2009.

22. Public health workforce study. Health Resources and Services Administration Web site. http://bhpr.hrsa.gov/healthworkforce/reports/publichealth/default.htm. Published Washington, DC; 2005. Accessed April 28, 2009.

23. The local health department workforce: findings from the 2005 national profile of local health departments study. National Association of County and City Health Officials Web site. http://www.naccho.org/topics/workforce/upload/LHD_WorkforceFinal.pdf (pp. 1–14). Published Washington, DC; 2007. Accessed April 28, 2009.

20

Evolving Challenges and Opportunities in Public Health Surveillance

LISA M. LEE AND STEPHEN B. THACKER

Problems can become opportunities when the right people come together.
—Robert South

Several definitions of surveillance have been quoted throughout this text. All capture the elemental characteristics of public health surveillance:

- Ongoing, systematic collection of health-related data
- Routine analysis and interpretation
- Essential tool for planning, implementation, and evaluation of public health practice
- Integrated with timely dissemination
- Application to disease and injury prevention and control, and health promotion

Despite many changes in the past decade, the way we define public health surveillance has remained constant. The 5th Edition of *A Dictionary of Epidemiology* summarizes surveillance as:

> [The] systematic and continuous collection, analysis, and interpretation of data, closely integrated with the timely and coherent dissemination of the results and assessment to those who have the right to know so that action can be taken. It is an essential feature of epidemiologic and public health practice. The final phase in the surveillance chain is the application of information to health promotion and to disease prevention and control. A surveillance system includes a functional capacity for data collection, analysis, and dissemination linked to public health programs (*1*).

Also constant in the midst of much change are the seven ongoing, systematic activities of any public health surveillance system:

- Planning and system design
- Data collection
- Data management

- Analysis
- Interpretation
- Dissemination
- Application to program to support actions to improve population health

All of the examples of public health surveillance systems described in the preceding chapters were built and operate on these seven activities. The responsibilities of the stewards of public health surveillance systems are to plan a system carefully with outputs in mind; to collect the necessary data; to collate, analyze, and interpret the data accurately; and to communicate the information to the right parties in a timely manner so that it will be used to support improvement of health in the community.

A key factor in understanding how public health surveillance differs from numerous other ways of knowing about health of a population lies in the purpose of the activity. The first of the systematic activities is to plan a system with defined outputs and a specific public health purpose—that is, to produce information about a population from which the data are collected to prevent or control disease or injury or to identify an unusual event indicative of public health importance. These defined public health outputs are then generated by a process of systematic data collection, management, analysis, interpretation, dissemination, and link to public health use.

The discipline and definition of public health surveillance have maintained their integrity over the past decade, even in the midst of numerous changes in information technology, demands on the data, and growth in related fields. Still, opportunities and challenges exist. Finding the discipline's right place under the broadly conceived umbrella of "health knowledge" in a community depends on finding a common lexicon for all health data collections. Advances in information technology promise to improve efficiency of data collection, collation, analysis, and dissemination, leaving crucial human inputs to the planning, interpretation, and application steps of a surveillance system. Understanding the role of public health surveillance as it relates to unstructured data scanning and mining leaves important ethical questions about data collection and use and leads to questions about protections afforded to public health data. It is a challenge for schools of public health and others to ensure an adequately large and well-trained public health workforce that allows us to do the surveillance system planning, data interpretation, and application of these findings to public health practice.

CHALLENGES AND OPPORTUNITIES FOR PUBLIC HEALTH SURVEILLANCE IN THE 21ST CENTURY

Surveillance As a Tool of Health Knowledge and Finding a Common Lexicon

Knowledge of the health of and health risks in a community or population depends on many inputs in addition to public health surveillance, including research studies that produce generalizable knowledge, health surveys, registries of vital events like births and deaths, medical and laboratory information systems, environmental monitoring systems, censuses, and many other data resources (Fig. 20–1). Finding a common lexicon across all disciplines that feed data and information into knowledge of a community's or a population's health has been challenging. The overarching goal of health knowledge is to maintain awareness of health outcomes and risks that impact health in a community to measure the extent or severity, causes, and means to control such events. Health, as defined by the World Health Organization, "is a state of complete physical, mental and social well-being and not merely the absence of disease or infirmity (2)." Maintaining knowledge about health of a community requires information from numerous disparate data sources.

Each discipline or type of data collection shown in Figure 20–1 has distinct and useful contributions to knowledge of health in a community. Although distinct, these data collections interact with each other in some cases, providing data to one another or informing the interpretation of information gleaned from a particular data collection. Calling overall health knowledge "surveillance" is a misnomer, as public health surveillance is defined by its methodology and purpose, which differs from overall health knowledge or awareness, which is a more inclusive term reflecting many elements in the environment, understanding and projecting their meaning to health (3). Calling all forms of data collection "surveillance" is also inaccurate and misleading, as each type of collection contributing to health knowledge has its own body of validated methods and standards. If, however, any of these other forms of data collection described below are designed with defined outputs and a specific public health purpose that then generate outputs by a process of ongoing systematic data collection, management, analysis, interpretation, dissemination, and link to public health use, they are considered public health surveillance systems. In other words, often methods look quite similar, but the purpose and outputs help define the data collection as public health surveillance. For example, a survey without specific public health purpose (or that has numerous purposes for its data collection) that does not produce outputs by ongoing systematic process, would not be considered a public health surveillance system; however, a surveillance system could be designed with public health purpose that uses a survey to produce outputs by using an ongoing systematic process that collects data at regular intervals. Those data are then analyzed, and the information is interpreted, disseminated, and applied to public health program.

Sources of health information

Population health surveys such as the National Survey of Family Growth (4), the National Health Interview Survey (5), and the National Health and Nutrition Examination Survey (6) offer a mechanism to measure, sometimes at repeated or regular intervals, indicators of health on a statistically selected sample so information can be generalized to entire populations. These health indicators can be tracked over time, supplying important information about trends in health. Unlike surveillance, health surveys are not associated directly with planning, implementation, and evaluation of public health practice. Often these indicators provide baseline measures used to compare results of public health surveillance, registries, environmental monitoring, or research studies.

Registration, such as vital statistics (birth and death registration), cancer research registries, and exposure registries often provide longitudinal data and include numerous events observed across the "life" or duration of a case. When each case in a population is recorded, such a registry can provide measures of incidence of an event (e.g., registries of multiple births), information about progression of disease (e.g., cancer registries), or potential subjects for epidemiologic studies. Registries can be public health surveillance systems if they are conducted in an ongoing, systematic way, analyzed routinely, used for planning and implementation of public health practice, and integrated with timely dissemination of information applied to disease prevention and health promotion. However, although registry data can be used for public health surveillance, they often fail to meet all seven ongoing activities of surveillance, such as timely information dissemination or direct link to public health programs.

Information systems, such as medical and laboratory records and pharmacy data, can provide useful ancillary data on diagnoses or what the population is purchasing, supplying context for surveillance data. These systems are useful also as data sources for public health surveillance. With improvements in information technology tools and application of informatics science, further improvements in data acquisition from these sources for surveillance are anticipated (*see below*). Environmental monitoring, such as climate and pollution, offers a macro-view of exogenous factors that influence health. Like health surveys, information from environmental monitoring systems can provide crucial context and comparison baseline measures for the interpretation of public health surveillance data. Some environmental monitoring systems enact all seven activities of a public health surveillance system and serve as surveillance systems.

Clinical and public health research supply yet another source of data to inform health knowledge but are not public health surveillance. Targeted studies designed to test hypotheses and produce generalizable knowledge provide decision makers with answers to specific questions. Public health surveillance data are often used to generate hypotheses, which then are tested through thoughtfully designed public health or clinical research studies. Alternatively, research results can inform public health surveillance and assist in setting priorities for data collection. Finally, other data sources external to the public health system, including population census information, criminal justice records, and inventories of website search terms or news articles accessed, can be used for surveillance but more often are used to supplement health knowledge. Population and subpopulation counts supplied by census data can provide important information on age distribution and other demographic characteristics of a population of interest. These counts also serve as denominator data for calculation of rates in many public health surveillance systems (*see* Chapter 6). Other databases can provide necessary social context for interpretation of public health surveillance, especially as the interest in social determinants of health emerges (*see* Chapter 13).

Public health surveillance remains a separate and unique discipline informing health knowledge in a population. It offers data from which outbreaks are detected and characterized; temporal, spatial, and demographic trends are outlined; prevention and control recommendations are developed; risk and protective factors are identified; and public health programs are planned, implemented, and evaluated.

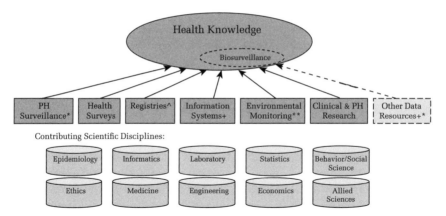

Figure 20–1 Conceptual framework for health knowledge: various data feeds to support health knowledge in a community or population.
[a]Systematic and continuous collection, analysis, and interpretation of data, closely integrated with the timely and coherent dissemination of the results and assessment to those who have the right to know so that action can be taken. Porta M. A *Dictionary of Epidemiology,* 5th *Ed.,* Oxford University Press, 2008.
^E.g., vital registration, cancer registries, exposure registries.
+E.g., medical and laboratory records, pharmacy records.
**E.g., weather, climate change, pollution.
+*E.g., criminal justice information, Lexis-Nexis.

The methods of public health surveillance differ from the other data collection efforts in ways described throughout this text. Designing, developing, and conducting surveillance demand rigorous and reliable methods. Analysis of surveillance data increases in complexity as demands on the data grow. There is an increasing demand for a variety of disciplines and areas of expertise as the need for breadth of analytic expertise grows (Fig. 20–1). Analysis of surveillance data has moved beyond descriptive epidemiology to guide policy development; appropriation and allocation of funding for prevention, care, and treatment; and measurement of the impact of health reform.

Advances in Information Technology and the Promise of Efficiency

Rapid development of information technology and increased computing capacity promise many improvements in efficiency, accuracy, and speed of several surveillance system activities, including real-time data collection, automated analysis, epidemic recognition, and dissemination of information products for immediate action (Fig. 20–2; ref. 7). Full implementation of electronic health records (EHRs) could revolutionize data collection (8), limiting the human input into this task to the routine clinical visit. Transcription errors could decline, and timeliness and accuracy could improve. In addition to automated programming for

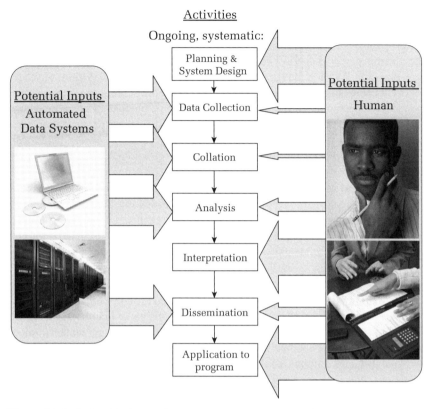

Figure 20–2 Optimal balance of human and automated inputs into ongoing, systematic public health surveillance system activities.

data management, expanding EHRs to a concept of personally controlled health records (PCHRs) (9), where a person collects his or her own data across health-care providers, could simplify the collation activities, removing inaccuracies in matching records of events in a person-based surveillance system. Automated analyses, including aberration detection and routine analysis to produce daily, weekly, monthly, annual, and even on-demand reports, could reduce human input substantially. Finally, using technology to disseminate public health surveillance information in an innovative and rapid manner could reduce both the human effort and the time between knowledge and action. Epi-X (10) and the Health Alert Network (11) are examples of attempts to automate the notification function of dissemination, and they meet this goal to varying degrees (12). Web-based communication to a variety of audiences, including policymakers, public health professionals, and the general public, could improve distribution and access to critical information, especially during an urgent public health event. Leveraging technology to improve four of the seven major routine activities of surveillance would free the human intellectual efforts for system design, data interpretation, and application to program where they are most needed.

In a fully functional system of EHR, the ideal outlined in Figure 20–2 could be achieved. However, there are several challenges that prevent the realization of these benefits in the United States. Despite the goal of complete adoption of the electronic medical office by 2001 (*13*), preliminary estimates for 2009 indicate that only 20.5% of physicians reported having basic EHR systems and 6.3% reported using fully functional systems (*14*). In the United States, there is strong governmental support for the update of the electronic medical office as evidenced by President Obama's 2009 $19 billion investment in health information technology (*15*), but it remains a less effective "push" concept, where health-care providers are provided incentives to adopt the technology rather than a "pull" commodity that providers are demanding (*16*).

The potential of the EHR is illustrated by the health information exchange (HIE), which mobilizes health information electronically across organizations within a region or community. An HIE enables electronic sharing of clinical information among disparate health-care information systems while maintaining the accuracy of the information being exchanged. Participants would include primary care physicians, specialists, ambulatory care centers, managed care organizations, hospitals, laboratories, pharmacies, payers, and public health authorities. The goal of an HIE is to facilitate access to and retrieval of clinical data to provide safer, more timely, efficient, effective, equitable, patient-centered care while assuring privacy and confidentiality with the use of data use agreements among participants. Public health authorities will have more complete and timely access to clinical data for public health surveillance and other important population-based activities such as timely physician notification of current public health recommendations (*17*).

The limited penetration of EHR, as well as the lack of standard software and perceived barriers by health-care providers (*18*), present concrete operational limitations for electronic data exchange (*19*). In addition, diagnostic coding algorithms are idiosyncratic and vary by health-care practice and setting (*20,21*). Coding is often tied to reimbursement, which can lead to up-coding to a better reimbursed diagnosis (*22,23*) Inaccurate coding leading to identification of false cases and an overload of previously unidentified cases have the potential to overwhelm understaffed public health surveillance programs. This aspect of EHR implementation must be considered. Finally, EHR's clinical, diagnostic, and billing orientations omit many pieces of information necessary for complete public health surveillance, including risk behaviors and exposure data. Until these logistical issues are resolved, the potential benefits of EHRs will remain out of reach.

Amassing Data and Ethical Considerations for Public Health Surveillance

Continued recognition of public health surveillance as a distinct and separate discipline that develops a data collection system with a public health purpose and an *a priori* question in mind remains a challenge when amassing health data from numerous sources is possible.

A fundamental principle of surveillance system design is to delineate intended uses of the data. This principle stems from fact that often public health surveillance, by its nature, is an unconsented process. Amassing and holding data, often personal and private in nature, without specific purpose is a breach of public trust. Without public trust, public health surveillance ceases to be possible.

A constant over many decades is that nearly always, and by necessity, the activities of public health surveillance are undertaken without individual patient consent. Public health surveillance is a function of states' police powers, and citizens cede to their legislative bodies their consent to be reported with a notifiable condition. Elected state or local governments make laws and regulations to protect the public's health on behalf of their constituents. Most citizens are unaware of disease reporting laws, and when informed of them, they typically are not concerned that their cases are reported to the local health authorities, even with highly sensitive conditions (24).

Although some researchers have suggested a consent-based model for public health surveillance (25), such a model is untenable for achieving the purposes and outcomes of public health surveillance. Requiring consent could lead to dangerous disruptions, delays, and unmanageable logistical burdens on health-care providers and laboratories (26)—all of which would impede the primary purpose of public health surveillance, which is a timely response to a health threat in a community or population.

The development of a data use plan is key in the planning step of a surveillance system. As part of the agreement with the public, appropriate use of data collected for public health is imperative. Herman Biggs, a New York physician who pioneered public health surveillance in the late 19th century, adamantly insisted that data were collected to be used to improve health—not to keep adding machines busy (27). This principle stood throughout the 20th century, when William Foege, a former director of the U.S. Centers for Disease Control and Prevention (CDC), stated in 1976, "The reason for collecting, analyzing, and disseminating information on a disease is to control that disease. Collection and analysis should not be allowed to consume resources if action does not follow (28)." In other words, the risk of collecting and holding the data must be worth the expected outcome of the use of the data (29). This principle remains a fundamental ethical consideration for all public health data collection (30).

Advances in technology and increased availability of electronic data have made collecting, storing, sharing, and disclosing private information much easier than in times past when manual collection and collation were the standard. President Obama has called for increased accountability of all U.S. government agencies in terms of how data are handled (31). Currently, no consistent enterprise-wide standards exist for collection, storage, and use of public health surveillance data; privacy safeguards are inconsistent and vary by state (32). An enterprise-wide guidance for ethical collection, storage, and use of public health data has been proposed, outlining 10 foundational guidelines that should be used to cover data from entry into the smallest local jurisdiction and apply through the life of the data, regardless of where they ultimately reside (33). Issues of appropriate use and sharing of sensitive health data are magnified when public health surveillance is being done across national borders when numerous donor agencies—some of which might not be traditionally health-oriented—are involved with funding public health surveillance activities.

Calls for public ownership of medical data (*34*), obligatory participation in biomedical research (*35*), and the way other types of private data (e.g., financial and location tracking) are collected and used might change the way Americans feel about the collection, storage, and use of private data. Currently, the overwhelming majority of Americans feels strongly that their medical information is private and should not be shared with others for purposes other than medical care (*36*). Ensuring the safety, privacy, and confidentiality of data collected, stored, and used by public health is one of our most important ethical obligations.

Ensuring the Future of the Public Health Workforce

Public health has enormous challenges ahead. We face urgent threats, such as weather events and influenza pandemics, as well as person-made disasters and war that cause massive morbidity and mortality in a short span of time and space. We also face urgent realities that cause the majority of disease and death but in a far less dramatic fashion, such as the obesity epidemic, smoking-related illness, extreme poverty, HIV/AIDS and other neglected infectious diseases. Public health personnel must be versatile and agile, equipped to deal with many aspects of measuring and responding to health problems in a community. Training, recruiting, and retaining public health surveillance professionals requires a systematic approach, as serious shortages exist both in the United States and globally.

Developing interest in science and public service must start early in academic life. These "pipeline" activities are critical to meet future needs for the diversity of scientific fields that populate public health. CDC began its work in 1946 with approximately 400 entomologists and engineers; 60 years later it employs thousands of scientists from approximately 25 disciplines (*37*). The accomplishment of public health goals has taken expertise from those initial fields of entomology and engineering at the start to the addition of epidemiology; statistics; laboratory sciences such as virology, microbiology, and clinical chemistry; and veterinary and clinical medicine throughout the 1970s followed by a wide range of others sciences such as social and behavioral sciences, economics, health services research, urban planning, toxicology, genomics, and informatics in the recent past. Maintaining interest in science is a first step in ensuring the future of public health, but it also requires creating a desire for public service on the part of bright scientists and the development of specific core competencies in surveillance and epidemiology (*38*). Generating interest in public health science in middle and high school is a priority. CDC engages middle and high school teachers and students in programs to develop interest in public health as a career (*39*). Overcoming the predicted shortfalls in public health professionals (*40*) will take broad efforts from education, health, and public sectors.

CONCLUSIONS

Public health surveillance as a distinct discipline continues to lay the foundation of public health action. Its characteristics, purposes, and outputs differ from health surveys, medical record and laboratory information systems, vital registration systems, and research studies. Public health surveillance plays a unique role in providing information to the overall health knowledge. It also requires a carefully considered ethical framework to ensure that we protect data adequately and make effective use of the information we glean. It requires a multidisciplinary expertise to meet the increasing demands on the data. A well-prepared public health workforce is critical for the future of public health surveillance. Technology provides countless opportunities for improvement in efficiency and productivity in many activities of public health surveillance; however, it will never replace the key human and ethical inputs at the planning and design, interpretation, and application to program activities.

REFERENCES

1. Porta M, ed. *A Dictionary of Epidemiology*, 5th ed. New York: Oxford University Press; 2008.
2. Preamble to the Constitution of the World Health Organization as adopted by the International Health Conference, New York, 19–22 June, 1946; signed on July 22 1946 by the representatives of 61 States (Official Records of the World Health Organization, no. 2, p. 100) and entered into force on April 7 1948.
3. Endsley MR. Design and evaluation for situation awareness enhancement. In: *Proceedings of the Human Factors Society 32 Annual Meeting.* Santa Monica, CA: Human Factors Society;1988:97–101.
4. Groves RM, Benson G, Mosher WD, *et al.* Plan and operation of cycle 6 of the National Survey of Family Growth. National Center for Health Statistics. *Vital health statistics.* 2005;1(42). http://www.cdc.gov/nchs/data/series/sr_01/sr01_042.pdf. Accessed August 15, 2009.
5. National Center for Health Statistics. Data File Documentation, National Health Interview Survey, 2007 (machine readable data file and documentation). Hyattsville, MD: National Center for Health Statistics, Centers for Disease Control and Prevention; 2008.
6. National Center for Health Statistics. National Health and Nutrition Examination Study. http://www.cdc.gov/nchs/nhanes/about_nhanes.htm. Updated July 21, 2009. Accessed August 14, 2009.
7. Institute of Medicine. *The Future of the Public's Health in the 21st Century.* Washington, DC: National Academy Press; 2003.
8. Lazarus R, Klompas M, Campion FX, *et al.* Electronic support for public health: validated case finding and reporting for notifiable diseases using electronic medical data. *J Am Med Inform Assoc* 2009;16:18–24.
9. Mandl KD, Kohane IS. Tectonic shifts in the health information economy. *N Engl J Med* 2008;358:1732–1737.
10. Epi-X: The Epidemic Information Exchange. Centers for Disease Control and Prevention. http://www.cdc.gov/epix/. Accessed July 20, 2009.

11. HAN: Health Alert Network. Centers for Disease Control and Prevention. http://www2a.cdc.gov/han/Index.asp. Accessed July 20, 2009.

12. M'Ikanatha NM, Rohn DD, Robertson C, *et al.* Use of the interet to enhance infectious disease surveillance and outbreak investigation. *Biosecur Bioterror* 2006;4:293–300.

13. Institute of Medicine. *The Computer-based Patient Record: An Essential Technology for Health Care.* Washington, DC: National Academy Press; 1991.

14. Hsiao CJ, Beatty PC, Hing E, Woodwell DA, Rechtsteiner E, Sisk JE. Electronic medical record/electronic health record use by office-based physicians: United States, 2008 and preliminary 2009. Health E-Stat. National Center for Health Statistics. 2009. http://www.cdc.gov/nchs/data/hestat/emr_ehr/emr_ehr.htm. Accessed March 8, 2010.

15. American Recovery and Reinvestment Act of 2009. Pub.L. 111-5. Signed February 17, 2009.

16. Lohr S. How to make electronic medical records a reality. *New York Times.* February 28, 2009. http://www.nytimes.com/2009/03/01/business/01unbox.html. Accessed July 20, 2009.

17. McDonald CJ, Overhage JM, Barnes M, Schadow G, Blevins L, Dexter PR, Mamlin B. The Indiana network for patient care: a working local health information infrastructure. An example of a working infrastructure collaboration that links data from five health systems and hundreds of millions of entries. *Health Aff (Millwood)* 2005;24:1214–1220.

18. Burdyny C, Findlater S, Caron M-P, Ajaz M. Strategies to increase familiarization and acceptance of electronic health records among health professionals and consumers. *Adv Inform Technol Commun Health* 2009;143:419–425.

19. Anderson JG. Social, ethical and legal barriers to E-health. *Int J Med Inform* 2007;76:480–483.

20. Dixon J, Sanderson C, Elliott P, Walls P, Jones J, Petticrew M. Assessment of the reproducibility of clinical coding in routinely collected hospital activity data: a study in two hospitals. *J Public Health Med* 1998;20:63–69.

21. Kljakovic M, Abernethy D, de Ruiter I. Quality of diagnostic coding and information flow from hospital to general practice. *Inform Primary Care* 2004;12:227–234.

22. Hsia DC, Ahern CA, Ritchie BP, Moscoe LM, Krushat WM. Medicare reimbursement accuracy under the prospective payment system, 1985–1988. *JAMA* 1992;268:896–899.

23. Hightower RE. Prevention of hospital payment errors and implication for case management: a study of nine hospitals with a high proportion of short-term admissions over time. *Prof Case Manag* 2008;13:264–274.

24. Hecht FM, Chesney MA, Lehman JS, *et al.* Does HIV reporting by name deter testing? *AIDS* 2000;14:1801–1808.

25. K Mandl, Presentation at CDC, Atlanta GA, June 19, 2009.

26. Verity C, Nicoll A. Consent, confidentiality, and the threat to public health surveillance. *BMJ* 2002;324:1210–1213.

27. Fairchild AL, Bayer R, Colgrove J. *Searching Eyes: Privacy, the State, and Disease Surveillance in America.* Berkeley, CA: University of California Press; 2007.

28. Foege WH, Hogan RC, Newton LH. Surveillance projects for selected diseases. *Int J Epidemiol* 1976;5:29–37.

29. The Turning Point Public Health Statute Modernization Collaborative. *The Turning Point Model State Public Health Act: A Tool for Assessing Public Health Laws.* September 2003. http://www.turningpointprogram.org/Pages/pdfs/statute_mod/MSPHAfinal.pdf. Accessed July 20, 2009.

30. CDC/ATSDR Policy on Releasing and Sharing Data. Centers for Disease Control and Prevention. http://www.cdc.gov/od/foia/policies/sharing.htm. Updated September 7, 2005. Accessed July 20, 2009.

31. Obama BH. Memorandum for the Heads of Executive Departments and Agencies, Subject: Scientific Integrity. White House Web site. http://www.whitehouse.gov/the_ press_office/Memorandum-for-the-Heads-of-Executive-Departments-and-Agencies-3-9-09/. Updated March 9, 2009. Accessed July 20, 2009.

32. Gostin LO, Lazzarini Z, Neslund VS, Osterholm MT. The public health information infrastructure. A national review of the law on health information privacy. *JAMA* 1996;275(24):1921–1927.

33. Lee LM, Gostin LO. Ethical collection, storage, and use of public health data: A proposal for a national privacy protection. *JAMA* 2009;302:82–84.

34. Rodwin MA. The case for public ownership of patient data. *JAMA* 2009;302:86–88.

35. Schaefer GO, Emanuel EJ, Wertheimer A. The obligation to participate in biomedical research. *JAMA* 2009;302:67–72.

36. California HealthCare Foundation. National Consumer Health Privacy Survey 2005. Forrester Research Inc., November 9, 2005. http://www.chcf.org/documents/healthit/ ConsumerPrivacy2005Slides.pdf. Accessed August 16, 2009.

37. Lee LM, Popovic T. Preface: 60 Years of Public Health Science at CDC. *MMWR* 2006;55(Suppl):1.

38. Core Competencies for Public Health Professionals. Council on Linkages between Academia and Public Health Practice. Public Health Foundation Web site. http:// www.phf.org/link/corecompetencies.htm. Accessed August 14, 2009.

39. Thacker SB, Koo D, Delany JR. Career paths to public health: programs at the Centers for Disease Control and Prevention. *Am J Prev Med* 2008;35:279–283.

40. More than 250,000 Additional Public Health Workers Needed by 2020 to Avert Public Health Crisis (Press Release). Association of Schools of Public Health Web site. http://www.asph.org/userfiles/finalasphworkforcerelease.pdf. Released February 27, 2008; Washington, DC. Accessed August 14, 2009.

Index

Note: Page numbers followed by "*b*," "*f*," and "*t*" denote boxes, figures, and tables, respectively.